Advanced MR Imaging Techniques

Advanced MR Imaging Techniques

Edited by

William G Bradley Jr, MD PhD FACR

Medical Director, Memorial MRI Center, Long Beach Memorial Medical Center,
Long Beach CA, USA

Graeme M Bydder, BSc MB ChB FRCR FRCP

Professor of Diagnostic Radiology, The Robert Steiner MR Unit,
Royal Postgraduate Medical School, Hammersmith Hospital, London, UK

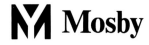 Mosby

St. Louis Baltimore Boston Carlsbad Chicago Naples New York Philadelphia Portland
London Madrid Mexico City Singapore Sydney Tokyo Toronto Wiesbaden

Martin Dunitz

© Martin Dunitz Ltd 1997

First published in the United Kingdom in 1997
by Martin Dunitz Ltd, The Livery House,
7–9 Pratt Street, London NW1 0AE

A CIP catalogue record for this book is available
from the British Library.

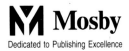 **Mosby**
Dedicated to Publishing Excellence

A Times Mirror
Company

Distributed in the U.S.A. and Canada by
Mosby–Year Book   Times Mirror Professional Publishing Ltd
11830 Westline Industrial Drive   130 Flaska Drive
St. Louis, Missouri 63146   Markham, Ontario L6G 1B8

ISBN 1-85317-024-0

Composition by Scribe Design, Gillingham, Kent,
United Kingdom
Origination, printed and bound in Singapore by
Toppan Printing Company (S) Pte Ltd

The editors and publishers wish to acknowledge
that the cover image is Figure 14.21 from
Chapter 14 "Interventional MRI" by George J So,
Gasser Hathout, Keyvan Farahani, et al.

We dedicate this book to our wives, Rosalind Dietrich and Patricia Hamilton, who have been putting up with our working nights, weekends, holidays and vacations for most of our professional lives. Without their support, you would not be reading this book.

Contents

List of contributors

Dennis J Atkinson MSc
Senior MR Scientist, Siemens Medical Systems, Iselin NJ 08830, USA.

Keith Black MD
Professor of Neurosurgery, Department of Neurosurgery, UCLA School of Medicine, Los Angeles CA 90095, USA.

William G Bradley MD PhD FACR
Medical Director, Memorial MRI Center, Long Beach Memorial Medical Center, Long Beach CA 90806, USA.

Graeme M Bydder
Professor of Diagnostic Radiology, the Robert Steiner Magnetic Resonance Unit, Royal Postgraduate Medical School, Hammersmith Hospital, London W12 8NN, UK.

Daniel Castro MD
Associate Professor in Head and Neck Surgery, UCLA School of Medicine, Los Angeles CA 90095, USA.

Dar-Yeong Chen PhD
Memorial MRI Center, Long Beach Memorial Medical Center, Long Beach CA 90806, USA.

Mark S Cohen PhD
Director, Functional MR Laboratory, UCLA School of Medicine, Departments of Neurology and Radiology, Psychology and Behavioural Sciences, Los Angeles CA 90095, USA.

Antonio A F deSalles MD PhD
Associate Professor of Neurosurgery, UCLA School of Medicine, Los Angeles CA 90095, USA.

Frank J Davies MA(Oxon)
Director of Research, Oxford Magnet Technology, Eynsham, Oxford OX8 1BP, UK.

Keyvan Farahani PhD
Assistant Professor of Radiological Sciences, UCLA School of Medicine, Los Angeles CA 90095, USA.

Joseph V Hajnal PhD
Senior Research Scientist and Honorary Senior Lecturer, Robert Steiner MR Unit, Hammersmith Hospital, Royal Postgraduate Medical School, London W12 0NN, UK.

Alasdair S Hall PhD
Senior Research Associate, GEC-Marconi Materials Technologies Ltd, Hirst Division, Borehamwood, Herts WD6 1RX, UK.

Gasser Hathout MD
Fellow, Department of Radiological Sciences, UCLA School of Medicine, Los Angeles CA 90095, USA.

Jeffrey David Lewine PhD
Director, Magnetic Source Imaging and Neuroscience Divisions, The New Mexico Institute of Neuroimaging, the New Mexico Regional Federal Medical Center; Clinical Research Assistant Professor of Radiology and Adjunct Assistant Professor of Psychology, The University of New Mexico, Albuquerque NM 87131-5336, USA.

Robert B Lufkin MD
Professor of Radiological Sciences, Department of Radiological Sciences, UCLA School of Medicine, Los Angeles CA 90095, USA.

Surya N Mohapatra PhD
Senior Vice-President, Picker International Inc, Cleveland OH 44143, USA.

William W Orrison Jr, MD
Chief, Division of Neuroradiology, The New Mexico Regional Federal Medical Center; Director, The New Mexico Institute of Neuroimaging; Professor of Radiology and Associate Professor of Neurology, The University of New Mexico, Albuquerque NM 87131-5336, USA.

Martyn Paley BSc PhD CPhys FInstP
Senior Lecturer, MRI Unit, Department of Imaging, The Middlesex Hospital, University College London Hospitals, London W1N 8AA, UK.

Shantanu Sinha PhD
Assistant Professor of Radiological Sciences, UCLA School of Medicine, Los Angeles CA 90095, USA.

George J So MD
Resident, Department of Radiological Sciences, UCLA School of Medicine, Los Angeles CA 90095, USA.

Robert M Weisskoff PhD
Director, High Speed Imaging Laboratory and MR Physics Research, Massachusetts General Hospital NMR Center, Department of Radiology, and Assistant Professor of Radiology, Harvard Medical School, Charlestown MA 02129, USA.

Ian R Young PhD
Professor, the Robert Steiner Magnetic Resonance Unit, Royal Postgraduate Medical School, Hammersmith W12 8NN, UK.

Preface

Several years ago, Martin Dunitz asked us to consider revising our 1990 volume *MRI of the Brain: A Text Atlas*. We said that the world already had enough brain MRI books, but we would be interested in doing something new and different. Now that MRI has been used clinically for over 15 years, there are quite a few radiologists who are using more sophisticated approaches than in the past. Therefore, we planned a book focused on these more advanced MR techniques. When asked for a deadline we hedged (a favourite ploy for radiologists) and preferred to wait and see when the timing was right.

Hopefully, the time is now. Over the last two years, several advanced applications have gained maturity (e.g. fast spin echo and inversion recovery), others have begun to mature (e.g. diffusion, CSF flow, magnetization transfer, EPI, spectroscopy) and several are just now coming into the mainstream (e.g. magnetic source imaging, registration and interventional MRI). *Advanced MR Imaging Techniques* deals with these and other advanced MR topics.

Specific topics have been chosen to reflect current research interests and our expectations of what is likely to be important in the future and we have targeted the book at experienced MR radiologists. We have not attempted to cover the entire field of MRI techniques. We hope you enjoy reading it as much as we enjoyed writing it.

WGB
GB
Long Beach and London, 1997

Acknowledgements

It is a pleasure to acknowledge the help and encouragement of Professor Robert Steiner during the whole period in which MRI has been in clinical use.

Venita Lombard-Smith, Lisa Slocum, Lillian Cayetano, Ed Gill, Eileen Wampler, Angela Oatridge, Jacqueline Pennock, Elaine Williams, Nadeem Saeed and Mary Rutherford have all made a major contribution to the specific studies described in *Advanced MR Imaging Techniques*. On the clinical front, Drs Paul Berger, Lou Teresi, John Jordan, Jay Amster, Daffyd Thomas, Basant Puri, Anita Holdcroft, David Harris, Frances Cowan, Lilly Dubowitz and Nandita de Souza have also been of considerable help.

In addition to our in-house scientists, Dar-Yeong Chen and Dennis Atkinson, we are also grateful for scientific discussion/support from Dave Weber of General Electric, Paul Finn of Siemens, and Neil Palmer, Paul Margossian, Rao Gullapalli, Surya Mohapatra and David Waldron of Picker International. Dar-Yeong gets additional thanks for help with computer graphics and computer support in general. We would like to thank Steve Henman and Leno Hansen from Nycomed, as well as Chris Soleimanpour and Trevor Thomas from Lister Bestcare for their help.

The manuscripts were prepared by Dulcie Rodrigues, Margarete Hayward and Patricia Hamilton, and we thank them. We would especially like to thank and acknowledge Kaye Finley, Bill Bradley's personal assistant of some 13 years, for her unstinting help in administering the grants and Fellows, and for preparing the manuscripts.

Finally, we would both like to thank Alan Burgess and Martin Dunitz for their continuous encouragement and motivation.

WGB
GMB

1

Fast spin echo

William G Bradley, Dar-Yeong Chen and Dennis J Atkinson

One of the most important recent advances in MRI has been a technique that was originally called RARE (rapid acquisition with relaxation enhancement) by Hennig when he described it in 1986.[1] Today it is more commonly called fast spin echo (by GE, Picker, Toshiba and Hitachi) or turbo spin echo (by Siemens and Philips). (For ease of discussion, it will be called fast spin echo or FSE hereinafter.)

The primary advantage of FSE is speed, without the usual concomitant loss of signal-to-noise ratio (S/N). In a conventional spin echo (CSE), S/N is proportional to the square root of the number of signal averages (also called N_{ex}, N_{ac} and repetitions). Everytime the number of signal averages is halved, the acquisition time is reduced by 50 percent, but the S/N is also reduced by 2 or 40 percent. In FSE, the S/N penalty for going faster is minimal. In order to understand how FSE is performed and how it differs from CSE, it is useful to introduce the concepts of the Fourier transform and k-space.[2,3]

The basic idea behind *Fourier analysis* is that any shape can be approximated by a weighted sum of sines and cosines.[3] Low fequency sine waves describe the bulk outline and high frequency sine waves fill in the details. (Since these sine waves describe an object in the x–y plane, the axes have units of 'spatial frequency' or cycles/cm).

A *Fourier transform* is a mathematical procedure that breaks any complex signal into its component frequencies, In NMR spectroscopy, the signal is an FID coming from a compound containing different chemical species—each with its own characteristic resonant frequency or chemical shift. The Fourier transform of this signal is the spectrum. This representation of the data as amplitude versus frequency amounts to a transform from temporal space to k-space. (The k comes from a variable in the mathematical formula for the Fourier transform.) In MR imaging, the signal of a sample with a single chemical shift, i.e. water, is acquired in the presence of a gradient so that the component frequencies of the FID or spin echo indicate position. (Again, since these represent an object they are *spatial* frequencies.) The process of MR imaging frequency-encodes the spatial coordinates of an object. Thus the FID or spin echo is actually *in* k-space. To form an image requires reverse Fourier transforming this data back into x–y space.

Figure 1.1a shows a one-dimensional Fourier transform in spectroscopy. A free induction decay (FID) is represented as an oscillating signal of decreasing amplitude versus time. There are many frequencies included in the signal. Some are strong (high amplitude); others are weak (low amplitude). The data in the FID can also be represented as amplitude versus frequency. Spectroscopic data in its original form is in the 'time domain', i.e. the x axis has units of time. The transformed data is in 'frequency domain' or 'k-space'. The units along the x-axis are frequency, i.e. cycles/sec. This transformation of one axis of data is called a 1-Dimensional Fourier Transform (1DFT). Transformation of two axes of data (e.g. the x and y axes of an MR image) is a 2DFT. The representation of the image data in k-space also has two axes (with units of spatial frequency), corresponding to phase and frequency (see, for example, Fig. 1.9). Similarly, a 3D (volume) acquisition would have three axes of k-space: frequency, phase I, and phase II (slice

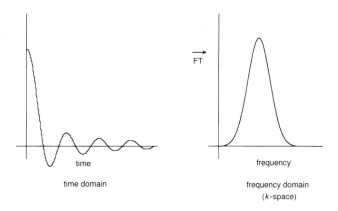

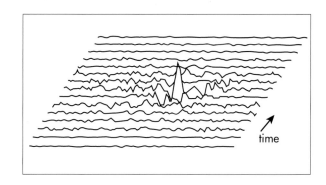

a

b

Figure 1.1

Fourier transform. (a) One-dimensional Fourier transform (1DFT). The free induction decay (FID) on the left is a plot of amplitude versus time. The signal is composed of multiple frequencies. The same data can be replotted as amplitude versus frequency (on the right), the central peak being the dominant

frequency in the FID. The x-axis of this new representation has units of spatial frequency and is in *k*-space. (This is the spectrum in MR spectroscopy.) (b) Temporal stack of spin echoes from beginning (bottom) to end (top) of acquisition.

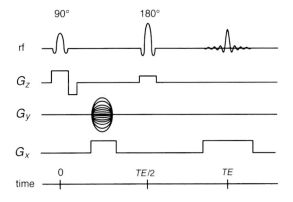

Figure 1.2

A spin echo pulse sequence diagram. The top line demonstrates rf transmission and reception. The spin echo is formed by the combination of a 90° and 180° pulse. The time between the 90° and 180° rf pulses (*TE*/2) is the same as the time between the 180° and the echo. The slice select gradient (G_z in this case) is applied at the same time as the rf pulses, so that only the desired slice is excited. The phase encode gradient (G_y in this case) is activated after the 90° pulse. Each time we cycle through the sequence, the phase encode gradient is changed. The readout gradient G_x is applied during readout of the spin echo. The initial gradient prepulse dephases the spins so that they can be perfectly rephased along the x-axis at the midpoint of the spin echo. Thus the spin echo is rephased in time (by the 180° pulse) and in space by the initial prepulses of G_x and G_z.

select). Just as there was no similarity between the shape of the FID in the time domain and its representation in the frequency domain, so there is no correspondence between an MR image as we see it in (x, y, z)-space and its representation in *k*-space. In a sense, the *k*-space representation of an object consists of a temporal stack (Fig. 1.1b) of multiple (e.g. 256) spin echo or FID signals viewed from above. Low spatial frequencies (e.g. 0.01/mm) are found in the center of *k*-space and high spatial frequencies (0.5/mm) are found at the periphery.[2,3]

In order to understand more about *k*-space, it is useful to consider the interplay between the rf pulses and the x, y and z gradient pulses that are needed to produce a conventional spin echo image. This representation is called a pulse sequence diagram (PSD). Figure 1.2 shows a 90° rf pulse followed a time *TE*/2 later by a 180° rf pulse. An interval *TE*/2 after that (i.e. an interval *TE* after the 90° pulse), the spin echo forms. For a double echo technique, a second 180° pulse is added, producing a second echo (Fig. 1.3). In general, any number of rephasing 180° pulses can be added to produce a 'train' of echoes. The only limitation to the length of such an echo train is the T_2 decay, which results in ever-diminishing signal from the last echoes (Fig. 1.3).

In order to limit rf excitation to a single slice, the 90° and 180° rf pulses must be applied while the 'slice select' gradient is activated (Fig. 1.2). (For

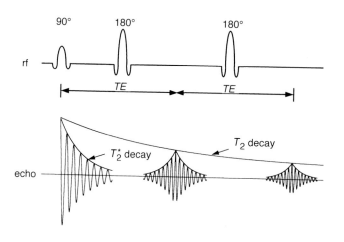

Figure 1.3

Double spin echo. Applying two 180° pulses after a 90° pulse produces two echoes with decreasing signal intensity owing to T_2 decay. (Also shown is the T_2^* decay of the FID resulting from the 90° pulse prior to initial rephasing by the first 180° pulse. This signal is usually not acquired.)

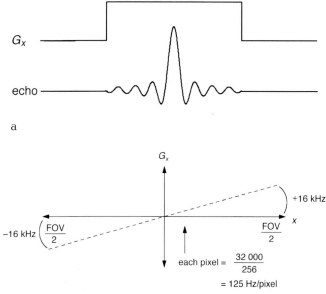

Figure 1.4

Frequency encoding. (a) The readout gradient G_x is applied during readout of the spin echo in order to provide spatial discrimination along that axis. (b) Activating the readout gradient changes the magnetic field (and therefore the resonance frequency) at each point along the readout axis. In this example, the maximum frequency offset at the borders of the field of view is ±16 kHz. This is also known as the bandwidth. Another way to represent the bandwidth is to divide the full bandwidth (32 kHz) by the number of pixels along the readout axis (256 in this example), giving a bandwidth of 125 Hz/pixel.

purposes of discussion, we shall assume we are producing an image in the transverse plane in a superconducting magnet, in which case G_z is the slice select gradient.) In addition to having the slice select gradient activated at the time of the 90° and the 180° rf pulses, it is also necessary for the spins along the thickness (z-axis) of the slice to be perfectly in phase at time *TE*. Hence there are additional negative pulses as shown for G_z in Fig. 1.2.

In order to obtain spatial information along the 'frequency encode' or 'readout' axis, another gradient (e.g. G_x) must be activated while the spin echo is being read out (Figs 1.2 and 1.4). Again, a prepulse is needed to initially dephase the spins along the x-axis so that they come perfectly into phase at time *TE*, in the middle of the spin echo readout (Fig. 1.2). (For gradient echo techniques, the prepulse has negative polarity, i.e. it is below the line in Fig. 1.2. For spin echoes, the prepulse is positive but becomes 'negative' as a result of the subsequent 180° pulse.)

In order to provide spatial information along the remaining 'phase encode' axis in the MR image, the phase encode gradient is activated once between the 90° and 180° pulses (Figs 1.2 and 1.5). On each pass through the sequence, i.e. following each 90° pulse, the phase encode gradient is advanced. In order to distinguish 256 points along

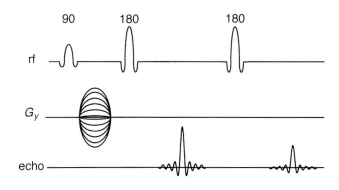

Figure 1.5

In conventional spin echo, the phase encode gradient is applied once following the 90° pulse regardless of the number of echoes produced (two in this example).

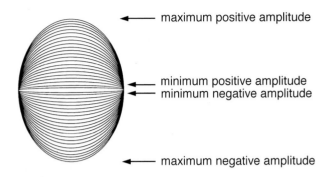

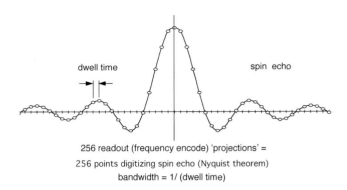

256 readout (frequency encode) 'projections' =

256 points digitizing spin echo (Nyquist theorem)

bandwidth = 1/ (dwell time)

Figure 1.6

Phase encoding. The maximum negative amplitudes of the phase encode gradient are generally applied first, passing through the lowest amplitudes to the maximum positive amplitude on each cycle through the pulse sequence of a conventional spin echo.

Figure 1.8

Routine frequency encoding. This plot of amplitude versus time indicates a spin echo (solid black line) digitized 256 times to provide frequency discrimination of 256 points along the readout axis (according to the Nyquist theorem). The sampling interval is known as the dwell time (which is the inverse of the bandwidth). The sampling is performed by a piece of equipment called the analog-to-digital (A/D) converter, which converts the continuous variation of voltage versus time of the spin echo to a stream of digits that can be handled by a digital computer.

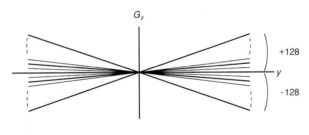

256 phase encode 'projections' N_p = 256 different values
of phase encode gradient G_y

$t = TR \times N_p \times NEX$

Figure 1.7

Phase encoding for conventional spin echo. This plot of gradient strength versus position along the phase encode axis demonstrates the most negative applications of the phase encode gradient passing through the weakest to the most positive.

the phase encode axis, 256 different values of the phase encode gradient are required on 256 separate passes (each taking time TR) through the sequence. Typically, the first pass is with the most negative value of the phase encode gradient (–127), followed by the next most negative up to zero (Figs 1.6 and 1.7). After zero, the phase encode gradient increases up to its most positive value (+128).

The process of reading out a spin echo involves converting a continuous (analog) signal to a stream of digits that can be processed by a digital

computer (Fig. 1.8). The computer hardware that performs this task is called an analog-to-digital (A/D) converter. In order to be able to distinguish 256 frequencies along the readout axis, the A/D converter must sample the spin echo 256 times, i.e. it must produce a stream of 256 digits. The time between samplings is called the sampling interval or the dwell time (Fig. 1.8). In fact, the dwell time is the primary determinant of noise in the MR image. (Noise is proportional to the square root of the receiver bandwidth, and the bandwidth is inversely proportional to the dwell time. Thus the longer the dwell time, the lower the noise and the greater the S/N.) Prolonging the dwell time also prolongs the total echo sampling time, which is simply the product of the number of readout projections (e.g. 256) and the dwell time. As the dwell time is increased to improve S/N, the total echo sampling time begins to encroach upon the 180° pulse, requiring that the entire echo sampling process be shifted to a later time, i.e. a longer TE. This is why the low-bandwidth techniques that are so prevalent at lower field strengths are associated with longer TE values than are typically seen at higher fields.)

Each time a spin echo is read out along the frequency encode axis, 256 points are filled in k-space (Fig. 1.9a). These are all at one spatial

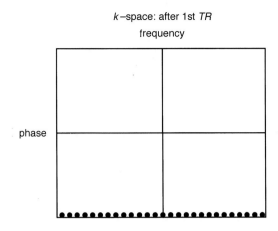

a

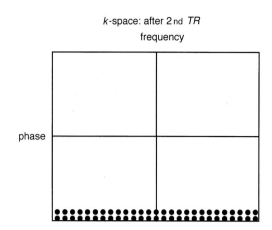

b

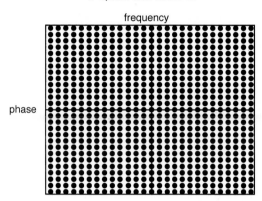

c

Figure 1.9

Conventional spin echo representation in k-space.
(a) Following sampling of the first echo after the first
TR interval, 256 points fill a single line in k-space at a
single value of the phase encode gradient. (b) After
the second TR interval, 256 additional points are
produced by a single spin echo at another value of the
phase encode gradient, filling another line in k-space.
(c) This process continues until 256 values of the
phase encode gradient have been applied, filling 256
lines in k-space, completing the k-space representation
of a 256 × 256 spin echo image. Most of the signal
and therefore most of the contrast come from the
center of k-space, where the values of the phase
encode gradient are weakest.

frequency along the phase encode axis. On the
next pass through the sequence, after another 90°
pulse and another interval TR, a second frequency
line is filled in at another spatial frequency along
the phase encode axis in k-space (Fig. 1.9b), and
so on up to 256 lines (Fig. 1.9c) (and 256 phase
steps/256 TR intervals).

k-space has some interesting properties, which
have led to modifications of the basic spin echo
sequence. For a start, k-space is symmetric. The
upper right-hand corner is symmetric with the
lower left-hand corner, and the upper left-hand
corner is symmetric with the lower right-hand
corner (this is called Hermitian symmetry). Thus the
top half of k-space is the mirror-image reflection of
the bottom half and the right half is the mirror-
image reflection of the left half. This k-space
symmetry reflects the physical symmetry of the spin
echo about the midpoint at TE (Fig. 1.4) and the fact
that the negative 128 phase encode steps are
symmetric with the positive 128 phase encodes (Fig.
1.7). Because of this symmetry, it is possible to
acquire half of k-space and calculate the other half.

When the bottom half of k-space is acquired, i.e.
half the phase steps, the acquisition time is halved
(at a reduction of S/N by $\sqrt{2}$). This has been called
a 1/2 Nex acquisition to emphasize the halving of
the acquisition time (Figs 1.10a,b). (Actually, there
is no such thing as 'half excitation'; however,
perfect truth in advertising would require that the
manufacturer point out that it is, in fact, one Nex
and 128 phase steps all in one half of k-space
(rather than being *centered* in k-space as usual).
The spatial resolution is thus the same as a 256^2
acquisition and not a lower-resolution 128^2 acquisition. Given the length of these last sentences, it
is easy to see why the designation '1/2 Nex' has
caught on!)

k-space is also symmetric about a vertical axis,
so that the right half can be sampled and the left
half calculated (Fig. 1.10c). Physically, this corresponds to sampling one-half of the spin echo.
When the second half of the spin echo (after TE)
is sampled, the front half can be ignored and the
TE moved to a shorter value. This has been called
a fractional echo, and is utilized for fast gradient

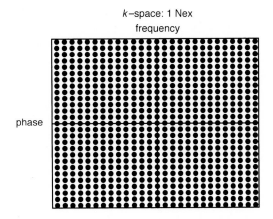

a

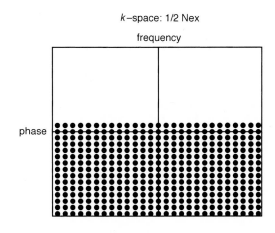

b

Figure 1.10

Properties of k-space. (a) k-space has Hermitian symmetry, which means that the top right-hand corner is symmetric with the lower left-hand corner, and the top left-hand corner is symmetric with the lower right-hand corner. Thus only the top half or the right half of k-space need be acquired, and the other half can be calculated. This 1 Nex acquisition fills k-space completely. (b) This 1/2 Nex acquisition fills slightly more than the bottom half of k-space in slightly more than half the usual time for a 1 Nex acquisition. The advantage of this 'half Fourier acquisition in phase' is the spatial resolution of a 256×256 matrix in half the time (with a concomitant loss of $\sqrt{2}$ in signal-to-noise). (c) This 'fractional echo' acquisition samples just over half of the right side of k-space, allowing the use of shorter TE for ultra-fast gradient echo techniques such as turboFLASH and fast SPGR. This 'half Fourier in frequency' acquisition is also known as 'asymmetric sampling of the echo' or 'fractional echo'.

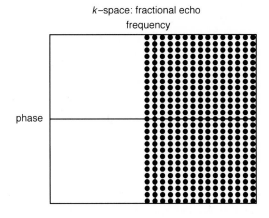

c

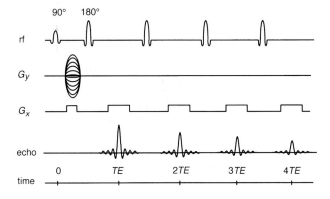

Figure 1.11

Conventional spin echo train. This pulse sequence diagram demonstrates a conventional four-echo train spin echo. Notice the single application of the phase encode gradient following the 90° pulse prior to production of four echoes, which decrease in amplitude owing to T_2 decay.

echo techniques such as turboFLASH. (Actually, the correct terms for these techniques are 'partial Fourier in phase' and 'partial Fourier in frequency' respectively.) Slightly more than 50% of k-space must be sampled in each of these techniques to provide phase information. This oversampling is typically eight lines of k-space for a 256^2 acquisition; i.e., instead of halving 256 to 128, 136 lines would be acquired. Although these partial Fourier techniques each have their advantages, they also have the disadvantage that any errors in the part that is acquired will propagate to the half of k-space that is calculated. ('Full' Fourier techniques, although they include a certain redundancy, tend to self-correct many errors.)

The spacing of the lines and the area occupied by k-space corresponds physically to the field of

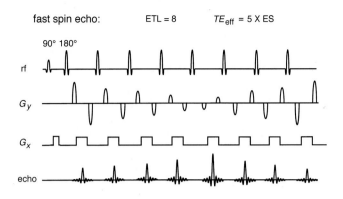

fast spin echo: ETL = 8 TE_{eff} = 5 X ES

Figure 1.12

Fast spin echo. The essential difference between
conventional spin echo and fast spin echo is that in
the latter, each echo is preceded by a different value
of the phase encode gradient (G_y in this example). As
a result, each echo in the echo train fills a separate
line in k-space, and (in this example) eight lines of k-space
are filled following a single 90° pulse during a
single interval TR. Unlike the conventional spin echo,
where the echoes following the 90° pulse continue to
decrease in amplitude owing to T_2 decay, in fast spin
echo, the amplitude of the echo is also determined by
the magnitude of the phase encode gradients
preceding it. (Weaker phase encode gradients result in
stronger echoes.) The TE of the strongest echo thus
produced is termed the 'effective TE', and is equal to
the product of the echo number (5 in this case) and
the echo spacing (i.e. the time between the 180°
pulses or the time between the echoes produced).

view and the spatial resolution respectively. The
more closely spaced the lines, the larger the FOV.
The greater the number of lines for a fixed
spacing, the better the spatial resolution. This is
discussed in greater detail in Chapter 2

Having now set the stage, it is finally possible to
discuss fast spin echo. The essential difference
between CSE and FSE is the following. In CSE, one
or more echoes is preceded by a *single* value of the
phase encode gradient on each pass or TR (Fig.
1.11). In FSE, *each* echo in an echo train is
preceded by a *different* value of the phase encode
gradient[4] (Fig. 1.12). Since each value of the phase
encode gradient corresponds to a separate line in
k-space, the result is that k-space is filled in that
much more rapidly (Figs 1.13a,b). For the eight-echo
train, eight lines of k-space would be filled in
during one TR, reducing the scan time by a factor
of eight (Fig. 1.13a). For a 16-echo train, the acqui-sition
time would be reduced by a factor of 16 (Fig.
1.13b). The only limitation on the total number of
echoes is the speed and strength of the gradients
and signal remaining following T_2 decay at long TE.

By sampling k-space more efficiently, FSE can
afford to increase TR, increase the matrix (improv-ing
spatial resolution), or increase the number of
averages (improving signal-to-noise ratio) without
unduly prolonging the acquisition.[4] In the brain,
increasing the TR to 4000–5000 ms decreases the
T_1 contribution to contrast, improving gray–white

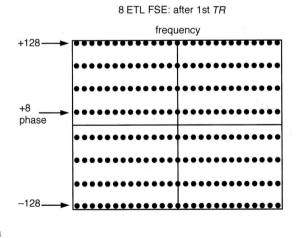

8 ETL FSE: after 1st TR

a

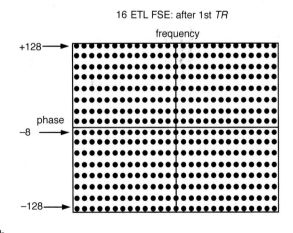

16 ETL FSE: after 1st TR

b

Figure 1.13

Fast spin echo in k-space. (a) An eight-echo train fast
spin echo fills eight lines in k-space for each 90° pulse
or TR interval. Thus the total acquisition time is one-eighth
that of a conventional spin echo. (b) With an

echo train length of 16, 16 lines in k-space are filled in
one TR interval, taking 1/16 of the time of a
conventional spin echo.

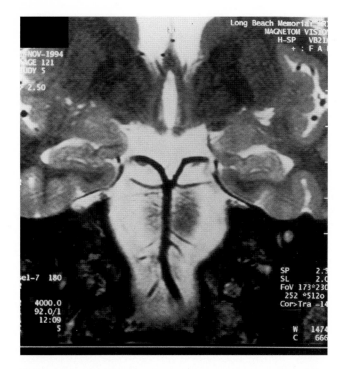

a

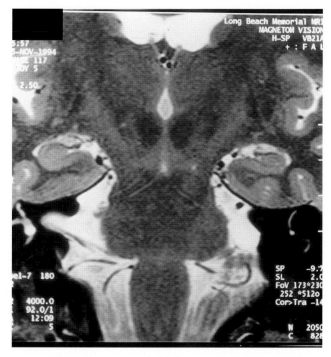

b

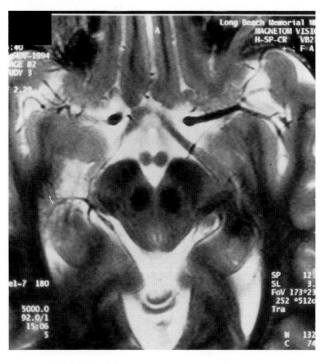

c

Figure 1.14

Long-*TR* capability. Using an ETL = 7, these images were acquired with *TR* = 4000 ms (a,b) or 5000 ms (c) in reasonable acquisition times, despite the relatively large matrix required to achieve 0.5 mm in-plane spatial resolution.

matter differentiation on proton density and T_2-weighted images (Fig. 1.14). Given the longer time spent at each slice position during a long echo train, fewer slices can be acquired for a given *TR*. A long *TR* is therefore not only desirable for contrast but also required for coverage.

The acquisition matrix can be increased to 512^2 (Fig. 1.15), improving spatial resolution. Increasing the number of averages improves S/N. In fact, FSE can utilize a higher *TR*, larger matrix and more averages than CSE *and* still do it in half the time (Fig. 1.16).

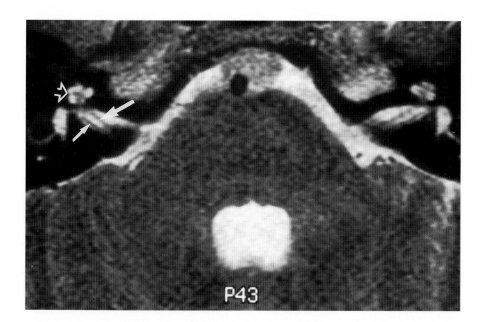

Figure 1.15

Large matrix acquisition. This 512^2 FSE image (ETL = 8) acquired through the seventh and eighth nerves clearly demonstrates the facial nerve (large arrow) and the superior vestibular nerve (small arrow) within the internal auditory canals. Also noted are the basal and secondary turns of the cochlea (open arrow).

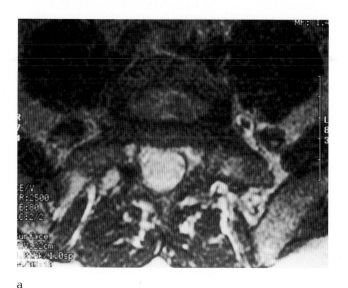

a

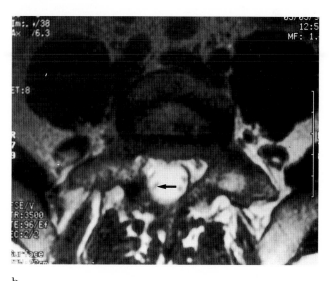

b

Figure 1.16

Comparison of CSE and FSE in the lumbar spine. (a) Conventional spin echo (CSE) acquired with 192×256 matrix barely demonstrates nerve roots. This acquisition took 9 min 10 s. (b) This fast spin echo image clearly demonstrates the nerve roots (arrow), has greater signal-to-noise ratio than the CSE image, and was acquired in approximately one-half the time (5½ min).

Several new parameters are required to describe FSE. The echo train length (ETL) or 'turbo factor' is a measure of the time efficiency of the sequence. The acquisition time for a CSE is the product of the *TR*, the number of phase encode steps and the number of excitations. The acquisition time for a single echo FSE is this number divided by the ETL.[4]

The echo spacing ES is the time between 180° pulses and therefore the time between echoes (Fig. 1.12). It is determined by the duration of the 180° pulses and the echo sampling time. To shorten the

ES, either the 180° pulse and/or the echo sampling time must be shortened (or both). As the 180° pulses shorten, they become less slice-selective and more 'broadbanded'. Rather than exciting a well-defined slice, i.e. a rectangular pulse profile, the slice becomes less well defined, i.e. more Gaussian. Crosstalk between slices increases, and the interslice gap must be increased accordingly. As the echo sampling time decreases, noise increases because of the higher bandwidth. Typical echo spacings are on the order of 16–20 ms at typical high field bandwidths of ±16 kHz (125 Hz/pixel).

The third (and most important) new parameter in FSE is the effective TE (TE_{eff}), since this parameter determines image contrast[4] (Fig. 1.12). TE_{eff} is the TE of one of the echoes in the echo train; therefore it is an integer multiple of the ES. To understand the concept of the effective TE, it is necessary to return to k-space.[2,3] Most of the signal and therefore most of the contrast come from the center of k-space. Physically, this reflects the effect of the phase encode gradient (Fig. 1.17). In the center of k-space, the phase encode gradient is weakest. This leads to the least dephasing along the phase encode axis and thus the strongest spin echo signal. Moving up or down from the center of k-space, the phase encode gradient gets stronger, causing spins at one end of the phase encode axis to be out of phase with spins at the other end, with partial cancellation of signal. With increasing gradient strength, there is more and more phase cancellation and a weaker and weaker signal.

Contrast in an FSE sequence is determined by matching the weakest value of the phase encode gradient with the echo to be emphasized (Fig. 1.12). The effective TE is that echo preceded by the weakest value of the phase encode gradient,[4] resulting in the least dephasing. To minimize adverse contrast averaging, the echoes on either side of the one with the effective TE are matched to the *next* weakest phase encode gradients. Those echoes with TE values furthest from the effective TE are assigned the strongest values of the phase encode gradient, thereby minimizing their overall contribution to the signal coming from the entire echo train (Fig. 1.12). Given this weighted averaging together of multiple echoes to form an image, FSE contrast is clearly going to be different from CSE contrast. Because the averaging of late echoes will enhance long-T_2 substances, CSF tends to be relatively brighter on a proton-density-weighted FSE image than on a CSE image with the same TR and TE (Fig. 1.18). Because fat makes a relatively strong contribution

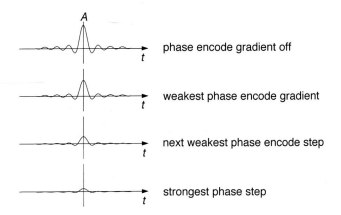

Figure 1.17

Signal strength versus phase encode gradient. With the phase encode gradient off, a strong spin echo is produced. As the phase encode gradient is increased in strength, protons at one end of the phase encode axis become 180° out of phase with protons at the other end, leading to phase cancellation and a decreased signal. As the strength of the phase encode gradient is increased, more and more auto-cancellation occurs, resulting in decreasing signal amplitude. This is why the strongest signal comes from the center of k-space, where the strength of the phase encode gradient is weakest.

to early echoes in the echo train, it is relatively brighter on T_2-weighted FSE images than it would be on a CSE image of the same TR and TE (Fig. 1.19). Actually, adipose tissue is artifactually dark on CSE images. Adipose tissue is 50% water and 50% fat. Fat and water resonate at different frequencies. As the spins diffuse through these different magnetic environments, they get out of phase. The amount of dephasing (and signal loss) depends on the time it is allowed to occur, i.e. the time before the rephasing 180° pulse is applied. The dephasing is minimized by the closely spaced 180° pulses in FSE, which minimize diffusion effects.[5] Thus the signal of fat on a T_2-weighted FSE image is 'truer' than on a CSE image, where it is decreased owing to diffusion-mediated dephasing.

Contrast averaging is one of the limitations of FSE. It can be minimized by reducing the number of echoes averaged together. In addition to

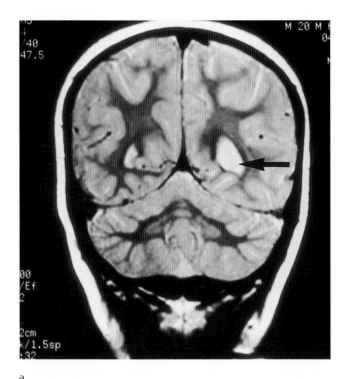

a

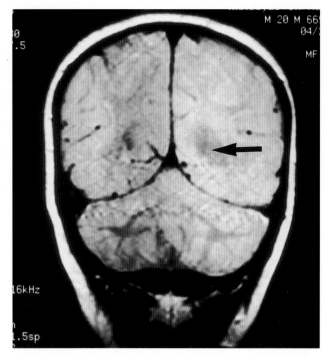

b

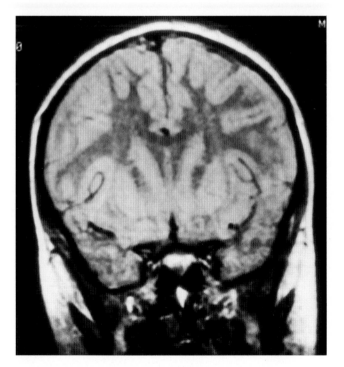

c

Figure 1.18

CSF intensity on proton-density-weighted image.
(a) FSE image acquired with $TR = 4000$ ms and minimum possible TE (17 ms at ±16 kHz bandwidth) demonstrates high intensity CSF (arrow).
(b) Conventional spin echo (SE 3000/30) demonstrates desired CSF isointensity to brain (arrow), despite longer TE. (c) In order to make the intensity of CSF equal to that of brain on an FSE image at the minimum effective TE of 17 ms, the TR could be reduced to approximately 2500 ms. This adds significant (undesirable) T_1 weighting to what should be a proton-density-weighted image, particularly at high field.

contrast (or k-space) averaging, there are two additional differences in contrast between FSE and CSE images. The multiple, rapidly repeated 180° pulses leave little time for spins to dephase as they diffuse through regions with different magnetic fields. This dephasing leads to signal loss associated with so-called magnetic susceptibility effects on T_2-weighted CSE images. In FSE images, the signal loss is minimized owing to the rephasing effects of the multiple 180° pulses.[4] Thus T_2-weighted FSE images are relatively less sensitive to the magnetic susceptibility effects of

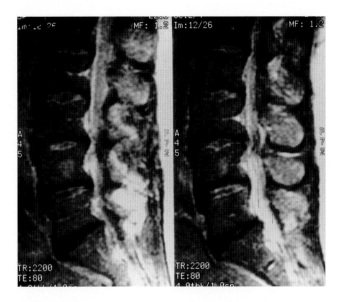

a

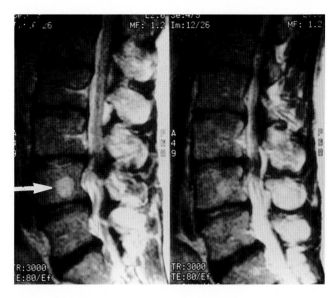

b

Figure 1.19

Intensity of fat: FSE versus CSE. (a) Conventional T_2-weighted image barely demonstrates a 'fat island' because of relatively low signal. (b) On T_2-weighted FSE image, the intensity of the fat island is significantly increased (arrow).

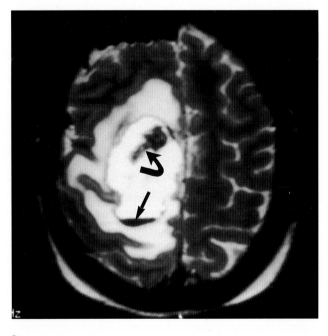

a

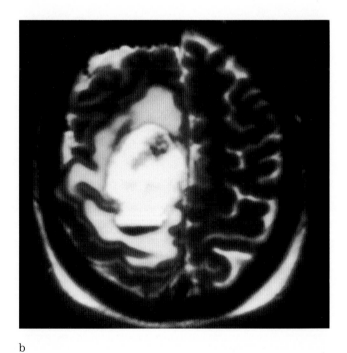

b

Figure 1.20

Relative sensitivity to magnetic susceptibility effects: CSE versus FSE. (a) CSE image demonstrates low signal in the recently operated tumor bed from deoxyhemoglobin (straight arrow) and gel foam (curved arrow). (b) On the FSE image, the low signal intensity from the diamagnetic susceptibility effects of the gel foam is somewhat reduced; however, the low intensity from the deoxyhemoglobin is maintained.

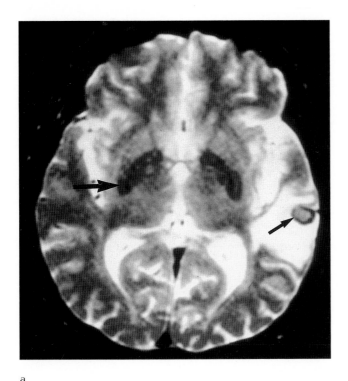
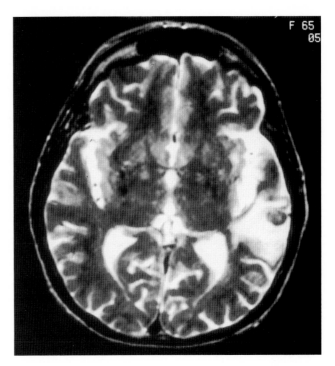

a   b

Figure 1.21

Sensitivity to hemosiderin. (a) On T_2-weighted CSE image, hemosiderin ring surrounding hemorrhagic metastasis (small arrow) is quite noticeable, as is the magnetic susceptibility effect from the ferritin in the globus pallidus (large arrow). (b) On FSE image, the hemosiderin rim is much more subtle, as is the low intensity of the globus pallidus due to increased sensitivity of FSE sequences to magnetic susceptibility effects.

hemorrhage (e.g. deoxyhemoglobin and hemosiderin) than T_2-weighted CSE images (Figs 1.20 and 1.21).

One FSE variant that increases sensitivity to magnetic susceptibility effects is called GRASE (Fig. 1.22).[6,7] In this, some of the spin echoes are replaced by gradient echoes. This leads to greater gradient echo-like contrast and increased sensitivity to susceptibility effects (Fig. 1.23). Since gradient echoes are produced by gradient reversal alone without a 180° pulse, the number of 180° rf pulses is decreased as well in GRASE. This results in decreased rf power deposition. Since less time is required to produce a gradient echo than a spin echo, the echo spacing is reduced, potentially leading to longer echo trains and greater k-space coverage in the same acquisition time following a given 90° pulse. This additional time savings can be taken as longer TR or larger matrices[8] (Fig. 1.24) in the same overall acquisition time.

Another manifestation of the rapid. multiple, 180° pulses is an inadvertent magnetization transfer (MT) effect. *Intentional* MT is produced by an off-resonance rf pulse that saturates protein-bound water in the broad peaks on either side of the narrow bulk phase water peak (see Chapter 6). Because the short 180° pulses in FSE are more broadbanded, they also contain frequencies off the bulk water resonance. Thus protein-bound water is relatively suppressed on FSE images compared with CSE images.This effect is most noticeable in the spine, where normally hydrated disks are bright on T_2-weighted CSE images but somewhat darker on FSE images[9] (Fig. 1.25). Thus the contrast between normal (usually bright) disks and desiccated (usually dark) disks is diminished.

There are also some positive features resulting from the multiple 180° pulses. Because they are evenly spaced, there is a natural 'even echo rephasing' effect.[10] Thus CSF motion artifacts are much less severe than on non-flow-compensated

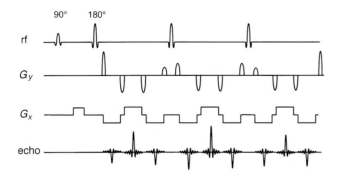

Figure 1.22

GRASE. In this variation of FSE, some of the spin echoes have been replaced by gradient echoes—hence the name GRASE for *gradient–spin echo*. In this example, there are two gradient echoes for each spin echo. Since there are 9 echoes in total, the sequence is as efficient as an FSE with an ETL of 9. However, contrast appears more like a gradient echo, with increased sensitivity to magnetic susceptibility effects. Also, there is less rf power deposition, since there are fewer 180° pulses than FSE.

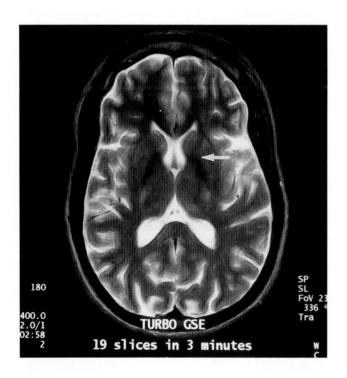

Figure 1.23

TURBO GSE (GRASE) image. This T_2-weighted TURBO GSE image through the globus pallidus demonstrates magnetic susceptibility effects to good advantage.

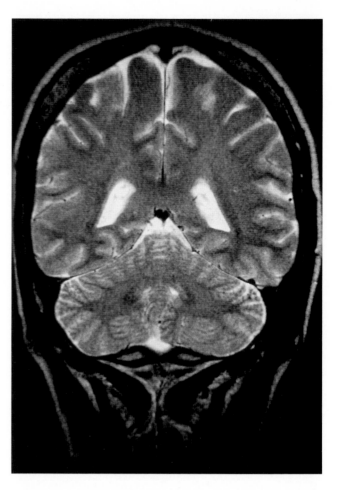

Figure 1.24

1024^2 GRASE image. With high-performance gradients, 1024^2 acquisition matrices are possible for sequences such as GRASE (or TURBO GSE). (Image provided by David Feinberg, MD PhD.)

T_2-weighted CSE images (Fig. 1.26). In addition, the rephasing resulting from the multiple 180° pulses leads to less distortion from metal on FSE images.[11] Finally, FSE images are much more tolerant of a poorly shimmed magnet than CSE images (Fig. 1.27).

On a conventional double spin echo acquisition, the first echo is 'free', i.e. it neither prolongs the overall acquisition time nor limits the total number of slices. In FSE, on the other hand, each 256^2 image requires filling a 256^2 matrix in *k*-space. Thus the time required to acquire a proton density and T_2-weighted FSE image is twice the time it would take to acquire either one alone (assuming the same *TR*: which is no longer a necessary requirement in FSE).[4]

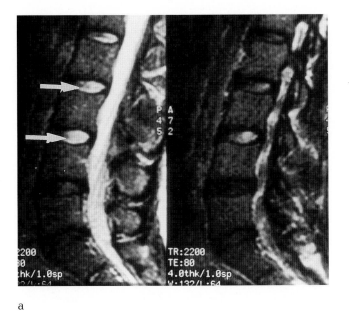
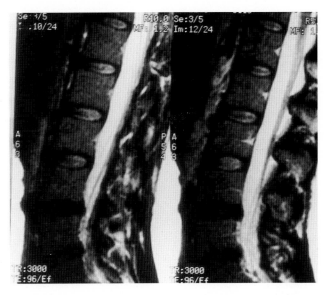

a   b

Figure 1.25

Magnetization transfer effect. Comparing the CSE image (a) to an FSE image (b), normal intravertebral disks are brighter on the T_2-weighted CSE image (arrows). This reflects a magnetization transfer effect that is intrinsic to the FSE sequence. Specifically, the protein-bound water in the normal disks is partially saturated by the off-resonant frequencies in the rapidly applied 180° rf pulses of which the FSE is composed. As a result of this, the contrast between normal disks and dehydrated disks (at L4–5 and L5–S1) is decreased.

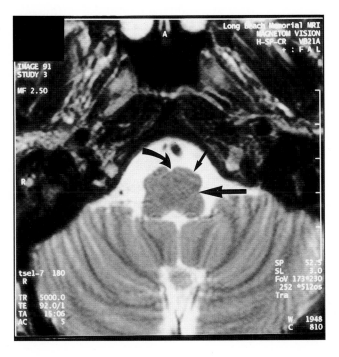

Figure 1.26

Natural flow compensation effect of FSE. Transverse FSE image through the medulla demonstrates boundaries distinctly, including the preolivary sulcus (small arrow), postolivary sulcus (large arrow) and ventral sulcus (curved arrow). The apparent 'flow compensation' in this example reflects the multiple 180° pulses and the 'even echo rephasing' effect.

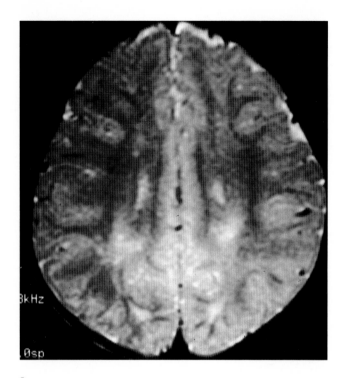

a

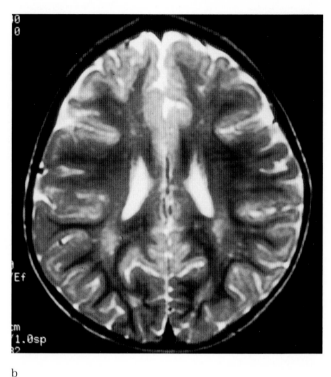

b

Figure 1.27

Benefit of FSE in a poorly shimmed magnet. CSE (a) and FSE (b) images were both acquired after the metallic wheel from a rolling i.v. pole somehow made its way into the bore of the magnet, leading to marked B_0 nonuniformity. The multiple rephasing 180° pulses of the FSE sequence are much more tolerant of a poorly shimmed magnet than the CSE sequence.

There are three ways to acquire a double echo image in FSE: a full echo train,[4] a split echo train[4] and a 'shared' echo approach[12] (Fig. 1.28). In a full echo train, all echoes in the train contribute to the image (Fig. 1.28a). For an ETL of 8 and a 256^2 image, 32 echo trains would be required ($8 \times 32 = 256$) for each image. In a split echo train, the first half of the echo train contributes to the image with the shorter effective TE, and the second half of the echo train contributes to the second effective TE (Fig. 1.28b). For an ETL of 8, only 4 echoes would be applied to each image from each train. Therefore 64 trains would be required to fill k-space ($4 \times 64 = 256$). In a shared echo approach,[12] the first and last echoes in the train are emphasized for TE_1 and TE_2 respectively, and the echoes in between are shared for both images (Fig. 1.28c). This has the advantage of a shorter ETL compared with a full or shared echo train approach, allowing more slices to be acquired for a given TR. (Since the number of slices is determined by the TR divided by the product of the echo spacing and the ETL, a shorter ETL allows more slices.) The example shown in Fig. 1.28(c) uses an ETL of 5. Four lines of k-space are filled per TR, three of which are the same for the first and second echo images. (Thus there is some overlap of the 'information' in the two images, compared with the split echo approach.) Filling four echoes per pass provides the same efficiency as a split echo approach, i.e. 64 echo trains total will be required to fill k-space ($4 \times 64 = 256$). On the other hand, the shorter ETL allows 60% more slices to be acquired in the same time:

$$\frac{\text{slices}_{\text{ETL}=5}}{\text{slices}_{\text{ETL}=8}} = \frac{TR/5 \times \text{ESP}}{TR/8 \times \text{ESP}} = \frac{8}{5} = 1.6$$

A variant of the shared echo approach is so-called keyhole imaging.[13] In this technique, k-space is covered completely on the first image, but only the central part (say 20%) of k-space is covered on subsequent images (Fig. 1.29), providing most of the contrast. This has the disadvantage that the high-frequency outer 80% of k-space is shared information; however, it has the advantage of speeding up the subsequent imaging by a factor

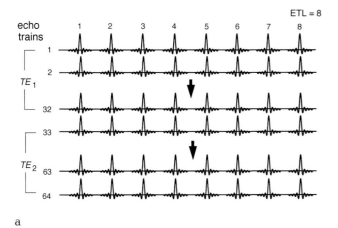

a

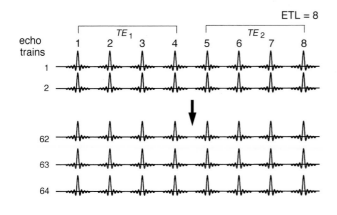

b

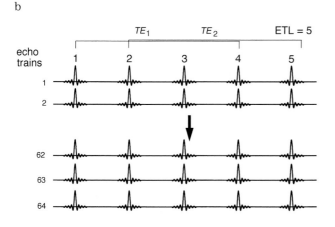

c

Figure 1.28

Double echo fast spin echo. (a) Full echo train. In this double echo fast spin echo technique, 256 lines in k-space are filled by 32 echo trains, each 8 echoes long. Two such sequences are applied sequentially, taking twice the time of a single sequence. The advantage of this approach is complete flexibility in the choice of the TE_{eff} for both sequences. The disadvantage is the contrast averaging that occurs when eight echoes are averaged together. (b) Split echo train double fast spin echo acquisition. In this example, the first four echoes in an eight-echo train contribute to the first TE_{eff}, and the second four echoes contribute to the second TE_{eff}. Since only four lines in k-space are filled for each image with each echo train, 64 echo trains in total must be acquired to fill 256 lines in k-space. The advantage of this approach is less contrast averaging with four echoes (as opposed to eight with the full echo approach). The disadvantage is restriction on the minimum TE_{eff} of the second echo image (five times the echo spacing in this example). (While not a significant restriction with an echo train length of 8, it does become significant with echo trains of 16 or longer.) (c) Shared echo train FSE. In this approach, the central three echoes are shared, i.e. they contribute to both echoes. For the first effective TE, the first echo is prioritized. For the second effective TE, the last is prioritized. The advantage of this approach is ETL = 8 efficiency (i.e. four lines of k-space filled for two images per pass) with a five-echo train, leading to more slices per TR. The disadvantage is some redundancy in the information.

of 5. Thus keyhole imaging is useful when fast repetitive imaging of the same slice is required, e.g. for perfusion imaging.[13]

There are advantages and disadvantages to these double echo FSE techniques. The split echo train has the disadvantage that the effective TE of the second echo is constrained (Fig. 1.28b). It can be no shorter than the first echo in the second half of the train. For short echo trains (i.e. those with an ETL of 8 or less), this is not a problem. However, for long echo trains (e.g. those with an ETL of 16 or larger), it could pose

a limitation. For example, for an ETL of 16 and ES of 20 ms, the minimum effective TE of the second echo image would be $9 \times 20 = 180$ ms, which might be longer than desired for a T_2-weighted image of the brain. This is not a problem with a full echo train, since there is complete flexibility in the choice of the second effective TE. An advantage of the split echo approach, however, is that there is less contrast averaging than for the full echo train; therefore, the images are sharper (Fig. 1.30). In practice, the split echo train is generally used for ETLs of 8 or less and

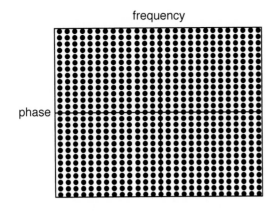

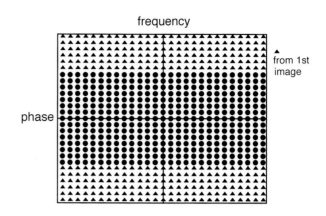

a

b

Figure 1.29

Keyhole imaging. (a) On the first pass, all of *k*-space is filled. (b) On subsequent passes, only the central 20% (or so) of *k*-space is filled and the outer 80% is 'borrowed' from the first pass. This has the advantage of decreasing the acquisition time by a factor of five, e.g. for perfusion studies.

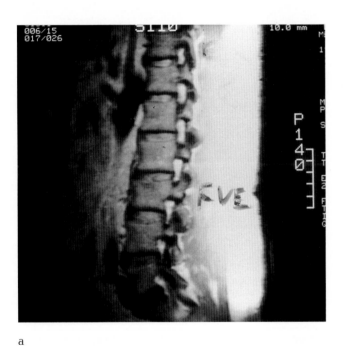

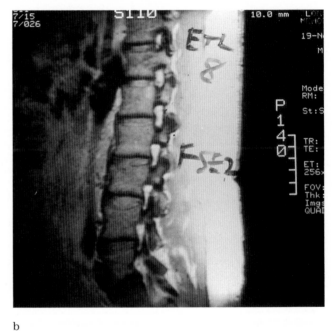

a

b

Figure 1.30

Comparison of full echo train (a) and split echo train (b) FSE. Both images were acquired with echo train lengths ETL = 8. The split echo train images (b) are clearly 'crisper' than the slightly blurred images in (a), which uses a full echo train acquisition.

the full echo train for ETLs greater than 8. The shared echo approach and keyhole imaging have the advantage of better coverage and faster scanning respectively; however, the information in the two images is not truly unique.

More recent versions of FSE with high performance gradients allow additional options, such as higher bandwidths, flow compensation and 3D acquisition (Fig. 1.31). With higher bandwidths, the echo sampling time can be

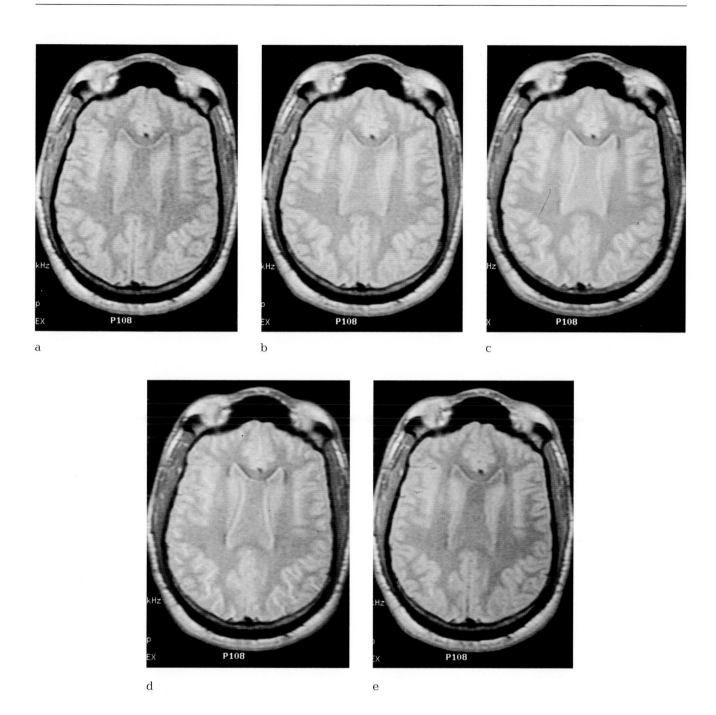

a   b   c

d   e

Figure 1.31

High-bandwidth FSE. In the series shown here, bandwidth, *TR*, minimum effective *TE*, and split versus full echo train are varied to ultimately produce a proton-density-weighted image in which the CSF intensity is the same as white matter. In the first nine images, the matrix has been reduced to 128×256 at 1 Nex to minimize the acquisition time. (a) In order to achieve the shortest possible *TE* (8 ms), the bandwidth must be increased to ±62 kHz. For an ETL = 8 (full echo train) and *TR* = 3000 ms, CSF is isointense to brain. (b) To recover some of the signal-to-noise ratio given up by the higher bandwidth in (a), the bandwidth has now been reduced to ±31 kHz, increasing the minimum effective *TE* to 10 ms, making the CSF slightly hyperintense to white matter. (c) Reducing the bandwidth further to ±16 kHz (standard) raises the minimum effective *TE* to 14 ms, which definitely results in hyperintense CSF. (d) Returning to a bandwidth of ±31 kHz (minimum effective *TE* = 10 ms), the ETL is increased to 16 (full echo). The averaging of twice as many echoes results in CSF hyperintense to white matter. (e) By splitting the 16-echo train at the same ±31 kHz bandwidth (minimum effective *TE* = 10 ms), the CSF returns to isointensity with white matter.

continued

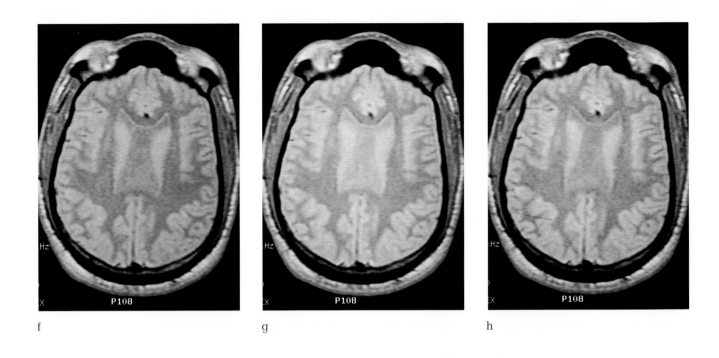

f   g   h

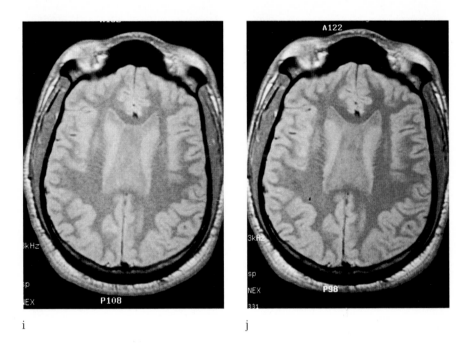

i   j

Figure 1.31 *continued*

(f) By reducing the ETL to 8 (split echo), there is even less *k*-space averaging, and the CSF remains isointense to white matter. (g) Keeping everything else the same but raising the *TR* to 4000 ms increases the intensity of CSF relative to white matter (as expected). (Note that for the first echo image, the contrast produced by a full echo train with ETL = 4 is the same as that produced by a split echo train with ETL = 8.) (h) Keeping everything else the same but reducing the

TR to 3500 ms results in CSF essentially isointense to white matter. (i) Increasing ETL to 8 with the split echo train approach leaves the CSF isointense to white matter (as expected), but adds a second echo image. (j) Leaving everything else the same but increasing the matrix to 256^2 and doubling the number of excitations leads to a high-resolution, high signal-to-noise ratio, double echo FSE technique with CSF isointense to white matter on the first echo.

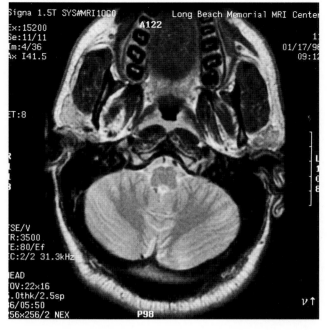

a

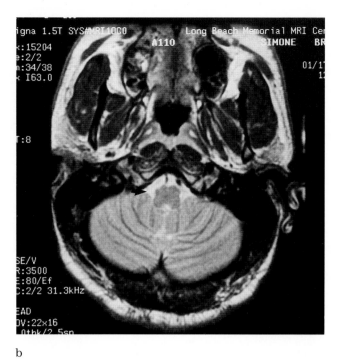

b

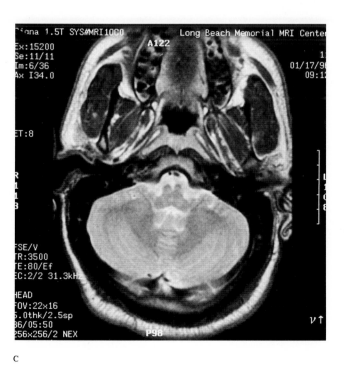

c

d

Figure 1.32

Flow-compensated FSE. (a,b) Comparison of non-flow-compensated (a) and flow-compensated (b) FSE acquisition at the level of caudal medulla. Note the increased intensity of the CSF in the medullary cistern (arrow) compared with the non-flow-compensated image. (c,d) Comparison of non-flow-compensated (c) and flow-compensated (d) FSE images in the upper medulla demonstrates higher-intensity CSF due to flow compensation (arrow) in basal cisterns as well as improved definition of cerebellar folia.

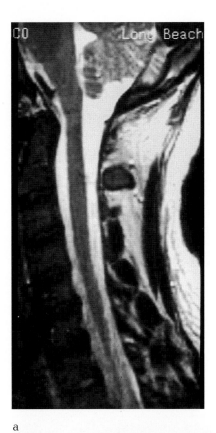

a

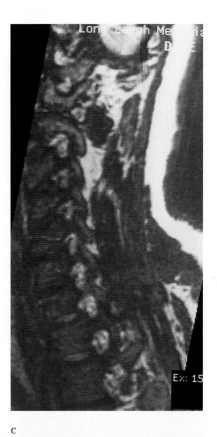

c

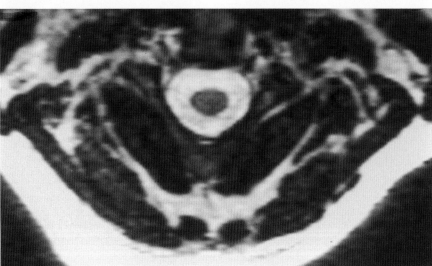

b

Figure 1.33

3D FSE of the cervical spine.
(a) Sagittal reformation of
primary axial acquisition.
(b) Primary 1 mm thick axial 3D
FSE acquisition. (c) Oblique 3D
FSE reformation demonstrating
neural foramina en face.

reduced, reducing the echo spacing ES. This
allows a lower minimum effective *TE* to be used,
reducing the intensity of CSF on the (suppos-
edly) proton-density-weighted first echo. With a
shorter ES, there is less contribution from later
echoes to bright CSF owing to their now-shorter
TE values. Thus the previously hyperintense CSF
on proton-density-weighted images can now be
made isointense to white matter (Fig. 1.31). Use
of a split (versus full) echo train approach also
minimizes unwanted T_2 contributions by only
averaging echoes from the early half of the echo
train. (This is the same principle that allows T_1-
weighted FSEs to be performed,[14] i.e. the use of

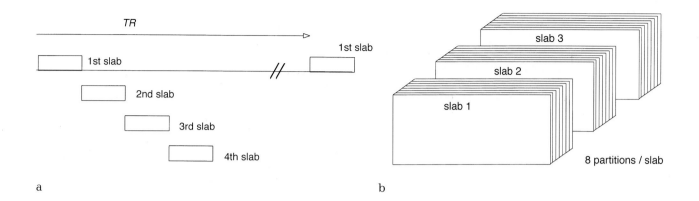

a

b

Figure 1.34

3D FSE schematic. (a) First step: multiple slabs are excited similarly to multislice imaging. Unfortunately, these slab profiles are more Gaussian than rectangular; thus there is a tendency for crosstalk. To obtain contiguous slabs, two acquisitions (with 100% gaps) can be interleaved or odd slabs can be excited, followed by even slabs within a given acquisition. (b) Second step: slabs are subdivided into contiguous partitions by second phase encode gradient.

higher bandwidths and shorter echo trains). Figure 1.31 demonstrates optimization of CSF–white matter isointensity while adjusting bandwidth, ETL, split versus full echo train and TR. Figure 1.32 demonstrates the additional CSF brightening in the basal cisterns resulting from flow compensation.

3D FSE is the newest enhancement to fast spin echo imaging.[15] In 3D FSE, the slice thickness is decreased to 1 mm, comparable to the in-plane spatial resolution. With isotropic resolution, a single acquisition can be reformatted into multiple planes. While 3D T_1-weighted gradient echo data sets have been used for some time (e.g. MP RAGE (Siemens), 3D SPGR (GE) and 3D rf spoiled FAST (Picker)), 3D T_2-weighted data sets have not hitherto been available. This is now possible with 3D FSE. A single, bright-CSF, 3D FSE acquisition can yield images in the reformatted planes (Fig. 1.33a) of near-comparable quality to the primary plane of acquisition (Fig. 1.33b). As an added bonus in the cervical spine, oblique en face views through the neural foramina can be obtained without increasing acquisition time (Fig. 1.33c).

3D FSE is like 2D FSE except that the multiple slices in 2D FSE are replaced by multiple slabs, each of which is subsequently partitioned into 1 mm slices (Fig. 1.34). The slab profiles are more Gaussian than rectangular, partly because of the

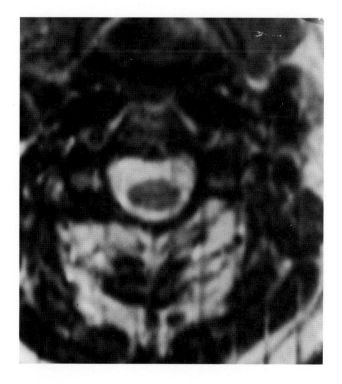

Figure 1.35

Misregistration artifact in 3D FSE. Axial reformation of primary sagittal acquisition demonstrates misregistration artifacts due to patient motion between two interleaved acquisitions.

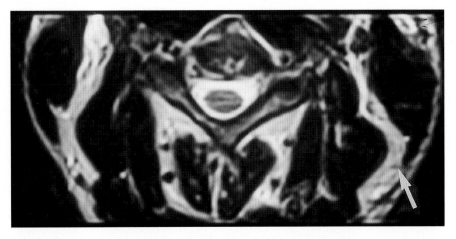

a

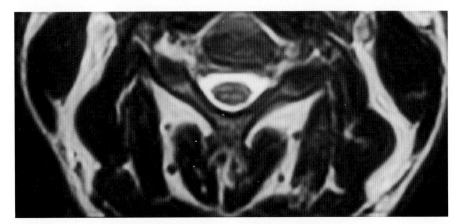

b

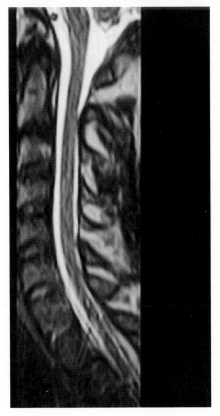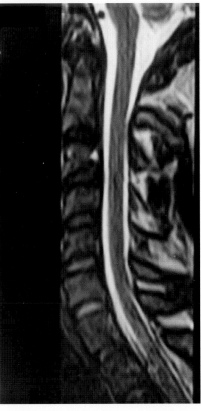

c   d

Figure 1.36

Non-slab-interleaved 3D FSE of the cervical spine. In this technique, the odd slices are excited first and then the even slices are excited within the same *TR* interval, thereby avoiding patient motion misregistration artifact. (a,b) Axial reformations of primary coronal acquisition using *TR* = 8000 ms with ETL = 16 (a) or *TR* = 16 000 ms with ETL = 32 (b), for the same acquisition time. Note the more prominent venetian blind artifacts due to saturation effects (arrows) in (a) than in (b). (c,d) Sagittal reformations of primary coronal acquisition using *TR* = 8000 ms/ETL = 16 (c) or *TR* = 16 000 ms/ETL = 32 (d).

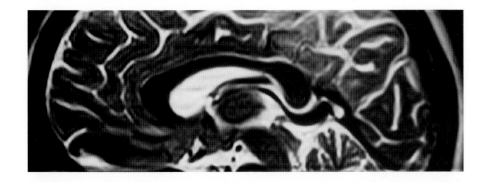

a

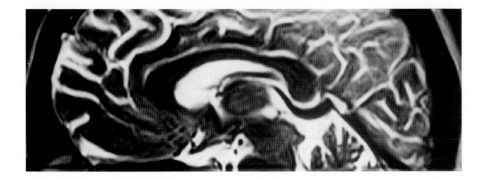

b

Figure 1.37

Non-slab-interleaved 3D FSE of the brain. Comparison of sagittal reformations of primary axial acquisition utilizing TR = 8000 ms (a) versus TR = 12 000 ms (b). The more prominent venetian blind artifacts in (a) reflect the saturation effects due to crosstalk from the interleaved slabs, which are largely eliminated in (b).

need to use extremely short rf pulses.[16] Gaussian slice profiles do not pose a serious problem on 2D (multislice) techniques, because 50% gaps can be inserted between slices without sacrificing image quality. For 3D techniques where perpendicular reformations are being contemplated, however, the slices/slabs must be contiguous. Forcing the slabs together results in crosstalk, leading to loss of signal on the edges of the slab. This is particularly prominent for long-T_1 substances such as CSF. One partial solution to this problem is to increase the gap to 100% and to interleave two separate acquisitions. This approach eliminates crosstalk, but runs the risk of slab misregistration due to patient motion between the two acquisitions (Fig. 1.35). Another potential solution involves exciting odd slabs first, and then exciting even slabs on a second pass within the same TR interval[17] (Figs 1.36 and 1.37). In either case, 'venetian blind' artifacts may be found on the reformations, as a result of either crosstalk or misregistration.

While this chapter has thus far only dealt with traditional T_1- and T_2-weighted FSE techniques, a 180° inversion pulse can be added to create a

fast inversion–recovery (IR) sequence[18] (see Chapter 7). The inversion time in 'fast IR' can be chosen to null specific tissues based on their respective T_1 values. Short-TI IR sequences (e.g. fast STIR) can be used to null fat or bone marrow. TI values on the order of 300–400 ms null gray matter, increasing gray–white differentiation in the brain. TI values on the order of 2000–2500 ms can be chosen to null CSF (e.g. fast FLAIR). Like traditional FLAIR, fast FLAIR is particularly useful to detect early parenchymal abnormalities in the brain, especially at the brain–CSF interface (e.g. the periventricular region). Unlike traditional FLAIR, however, fast FLAIR can be performed much more quickly. For example, we have developed a fast FLAIR technique that yields 30 slices in 8 min[19] (Fig. 1.38). When applied to 'rule out MS' patients, we reduce the slice thickness to 2 mm (to minimize partial volume effects) and scan in the sagittal plane (to visualize the undersurface of the corpus callosum) with a 50–100% gap (to cover all of the white matter). With this technique, we recently reported a series of 25 potential MS patients, 13 of whom would have been sent home with a

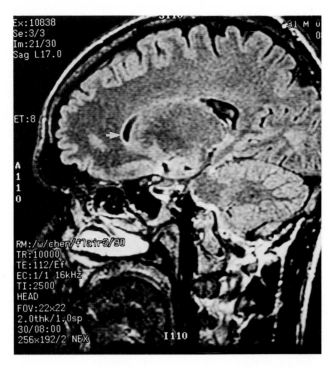

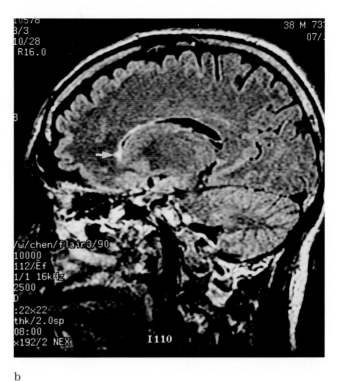

a   b

Figure 1.38

Fast FLAIR. This 2 mm thick sagittal acquisition features the contrast of FLAIR and the speed of fast spin echo. (a) Normal subject. Note the excellent gray–white differentiation and normal subependymal stripe (arrow). (b) In a patient with suspected multiple sclerosis, focal lesions are noted on the inner aspect of the corpus callosum (arrow) consistent with early diagnosis of multiple sclerosis. The conventional axial 5 mm thick spin echo images were normal in this patient.

'normal' diagnosis using a routine CSE 3000/30 and 80 technique. Of these patients, 43% had abnormalities on the fast FLAIR consistent with early MS[19] (Fig. 1.38).

FSE can also be combined with spectral pre-saturation pulses (e.g. fat saturation or water saturation). Fat-saturated T_2-weighted FSE is particularly useful for detecting early bone marrow abnormalities, such as metastases[20] and bone marrow contusions (Fig. 1.39).[12] In one recent series, fat-saturated T_2-weighted FSE was applied to a series of 73 knees with suspected internal derangement. It was found that 30% of the patients in this series who had ostensibly normal bone marrow on the routine 3 mmconventional T_2-weighted SE exam had clearly defined bone marrow contusions on the fat-saturated T_2-weighted FSE.[21] In another series of 29 patients with head and neck lesions,[22] fat-saturated T_2-weighted FSE was shown to be comparable to the 'gold standard', gadolinium-enhanced, fat-saturated, T_1-weighted spin echo in characterizing lesions (Fig. 1.40). By changing the frequency of the saturation pulse, water can be suppressed instead of fat. This has application in MRI of the breast. When examining breast implants for suspected extracapsular rupture, fast STIR is usually used to null the signal from the fat in the breast. Unfortunately, with this technique, breast parenchyma remains bright (like silicone). When a spectral water saturation prepulse is added to the fast STIR, the signal from the watery parenchyma is canceled. Thus the only substance with high signal is silicone, reducing potential ambiguities.

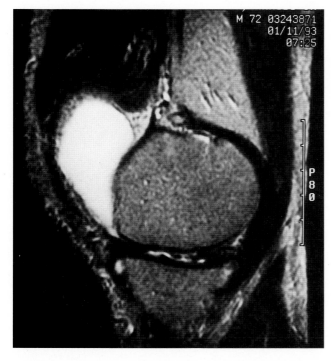

a

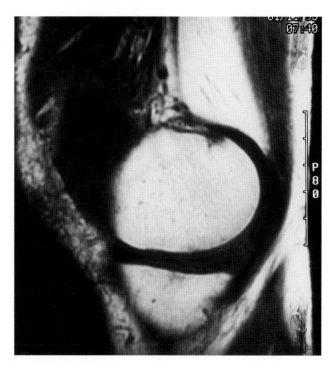

b

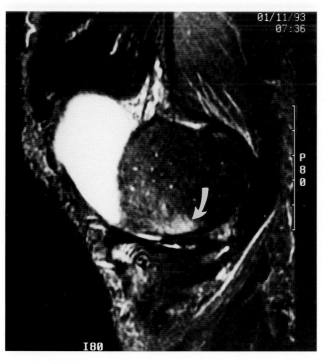

c

Figure 1.39

A 72-year-old male with recent history of fall and persistent medial knee pain. (a) T_2-weighted spin echo image (SE 2700/80). (b) T_1-weighted image (SE 500/16). (c) T_2-weighted fast spin echo images with fat suppression (FSE 4500/95). Focal site of bone contusion is not seen using conventional T_2- and T_1-weighted sequences. The site of bone contusion (arrow) is readily apparent using the T_2-weighted FS–FSE technique.

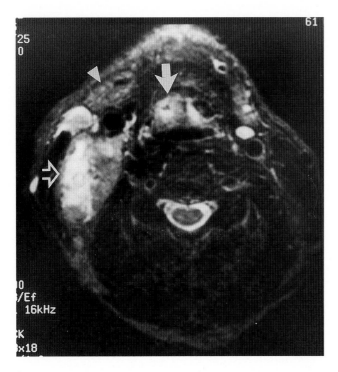

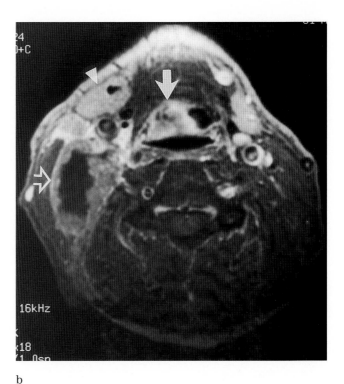

a   b

Figure 1.40

FS FSE in head and neck: a 61-year-old man with supraglottic squamous cell carcinoma. (a) Axial T_2-weighted fat-suppressed FSE (4700/108) MR image shows complex necrotic right supraglottic tumor (solid arrow), involving vallecula and anterior surface of epiglottis. In addition, a large complex necrotic lymph node in right internal jugular chain (open arrow) is readily apparent on this image. Again note the excellent contrast between both primary mass and metastatic node and their respective adjacent soft tissues. In addition, complexity of both masses is well defined, with a central cystic component exhibiting high signal intensity and a peripheral nodular solid component exhibiting intermediate signal intensity. Low-signal-intensity right submandibular gland (arrowhead) is also visible. (b) Axial contrast-enhanced T_1-weighted fat-suppressed SE (500/16) MR image at the same level as (a) clearly defines central cystic nonenhancing and peripheral nodular solid enhancing components of both primary tumor (solid arrow) and metastatic node (open arrow). However, the primary mass appears slightly less conspicuous relative to adjacent supraglottic tissues. Low-signal-intensity right submandibular gland (arrowhead) is also visible.

References

1. Hennig J, Nauerth A, Friedburg H, RARE imaging: a fast imaging method for clinical MR. *Magn Reson Med* 1986; **3:** 823.

2. Wehrli FW, Principles of magnetic resonance. In: *Magnetic resonance imaging*, 2nd edn (ed DD Stark, WG Bradley) 3–20. Mosby-Year Book, St Louis, 1992.

3. Wood, ML, Fourier imaging. In: *Magnetic resonance imaging*, 2nd edn (ed DD Stark, WG Bradley) 21–66. Mosby-Year Book, St Louis, 1992.

4. Jolesz RA, Jones KM, Fast spin-echo imaging of the brain. *Top Magn Reson Imaging* 1993; **5:** 1–13.

5. Henkelman RM, Hardy PA, Bishop JE et al, Why fat is bright in RARE and fast spin-echo imaging. *J Magn Reson Imaging* 1992; **2:** 533–40.

6. Oshio K, Feinberg DA, GRASE (gradient- and spin-echo) imaging: a novel fast MRI technique. *Magn Reson Med* 1991; **20:** 344–9.

7. Feinberg DA, Oshio K, GRASE (gradient- and spin-echo) MR imaging: a new fast clinical imaging technique. *Radiology* 1991; **181:** 597–602.

8. Feinberg DA, Kiefer B, Litt AW, High resolution GRASE MRI of the brain and spine: 512 and 1024 matrix imaging. *J Comput Assist Tomogr* 1995; **19:** 1–7.

9. Santyr GE, Magnetization transfer effect in multislice MR imaging. *Magn Reson Imaging* 1993; **11:** 521–32.

10. Waluch V, Bradley WG, NMR even echo rephasing in slow laminar flow. *J Comput Assist Tomogr* 1984; **8:** 594–8.

11. Tartaglino LM, Flander AE, Vinitski S, Friedman DP, Metallic artifacts on MR images of the postoperative spine: reduction with fast spin-echo techniques. *Radiology* 1994; **190:** 565–9.

12. Johnson BA, Fram EK, Drayer BP et al, Evaluation of shared-view acquisition using repeated echoes (SHARE): a dual-echo fast spin-echo MR technique. *AJNR* 1994; **15:** 667–73.

13. Kucharczyk W, Bishop JE, Plewes DB et al, Detection of pituitary microadenomas: comparison of dynamic keyhole fast spine-echo, unenhanced, and conventional contrast-enhanced MR imaging. *AJR* 1994; **163:** 671–9.

14. Weinberger E, Murakami JW, Shaw DW et al, Three-dimensional fast spin echo T_1-weighted imaging of the pediatric spine. *J Comput Assist Tomogr* 1995; **19:** 721–5.

15. Yuan C, Schmiedl UP, Weinberger E et al, Three-dimensional fast spin-echo imaging: pulse sequences and in vivo image evaluation. *J Magn Reson Imaging* 1993; **3:** 894–9.

16. Bradley WG, Atkinson DJ, Chen D-Y et al, Three-dimensional Turbo FLAIR sequence: comparison with the conventional SE sequence in the brain. Presented at the 1995 RSNA, Chicago, IL, 25 November–1 December.

17. Loncur M, Palmer N, Gullapalli R, Bradley WG, Non-slab-interleaved 3D fast spin-echo imaging of the brain and spine. Abstract, 4th Annual Meeting ISMRM, 27 April–3 May 1996, New York, NY.

18. Weinberger E, Shaw DW, White KS et al, Nontraumatic pediatric musculoskeletal MR imaging: comparison of conventional and fast-spin-echo short inversion time inversion–recovery technique. *Radiology* 1995; **194:** 721–6.

19. Hashemi RH, Bradley WG, Chen D-Y et al, Suspected multiple sclerosis: MR imaging with a thin-section fast FLAIR pulse sequence. *Radiology* 1995; **196:** 505–10.

20. Jones KM, Schwartz RB, Mantello MT et al, Fast spin-echo MR in the detection of vertebral metastases: comparison of three sequences. *AJNR* 1994; **15:** 401–7.

21. Kapelov SR, Teresi LM, Bradley WG et al, Bone contusions of the knee: increased lesion detection with fast spin-echo MR imaging with spectroscopic fat saturation. *Radiology* 1993; **189:** 901–4.

22. Dubin MD, Teresi LM, Bradley WG et al, Conspicuity of tumors of the head and neck on fat-suppressed MR images: T_2-weighted fast-spin-echo versus contrast-enhanced T_1-weighted conventional spin-echo sequences. *AJR* 1995; **164:** 1213–21.

2

Using high-performance gradients

William G Bradley, Dennis J Atkinson and Dar-Yeong Chen

Abbreviations

ADC   analog-to-digital converter
BW   receiver bandwidth
BW_ϕ bandwidth along phase encode axis (EPI)
BW_{ss} slice select bandwidth
CSE   conventional spin echo
Δk_x k-space spacing along k_x
Δk_y k-space spacing along k_y
Δt dwell time
Δt_{rf} duration of RF pulse
EPI   echo planar imaging
ESP   echo sampling period (EPI)
EST   total echo sampling time
ETL   echo train length
f_{max} maximum (Nyquist) frequency
FOV   field of view

FSE   fast spin echo
γ gyromagnetic ratio
G_{max} maximum gradient strength
GRASE   gradient spin echo
k_x frequency axis in k-space
k_y phase axis in k-space
N_{ex} number of excitations
N_p samples in phase
N_s number of slabs
N_x samples in read
SR   slew rate
t_{acq} acquisition time
t_{min} ramp time (EPI)
t_y time for which phase encode gradient is applied
T total readout time
V voxel volume

Introduction

While MR imaging technology has advanced steadily since the late 1970s, every five or ten years there is a quantum jump. In the beginning, there were only low field (0.15 T) resistive magnets such as the unit at the University of Nottingham. In the early 1980s, mid- and low-field superconducting systems were installed, including the 0.15 T system at the Hammersmith and the 0.35 T system at UCSF. In the mid 1980s, GE and Siemens introduced the first high-field systems at 1.5 T. The upper limit has remained at 1.5–2 T for all but a few 'boutique' research systems since that time.

Early whole body gradients had a maximum strength of 3–6 mT/m, with rise times on the order of 1.5–2 ms. In the mid 1980s, GE introduced shielded gradients with a maximum strength of 10 mT/m and a minimum rise time of 675 ms. The new 'high-performance' systems (Siemens VISION, GE EchoSpeed, Picker EDGE, Philips ACS-NT) feature gradient strengths as high as 27 mT/m with rise times as short as 180 µs.

With such gradient performance comes many benefits, one of which is smaller fields of view (FOV), leading to higher spatial resolution. Faster imaging is possible, including 2D and 3D versions of long-echo-train fast spin echo (FSE) (also called turbo spin echo or TSE), GRASE (also called turbo GSE or TGSE), multishot echo planar imaging

(EPI), and—faster yet—single shot EPI. With high-performance gradients, shorter *TE* values are possible, improving T_1 contrast and increasing the number of slices that can be acquired for a given *TR*. Strong gradients allow higher orders of flow compensation without unduly prolonging *TE*. Using phase contrast flow quantification techniques, strong gradients allow detection of much lower velocities of flowing blood and CSF. Stronger gradients allow phase-contrast MRA to be performed with reduced acquisition times, and excellent sensitivity to slow flow. Strong gradients are essential for dynamic MR techniques, which trade off spatial and temporal resolution. For example, in dynamic contrast-enhanced imaging of breast carcinoma, high spatial resolution is required to see spiculated borders, and high temporal resolution is desirable to determine the rate of enhancement.

In some cases, high-performance gradients are not only desirable but are *necessary*. Gradient-intensive techniques such as single shot EPI may *only* be possible with high-performance gradients. For screening studies (e.g. for breast cancer), some early diagnoses may *only* be possible using high-performance gradients. While this chapter clearly overlaps with others in this book, the purpose is to focus on the marginal benefits provided by strong, fast gradients.

High-resolution imaging

Spatial resolution is generally determined by dividing the field of view (FOV) by the number of projections/pixels along a particular axis. (See the potential exception to this statement in the EPI section of this chapter.) Since the FOV and number of pixels can be varied independently and can be different for different axes, spatial resolution along the three axes can vary as well. For 2D techniques, the spatial resolution along the slice select axis is typically about five times the in-plane spatial resolution. For thin-slice, 3D techniques, the spatial resolution may be isotropic, i.e. the same along all three axes. (An advantage of isotropic data is the ability to reformat a single acquisition into multiple planes without significant loss of resolution.)

In order to better appreciate the impact of high-performance gradients on spatial resolution, it is useful to review some of the basic aspects of MR

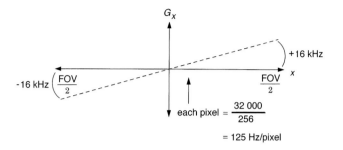

Figure 2.1

Routine frequency encoding. The readout gradient G_x is applied in order to provide spatial discrimination along the x-axis. Activating the readout gradient changes the magnetic field (and therefore the resonance frequency) at each point along the readout axis. In this example, the maximum frequency offset at the borders of the field of view is 16 kHz, which is also the bandwidth. Another way to represent the bandwidth is to divide the full bandwidth (32 kHz) by the number of pixels along the readout axis (256 in this example), i.e. 125 Hz/pixel.

image formation. The main function of the gradients is to encode spatial information. By activating the gradients, the local resonance frequencies are altered. For example, activation of the frequency encode gradient during readout imparts different resonance frequencies to spins at different locations along the frequency encode axis (Fig. 2.1). (The spin echo contains all of these frequencies.) Most gradients today are linear, i.e. the net magnetic field strength changes linearly with position. Thus each spin has a unique frequency, corresponding to its position along that axis. The *range* of frequencies in the spin echo covering a given FOV is known as the receiver bandwidth or simply the bandwidth (BW). A typical BW at high field is 32 kHz, usually represented as ±16 kHz, reflecting the fact that frequencies on either side of midline are 180° out of phase with each other. Regardless of phase, the highest frequencies received (e.g. +16 kHz and –16 kHz) originate at positions furthest removed from the center of the FOV. In a sense, these frequencies *define* the FOV limits along the frequency encode axis (Fig. 2.1).

Another way to represent the BW is on a 'per pixel' basis by dividing the total BW by the number of projections along the readout axis. For example, if there were 256 readout pixels and a BW of ±16 kHz, the BW could also be represented as 32 000 Hz/256 pixels = 125 Hz/pixel (Fig. 2.1). In general, the conversion between bandwidth in ±kHz and bandwidth in Hz/pixels is

$$BW(Hz/pixel) = 2 \times BW(\pm kHz) \times \frac{1000}{N_x} \quad (1)$$

Thus each pixel is 125 Hz wide or, stated differently, the pixel 'bin' contains 125 Hz of frequencies. An advantage of this representation is the lack of ambiguity if the '±' is deleted from the kHz measurement of BW. Another advantage of the Hz/pixel representation is that it allows a quick calculation of chemical shift. For this BW at 1.5 T, for example, the fat–water chemical shift of 220 Hz would be approximately 2 pixels.

The spin echo signal is received in analog form, i.e. it is a continuous variation in voltage versus time. In order for the signal to be processed by a digital computer, it has to be converted into a stream of digits. This is accomplished by a piece of equipment called the analog-to-digital converter (ADC). The number of points used to digitize the MR signal is the same as the number of pixels or frequencies that can be discriminated along the readout axis, e.g. 256 (Fig. 1.2). This is a consequence of the Nyquist sampling theorem, which states that a minimum of two points are required to represent a sine wave. Thus 256 points would

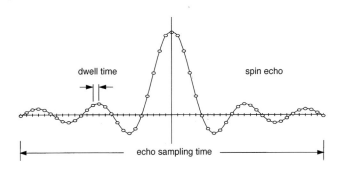

Figure 2.2

Routine frequency encoding. This plot of amplitude versus time indicates a spin echo (solid black line) being digitized 256 times to provide frequency discrimination of 256 points along the readout axis (according to the Nyquist theorem). The sampling interval, i.e. the echo sampling time divided by 256, is known as the dwell time (which is the inverse of the bandwidth). The sampling is performed by the analog-to-digital (A/D) converter, which converts the analog spin echo to a stream of digits that can be processed by a digital computer.

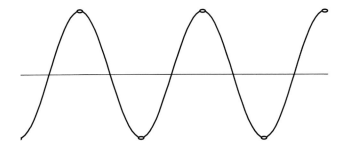

Figure 2.3

Nyquist theorem. It takes a minimum of two points to characterize the frequency of a sine wave (and slightly more to determine its phase).

allow the discrimination of 128 frequencies, each having a positive and negative polarity, i.e. 180° phase difference, for a total of 256 frequencies.

As an aside, you may have noticed that the number of phase encode projections can be almost anything, while the number of readout projections is always 128, 256, 512 or 1024. This is a consequence of the fast Fourier transform (FFT) algorithm, which requires that the frequency encode data be a power of 2, i.e. $2^5 = 128$, $2^6 = 256$, $2^7 = 512$, and $2^8 = 1024$.[1]

The time Δt between digital samplings of the echo is called the sampling interval or the dwell time (Fig. 2.2). By definition, the total BW is the inverse of the dwell time Δt. Since (by the Nyquist theorem), it takes two points (minimum) to represent the frequency of a sine wave (Fig. 2.3), the maximum frequency f_{max} that can be discriminated by a given dwell time is $1/(2\Delta t)$. This is called the Nyquist frequency.[1] (When the total BW is represented in ±kHz, e.g. ±16 kHz, the Nyquist frequency is also 16 kHz.) The total echo sampling time EST (i.e. the time the ADC is 'on') is the product of the dwell time and the number of readout projections N_x. Thus

$$BW_{tot} = \frac{1}{\Delta t} = \frac{N_x}{EST} \quad (2)$$

In general, Eqn (1) can be written as

$$BW_{per\ pixel} = \frac{BW_{tot}}{N_x}$$

Thus,

$$BW_{per\ pixel} = \frac{1}{EST} \quad (3)$$

The FOV is also determined from the Nyquist theorem. It is determined by the combination of position and gradient strength along the particular axis that results in the highest (Nyquist) frequency that can be discriminated, i.e. ±BW. For the readout axis, the highest f_{max} will simply be the product of the maximum gradient strength G_{max}, (mT/m), half the FOV (cm) and the gyromagnetic ratio γ for hydrogen (42.57 MHz/T):

$$f_{max} = \gamma G_{max}\ FOV/2 \qquad (4)$$

Since f_{max} (the Nyquist frequency) also equals the receiver bandwidth (in ±kHz), Eqn (4) can be rewritten as

$$BW(\pm kHz) = \gamma G_{max}\ FOV/2 \qquad (5)$$

Rearranging, we can derive a useful expression relating the minimum FOV achievable at a given maximum gradient strength as a function of BW:

$$FOV_{min} = \frac{(2/\gamma)\ BW}{G_{max}} \qquad (6)$$

When BW is expressed in ±kHz and the maximum gradient is in mT/m, the minimum FOV in cm is

$$FOV_{min} = \frac{4.67 \cdot BW_{kHz}}{G_{max}} \qquad (7)$$

Rearranging Eqn (1)

$$BW_{kHz} = BW_{Hz/pixel} N_x / 2000$$

Substituting, we can derive an expression for the FOV (in cm) as a function of the bandwidth (in Hz/pixel) and the number of readout projections N_x:

$$FOV = \frac{0.00233 BW_{Hz/pixel} N_x}{G_{max}} \qquad (8)$$

Thus Eqns (7) and (8) can be used to provide the minimum FOV as a function of the maximum gradient strength at a given BW represented in ±kHz or Hz/pixel respectively.

As TE is shortened, the time available for echo sampling decreases, increasing the bandwidth (Fig. 2.4). By Eqns (7) and (8), such increases in BW (at constant gradient) are accompanied by increases in FOV (Fig. 2.5). Thus short-TE sequences tend to have larger fields of view, and smaller fields of view tend to have longer TEs. Given the higher G_{max} of high-performance gradients, shorter TEs and smaller fields of view can both be accommodated. (As an added bonus for TE values on the order of 1–2 ms, flow-related dephasing is effectively eliminated, potentially obviating the need for flow compensation on MRA sequences.) Short TE values also allow more slices to be acquired per unit time, increasing coverage in multislice techniques.

Along the phase encode axis, the FOV is defined by that position where the incremental

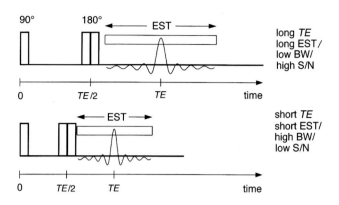

Figure 2.4

Bandwidth versus TE. The lower the bandwidth, the longer the echo delay time TE. This is a consequence of the bandwidth being inversely proportional to the echo sampling time EST. Longer echo sampling times (lower bandwidths) push TE to larger values, decreasing the degree of T_1-weighting.

phase encode gradient step ΔG_p leads to a 180° phase shift or, stated differently, it is the position of the highest (Nyquist) frequency that can be discriminated by the minimum two points (Fig. 2.3). The following describes this in more detail.

In order to better understand the relationship between FOV, BW and gradient strength, it is useful to review a few details of frequency and phase encoding in a 2DFT image.[1] Frequency

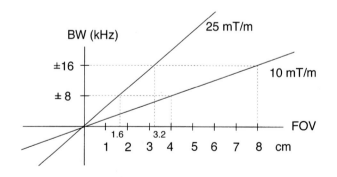

Figure 2.5

Bandwidth versus field of view. The higher the bandwidth BW, the larger the field of view FOV for a given readout gradient. Stronger gradients at a given bandwidth result in smaller fields of view—hence the need for strong gradients for high-resolution imaging.

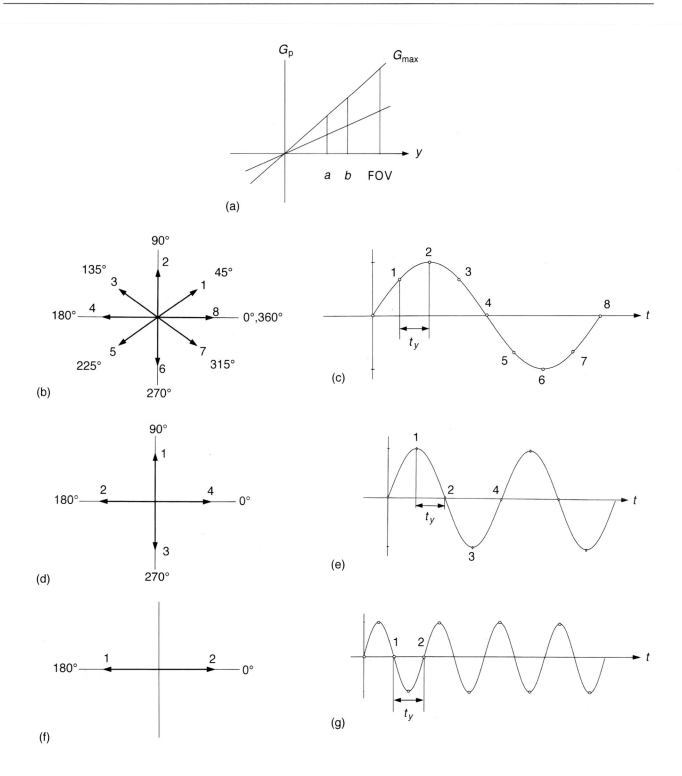

Figure 2.6

Phase encoding. (a) Position along phase encode axis versus strength of phase encode gradient G_p. Point a is 1/4 of the FOV away from the origin, and point b is FOV/2 away. (b) At point a, each application of the phase encode gradient advances the phase by 45°. (c) At point a, it takes eight applications of the phase encode gradient to describe a single sine wave. The time interval t_y is the time for which the phase encode gradient is applied. (d) At point b, the phase is advanced 90° with each application of the phase encode gradient. (e) At point b, four points describe a sine wave. (f) At the limits of the FOV, the phase is advanced 180° with each application of the phase encode gradient (by definition, according to the Nyquist theorem). (g) At the limits of the FOV, exactly two points describe a sine wave.

encoding is relatively simple: by adding or subtracting the local value of the gradient field from that of the main B_0 field, the *net* magnetic field can be shown to vary linearly along the frequency encode axis (Fig. 2.1). Since the Nyquist frequency (i.e. half the BW), is the highest frequency f_{max} that can be discriminated, the FOV is defined as shown in Eqn (6).

Phase encoding is a bit more difficult. Since frequency has units of phase per unit time, phase is the product (or integral) of frequency and time. In other words, activating the phase encode gradient for a brief time interval imparts a small amount of incremental phase to spins at a certain location. By keeping track of the amount of phase added (or subtracted) from 'baseline', position can be sorted out. In order for this phase value to be unambiguous, it must be less than ±180°. (For example, +190° is the same as –170°.)

Each time the phase encode gradient is activated, the phase at a specific point advances. Consider point *a* in Fig. 2.6(a). As shown in Fig. 2.6(b), the phase at point *a* advances 45° with each successive application of the phase encode gradient. Over eight applications (each separated by time t_y), the phase advances 360° and describes a sine wave (Fig. 2.6c). Now consider point *b*, which is further removed from the center of the FOV (Fig. 2.6a). Each successive application of the phase encode gradient advances the phase 90° (Fig. 2.6d). After four applications, the cumulative phase has been increased by 360°, and a sine wave is described (Fig. 2.6e). Since the sine waves in Figs 2.6(c,e) are plots of phase versus time, and since the gradient is activated for the same time interval t_y for each application, the temporal spacing t_y between points is the same. Since 360° is described by four points in Fig. 2.6(e) and eight in Fig. 2.6(c), the frequency at point *b* is twice that at point *a* (Fig. 2.6a). More peripherally still from the center, the phase is advanced 180° (Fig. 2.6f) each time the phase encode gradient is applied, and two points (the Nyquist minimum) just barely describe a sine wave (Fig. 2.6g). This is the highest frequency that can be discriminated, and it therefore defines the FOV (Fig. 2.6a). (In retrospect, point *a* was at position FOV/4 and point *b* was at position FOV/2 in Fig. 2.6a.) Note that it is the gradient *increment* and not the maximum gradient *strength* that defines the FOV. Clearly the stronger the gradient, the closer to the origin the marginal phase is advanced 180°. Thus stronger gradients at a given BW or Nyquist frequency result in a smaller FOV. This has the advantage of improving the spatial resolution, but also increases the risk of 'aliasing'.

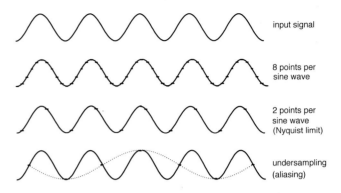

input signal

8 points per sine wave

2 points per sine wave (Nyquist limit)

undersampling (aliasing)

Figure 2.7

Aliasing due to undersampling. The input signal can be accurately digitized by as few as two points per sine wave (Nyquist limit). When *less* than 2 points are used, the sampling results in a wave of much lower frequency than the input signal. This lower frequency is mismapped along the aliased axis as a wave of lower frequency and opposite polarity. For this reason, aliased tissue appears on the *opposite* side of the FOV.

Aliasing or 'wraparound artifact' results when the phase is advanced more than 180° per gradient application at a point, resulting in phase ambiguity. As shown in Fig. 2.7, the high-frequency true input signal is undersampled, leading to a lower-frequency false signal of opposite sign. (Frequencies to the right of the center of the FOV have positive sign, i.e. zero frequency to $+f_{max}$, while those to the left of midline have negative sign, i.e. 0 to $-f_{max}$.) The frequency of the false signal is the frequency of the true signal minus the Nyquist frequency. Thus, for a 16 kHz Nyquist frequency, a true signal of 17 kHz would appear to have frequency 16–17 kHz = –1 kHz, while a true signal of 31 kHz would appear to have frequency –15 kHz. Thus aliased tissue just past the right-hand edge of the FOV wraps just to the left of midline; tissue further past the edge of the FOV wraps increasingly from the midline towards the opposite edge of the image.

There are two ways to increase spatial resolution along the frequency encode axis (Fig. 2.8): halve the FOV or double N_x (i.e. the number of samplings). There are two ways to halve the FOV: halve the BW at constant gradient (Fig. 2.8b) or double the gradient at constant BW (Fig. 2.8c). Let us examine the ramifications of these options.

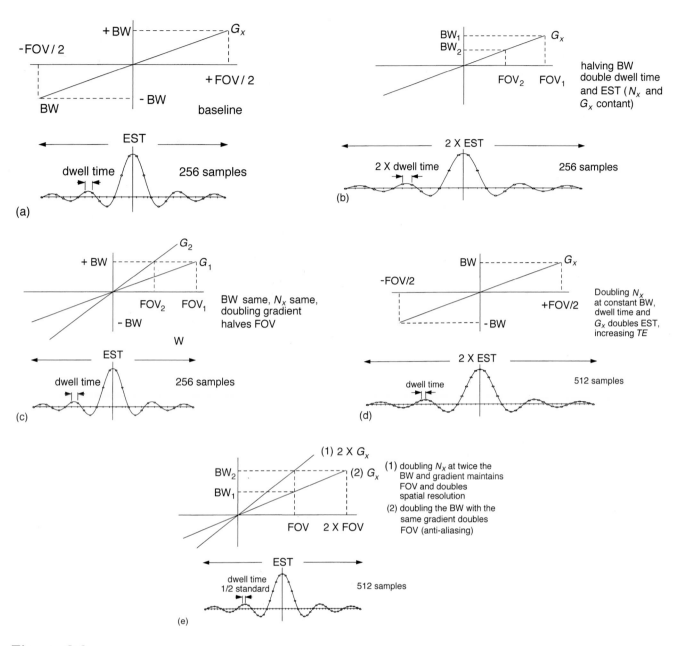

Figure 2.8

Increasing spatial resolution in the frequency encode direction. (a) In a standard baseline acquisition, 256 samples are taken during the echo sampling time EST, thereby defining the dwell time EST/256, which is the inverse of the bandwidth. The bandwidth in combination with the gradient G_x determines the FOV. (b) To increase the spatial resolution in the frequency encode direction, the bandwidth can be reduced to BW_2 (which entails doubling the dwell time and therefore the echo sampling time EST for the same 256 points). This increases the minimum TE, decreasing the degree of T_1 weighting, and increases the chance of aliasing due to the smaller FOV. (c) By doubling the strength of the readout gradient G_2 at constant bandwidth, the FOV is again halved (FOV_2), increasing spatial resolution. Since the bandwidth is unchanged, the dwell time (and therefore TE) are the same as in

(a). Increasing the gradient therefore allows improved spatial resolution without increasing TE—but still runs the risk of aliasing. (d) Holding the bandwidth constant and doubling the number of frequency encode steps N_x doubles the spatial resolution without changing the bandwidth or requiring a stronger gradient. This approach has the advantage that it only requires standard gradients and decreases the risk of aliasing but it has the disadvantage that it prolongs TE, decreasing T_1 weighting. (e) Doubling N_x at twice the bandwidth and twice the gradient maintains the FOV while doubling the spatial resolution. When the bandwidth is doubled at the same gradient, the FOV is also doubled which decreases the chance of aliasing. In both cases the EST and therefore TE are unchanged but the signal-to-noise ratio is reduced because of the higher BW.

Halving the bandwidth doubles the dwell time and the total echo sampling time (Fig. 2.8b). While this doubles spatial resolution without additional demands on the gradients, it also increases the minimum *TE* and reduces the FOV, increasing the chance of aliasing. Doubling the strength of the readout gradient at constant BW (Fig. 2.8c) keeps *TE* short (for better T_1 or proton density weighting) but places additional demands on the gradients (and still increases the chance of aliasing due to the smaller FOV).

Doubling the number of readout projections or samplings N_x can be done at the same BW (increasing *TE*) or at a higher BW (at constant *TE*). (Since noise is proportional to $\sqrt{BW}$, this later option also increases the noise, decreasing the signal-to-noise ratio S/N.) If the dwell time (and BW) as well as the readout gradient are left unchanged, doubling the number of samples will double the echo sampling time (Fig. 2.8d). This will push the *TE* to larger values (which may not be desirable for T_1-weighted sequences). This approach does not increase the chance of aliasing, and does not place excessive demands on the gradients. Alternatively, the number of samplings N_x can be doubled during the same sampling time (and *TE*) (Fig. 2.8e). This will halve the sampling interval (dwell time), doubling the BW. When the BW is doubled, the strength of the readout gradient also needs to be doubled in order to maintain the same FOV and double the spatial resolution (option 1, Fig. 2.8e). Without increasing the readout gradient, doubling the BW will double the FOV (option 2, Fig. 2.8e), which will decrease aliasing but leave spatial resolution unchanged. (Actually, this is the basis for 'no frequency wrap' or 'oversampling', a technique to decrease aliasing along the frequency encode axis.) These techniques and their ramifications are summarized in Table 2.1.

Equations (5)–(7) and Fig. 2.5 provide some insight into the best spatial resolution achievable at a given BW with high-performance gradients. At a standard high-field BW of ± 16 kHz (125 Hz/pixel), the usual maximum gradient strength of 10 mT/m would lead to a minimum FOV of just under 8 cm (Fig. 2.5). Keeping the BW at ± 16 kHz, increasing the gradient strength from the standard 10 mT/m to 25 mT/m will lead to a minimum FOV of 3.2 cm. At a lower BW of ± 8 kHz, the FOV would be further reduced to 1.6 cm. With a 256 × 256 matrix over this FOV, pixels 64 µm on a side would be produced, approaching the resolution of a low-power histologic slide. Of course, an FOV of 1.6 cm would only be appropriate for a sample of approximately the same size. Using such a small FOV for a larger sample would lead to aliasing—unless oversampling or spatial presaturation pulses were used to eliminate the signal from the aliased tissue.

Another potential problem with high-resolution imaging is the marked decrease in S/N. The signal-to-noise ratio is proportional to the product of voxel volume V and the square roots of the number of phase encode steps N_p, the frequency encode steps N_x, the number of excitations N_{ex}, and the inverse of the BW:

$$\text{S/N} \propto V \sqrt{N_p} \sqrt{N_{ex}} \sqrt{N_x} / \sqrt{BW}$$

By Eqn (2) at constant EST, N_x and BW drop out, thus:

$$\text{S/N} \propto V \sqrt{N_p} \sqrt{N_{ex}} \tag{9}$$

To compare the S/N for two techniques with the same EST but with different values of V, N_p and N_{ex}, the following equation can be used:[2]

$$\frac{(\text{S/N})_1}{(\text{S/N})_2} = \frac{V_1}{V_2} \sqrt{\frac{N_{p1}}{N_{p2}}} \sqrt{\frac{N_{ex1}}{N_{ex2}}} \tag{10}$$

Equation (10) can be used to determine the effect on S/N if the spatial resolution is doubled at constant acquisition time. For example, if technique '1' is a standard-resolution 256^2 matrix with $2N_{ex}$ and technique '2' is a high-resolution 512^2 matrix with $1N_{ex}$ (all with the same *TR*, slice

Table 2.1 Improving spatial resolution along readout axis

N_x	*FOV*	*BW*	G_x	*Δt*	*EST*	TE	Risk of aliasing	*Fig.*
1	1/2	1/2	1	2	2	↑	↑	2.8(b)
1	1/2	1	2	1	1	—	↑	2.8(c)
2	1	1	1	1	2	↑	—	2.8(d)
2	1	2	2	1/2	1	—	—	2.8(e)

thickness, and FOV), acquisition time ($TR \times N_p \times N_{ex}$) will be the same. However, halving the spatial resolution will *quarter* the pixel area, quartering the voxel volume (since the slice thickness is the same). Therefore the effect on S/N will be

$$\frac{(S/N)_1}{(S/N)_2} = \frac{1}{4} \sqrt{\frac{256}{512}} \sqrt{\frac{2}{1}} = 0.25$$

Thus doubling the spatial resolution at constant acquisition time reduces the S/N to 25% of its original value. The volume of isotropic voxels 64 µm on a side would be $(0.064)^3$ mm^3 = 0.000264 mm^3 or approximately 1/5000th of the volume of an isotropic 1 mm voxel (Fig. 2.9). To maintain S/N, it is necessary to increase N_p or N_{ex} or to improve the filling factor of the *rf* coil. For small specimens, improving the filling factor requires using smaller surface or volume coils, ideally with quadrature detection.

One potential clinical application of 'histologic'-resolution MRI is the evaluation of prostate carcinoma.[3] Pathologists currently use the Gleason grade to determine prognosis for prostatic carcinoma. The Gleason grading system is based on the gross pattern of the carcinoma as seen on a low-power H & E slide. A grade of 5 is assigned to the least well-differentiated prostatic carcinoma and a grade of 1 to the best-differentiated. The pathologist picks the two most prevalent patterns in the carcinoma, leading to a combined Gleason score that could vary between 2 and 10. Grades of 2 are associated with an excellent prognosis and very small likelihood of metastases. This is the Gleason grade that corresponds to prostate carcinoma most 80-year-old men take with them to the grave. Gleason scores of 8, 9 and 10, on the other hand, are associated with a poor prognosis and a much higher likelihood of metastatic disease.

Knowing the Gleason grade prior to surgery would influence patient management. For example, a high Gleason score would be less likely to result in aggressive treatment, i.e. a radical prostatectomy, chemotherapy and radiation, than an intermediate Gleason grade. (The lowest Gleason grades would not require any treatment at all.) Unfortunately, the ideal Gleason grading is based on evaluation of the complete specimen, presumably following radical prostatectomy. Thus the postoperative finding of a high Gleason score might have led to a decision *not* to do a radical prostatectomy in the first place. Clearly, MRI may have something to offer in the management of prostate carcinoma.

Figure 2.10 is a 3D FSE image of a prostate carcinoma specimen achieved with a small Helmholtz coil on a prototype GE Echo-Speed MR system (SR-230) with high-performance gradients.[3] The spatial resolution is 78 µm in-plane, with a 100 µm slice thickness. The acquisition time was under 30 min. Clearly, there is some correspondence between the pattern of low-signal-intensity carcinoma on this T_2-weighted fast spin echo and the dark basophilic stain on the low-power H & E slide. In the future, should such imaging be possible in vivo using an endorectal coil, Gleason grading can be performed preoperatively, saving unnecessary radical prostatectomies (with the associated morbidity, mortality and cost) in very high- or very low-grade lesions.

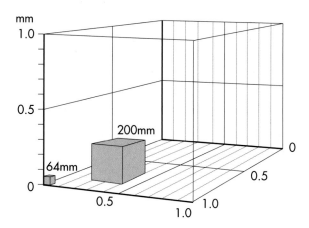

Figure 2.9

Signal-to-noise ratio of 'histologic-resolution' voxel. Compared with 1 mm isotropic MRA voxel, a voxel 200 µm on a side would have 1/125 of the signal-to-noise ratio. A voxel 64 µm on a side would have 1/5000 of the volume of a standard MRA voxel.

Thin slice/short *TE* imaging

The timing diagram for a spin echo sequence is shown in Fig. 2.11. The minimum *TE* depends on the duration of the rf pulses Δt_{rf}, the duration of the gradients, and half the echo sampling time. With stronger gradients, the duration of the gradients can be decreased; thus the sequence can be performed faster (with a shorter *TE* and more T_1-weighting). Alternatively, the duration of the rf pulse can be increased to produce thinner slices

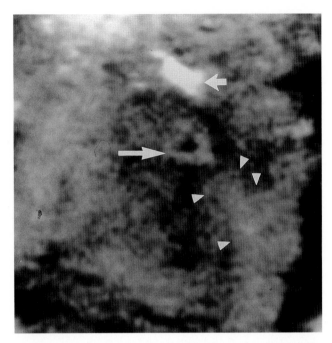

a

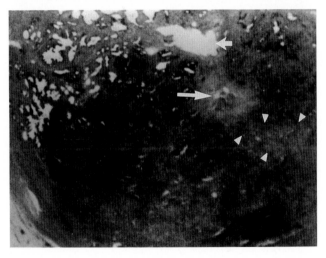

b

Figure 2.10

Histologic resolution imaging of the prostate. (a) 3D-FSE image of prostate carcinoma specimen scanned in a commercially available MR system (GE EchoSpeed) using a 2 cm volume coil. The 512 matrix and 4 cm FOV result in 78 μm in-plane spatial resolution. The slice thickness is 100 μm. (b) Low-power hematoxylin and eosin stain of the same prostate carcinoma specimen. Note the similarity between the (basophilic) cancer on the H&E slide and the low intensity on the T_2-weighted 3D-FSE. Although the images are rotated slightly with respect to each other, the hole (small arrow) appears bright, the collagen scar (large arrow) appears like a bull's eye, and the tongue of collagen (arrow heads) has intermediate signal.

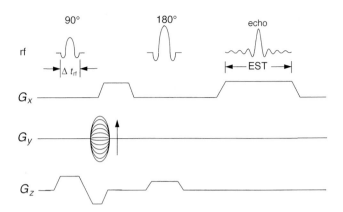

Figure 2.11

Conventional spin echo pulse sequence diagram. The top (rf) channel is both transmit and receive. The duration of the 90° rf pulse is Δt_{rf}. The 180° pulse could be applied for the same time as the 90° pulse, but with twice the power or with the same rf power for twice the time. The spin echo occurs an equal time after the 180° pulse as the 180° occurs after the 90° pulse. The spin echo must be read out in the presence of the readout gradient (G_x for an axial image). (The initial smaller prepulse dephases the spins so that they come into phase along the readout axis at the middle of the spin echo.) The phase encode gradient G_y is applied once after each 90° pulse in a conventional spin echo. The slice select gradient G_z is applied during the 90° and 180° pulses.

with the same *TE*. The tradeoff between the minimum *TE* and the minimum slice thickness is based on the slice-select BW_{ss} of the rf pulse (which is different from the receiver BW).[1]

As shown in Fig. 2.12, slice thickness is determined by the relationship between the strength of the slice select gradient and the BW_{ss} of the rf pulse. The stronger the slice select gradient (at a given BW_{ss}), the thinner the slice (Fig. 2.12a). The narrower the BW_{ss} at a given value of the slice select gradient, the narrower the slice (Fig. 2.12b). Unfortunately, narrower bandwidths require longer rf pulses. (The 'ideal' rf pulse is a sinc function: sinc x = (sin x)/x. The sinc function is a central peak with many side lobes. The Fourier transform of a sinc function is a rectangle. Thus prolonged sinc rf pulses—with lots of side lobes—produce rectangular slice profiles. The longer the duration of the sinc pulse, the lower its BW and the narrower the slice.) The longer the duration of the 90° and 180° rf pulses, the longer the *TE*. Thus

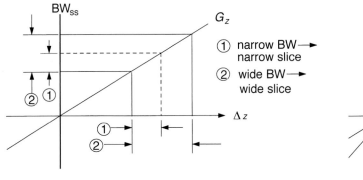

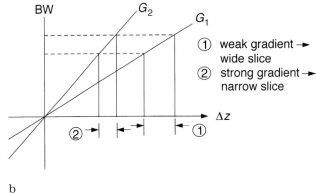

a   b

Figure 2.12

Slice thickness versus bandwidth of rf pulse. (a) At fixed slice select gradient G_z, the narrow rf bandwidth ① results in a narrow slice thickness while the wider bandwidth ② results in a wider slice

thickness. (b) When the bandwidth of the rf pulse is fixed, a weak gradient G_1 results in a wide slice, while a strong gradient G_2 results in a narrow slice.

on conventional gradient systems, thinner slices mean longer *TEs* and decreased T_1 contrast compared with high-performance gradient systems. Doubling the gradient strength at a fixed BW results in slices of half the thickness without changing *TE* (Fig. 2.12b). Alternatively, if a stronger slice select gradient is used without changing slice thickness, the BW_{ss} can be increased, *decreasing* the duration of the rf pulse, shortening *TE*, increasing the degree of T_1 contrast (Fig. 2.12c). This effect is illustrated in Fig. 2.13.

The ideal T_1-weighted image would have a short *TR* and the shortest possible *TE* (ideally zero). Any increase in *TE* beyond zero adds T_2 contrast to what should be a T_1-weighted image. These two types of contrast tend to cancel each other in a spin echo sequence. The contribution from T_2 contrast is reflected in the expression e^{-TE/T_2}. For *TE* = 0, this expression has a value of 1.0; for *TE* > 0, e^{-TE/T_2} has a value less than 1.0, decreasing the amount of T_1 contrast. This is plotted in Fig. 2.14. By using high-performance gradients, the minimum *TE* can typically be decreased from 15 to 5 ms at a fixed slice thickness. By decreasing the minimum *TE* from 15 to 5 ms, the signal from single dose gadolinium is increased by 33%. This is comparable to keeping *TE* fixed at 15 ms and tripling the dose of gadolinium (Atkinson DJ, Chen D-Y, Bradley WG, unpublished). Thus high-performance gradients can provide triple dose performance for

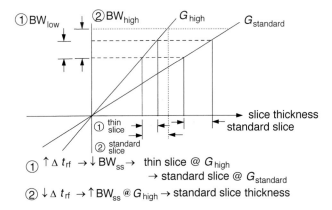

Figure 2.13

Slice thickness versus slice select bandwidth and rf pulse duration Δt_{rf}. The longer the duration of the rf pulse Δt_{rf}, the lower the slice select bandwidth BW_{ss}. When a narrow bandwidth BW_{low} is applied with a strong gradient G_{high}, a thin slice is produced ①. When it is applied with a standard gradient, the standard slice thickness is produced ②. When the duration of the RF pulse is short, the slice select bandwidth is high ② which would result in a standard slice thickness with a strong gradient G_{high} and a much wider slice with the standard gradient.

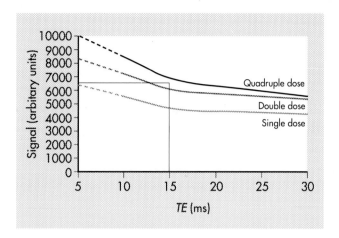

Figure 2.14

Plot of T_1 signal versus TE at various concentrations of Gd-DTPA.

a single dose of gadolinium—or, alternatively, provide single dose performance for half dose gadolinium.

Higher orders of gradient moment nulling

Gradient moment nulling is also known as flow compensation, GMR (gradient motion rephasing) or MAST (motion artifact suppression technique). It represents a series of techniques for eliminating motion artifacts by adding additional gradient pulses to rephase the spins at the time of the echo. As shown in Fig. 2.15, the magnitude, number and duration of the gradient pulses are adjusted so that spins moving with constant velocity have zero net phase gain at the time of the echo TE. This is known as first-order flow compensation.[4]

As illustrated in Fig. 2.15, the gradient pulses are balanced so that the area under the gradient-versus-time curves is equal at the center of the echo sampling time TE. Comparing (a) and (b) in Fig. 2.15, note that the additional gradient pulses have opposite signs for gradient echo imaging and the same sign for spin echo imaging. As shown in the phase diagrams, this reflects the phase reversal that results from the 180° pulse in the spin echo technique.[4]

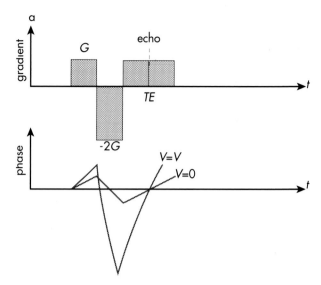

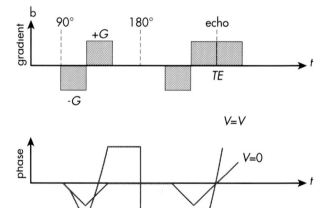

Figure 2.15

First-order (velocity) flow compensation (slice-select axis) for gradient echo and spin echo techniques. (a) First-order flow compensation for a gradient echo technique. Additional lobes of the G_x gradient result in both stationary and flowing material rephasing at time TE. (b) Velocity-compensated spin echo with variable TE. Because the gradients are balanced on either side of the 180° pulse, time may be added equally on either side of the 180° pulse to increase TE.

Figure 2.16 illustrates the additional gradient pulses needed for second-order flow compensation. This leads to rephasing of spins traveling at constant acceleration. Each additional order of

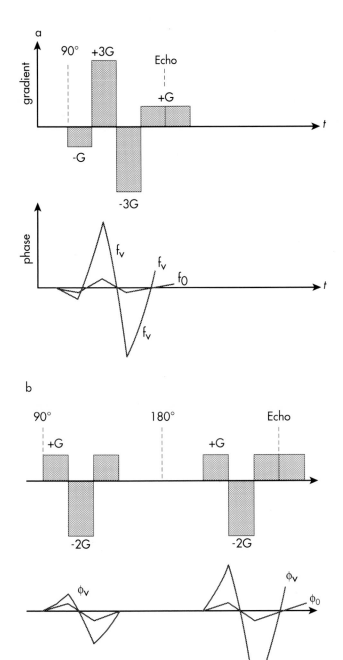

Figure 2.16

Second-order (acceleration) flow compensation. (a) Acceleration-compensated gradient echo image. Phase is gained as the third power of time, but returns to zero at time *TE*. (b) Spin echo image with third-order flow compensation (or second-order flow compensation with variable *TE*). Note the symmetry of the gradient lobes on either side of the 180° pulse, indicating the potential to vary *TE*. The phase plots are for constant acceleration, which results in zero phase angle at time *TE* (for both constant acceleration and constant velocity). Whenever zero phase also occurs at the time of the 180° pulse for the moving spins, the technique is also compensated for the next higher order of motion, in this case the 'jerk'.

flow compensation requires larger gradient moments. These can be produced by standard gradients running over a longer period of time or stronger gradients running in the same or slightly increased time. As shown in Figs 2.15(b) and 2.16(b), balancing the gradient lobes on either side of the 180° pulse allows for variable *TE*. When the phase of spins moving with a certain order of motion is zero at the initiation of the 180° pulse, the technique is also compensated in the next higher order of motion. Therefore the sequence shown in Fig. 2.16(b) is flow-compensated for both constant acceleration with variable *TE* and constant jerk at a fixed *TE*.

Higher orders of flow compensation can also be used for MR angiography. Since these require additional time, the minimum *TE* is increased. This also increases the time available for dephasing to occur, potentially decreasing luminal signal. Thus a tradeoff occurs: higher-order techniques compensate for additional motion but may lead to additional dephasing because of the longer *TE*. The *TE* is minimized if high-performance gradients are used, minimizing these dephasing artifacts.

Dynamic scanning

Dynamic scanning generally sacrifices spatial resolution for enhanced temporal resolution. TurboFLASH imaging, for example, typically uses a *TR* of 5 ms and a *TE* of 1.9 ms (with partial Fourier in read or 'fractional echo'), with a 128^2 matrix to acquire images in under 1 s ($7 \times 128 = 896$ ms). With high-performance gradients, *TE* can be shortened to 1 ms (at a given slice thickness), allowing shortening of *TR* to 3 ms. For a given matrix, this further shortens acquisition time, improving temporal resolution. Alternatively, a larger matrix can be applied over the same FOV, improving spatial resolution at a given temporal resolution (Fig. 2.17). In MR imaging of breast cancer, for example, *both* high temporal and high spatial resolution are desirable—the former to determine the rate of enhancement with gadolinium and the latter to evaluate lesion boundaries. High-performance gradients allow improvements in either spatial and temporal resolution—or both.

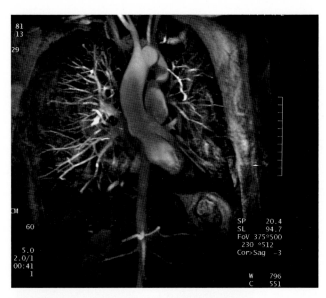

a

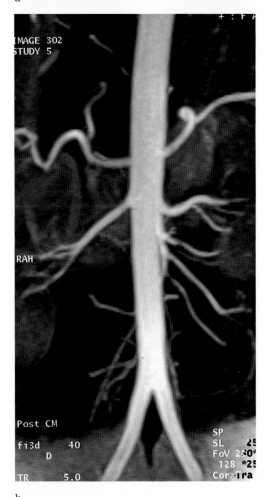

b

Figure 2.17

Ultrashort-*TE* turbo FISP. (a) Pulmonary angiogram.
(b) 3 Image/s aortogram.

Diffusion imaging

Diffusion imaging is discussed in Chapter 4.
Basically, diffusion-sensitizing gradient pulses can
be added to almost any sequence, from conventional spin echo to EPI. The sensitivity to diffusion
effects is proportional to the duration of these extra
gradient pulses and to their temporal separation;[5]
it is also proportional to the square of the gradient
strength. All other factors being equal, therefore,
increasing gradient strength and shortening rise
times lead to improved sensitivity to diffusion.

This may have important clinical ramifications,
since it is becoming increasingly apparent that
diffusion imaging is a particularly sensitive and
specific technique to diagnose an acute cerebral
infarct (Fig. 2.18).[6] In this era of 'outcomes analysis', early detection of stroke is likely to have a
major impact.

Diffusion imaging has also been shown to be
sensitive to local temperature changes.[7] Thus, for
example, in interventional MRI of the brain
(Chapter 14), high-performance gradients may
enable the radiologist and neurosurgeon to more
closely monitor thermal ablation of brain tumors.

Phase contrast MRA

Flow-sensitive MRA techniques based on phase
contrast benefit markedly from high-performance
gradients. Since the incremental phase gain is the
product (integral) of gradient strength, duration
and velocity, stronger gradients allow shorter *TR*
(faster scanning) or smaller 'aliasing' or 'encoding'
velocities, i.e. increased sensitivity to slow flow. A
standard phase-contrast MRA from a 10 mT/m
system acquired with an effective *TR* of 36 ms and
a 192 × 256 × 64 matrix takes 30 min to acquire.
Figure 2.19 is a 3D PC-MRA from a 25 mT/m unit
acquired with the same matrix but a *TR* of 13 ms,
decreasing the total acquisition time to 11 min.

The Holy Grail of MRA of the brain is a 1024[2]
matrix over a 22 cm FOV with good signal-to-
noise. The resultant 250 µm resolution is comparable to that of cut-film catheter angiography.
While most MRA to date has been based on time-
of-flight (TOF) techniques, high-performance
gradients may offer new advantages for phase-
contrast techniques. In TOF MRA, the minimum
TR is limited by the time for inflow of unsaturated

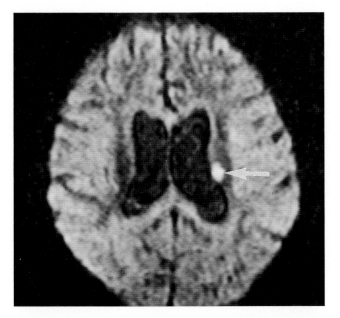

a

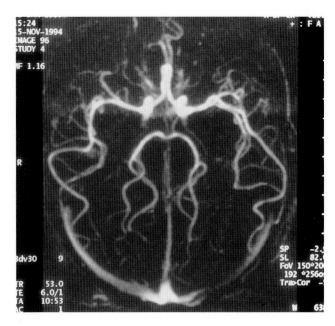

Figure 2.19

Rapid phase contrast MR angiography. This 3D phase-contrast MRA was acquired with a 192 × 256 matrix in just under 11 min. The *TR* shown (53 ms) is actually for four separate acquisitions (baseline and three axes of phase encoding) for an effective *TR* of just over 13 ms. Such short *TR* values are only possible with strong gradients.

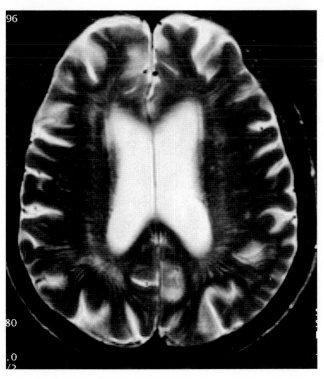

b

spins, i.e. flow-related enhancement. In PC-MRA, the duration of the flow-sensitizing gradient pulse (which determines the minimum *TR*) can be decreased if the strength of the flow encoding gradient is increased. To achieve 1024² resolution over a small FOV, short *TR* will be necessary—which will probably only be possible with high-performance gradients.

Figure 2.18

EPI diffusion imaging. 87-year-old woman with acute onset right hemiparesis. (a) EPI–diffusion image demonstrates high signal intensity in left corona radiata (arrow). This image was acquired with a *b* value of 1000, with diffusion sensitization in the slice select direction. (b) T_2-weighted image is normal in the same area.

Fast scanning

For conventional spin echo and gradient echo imaging, the acquisition time t_{acq} is the product of

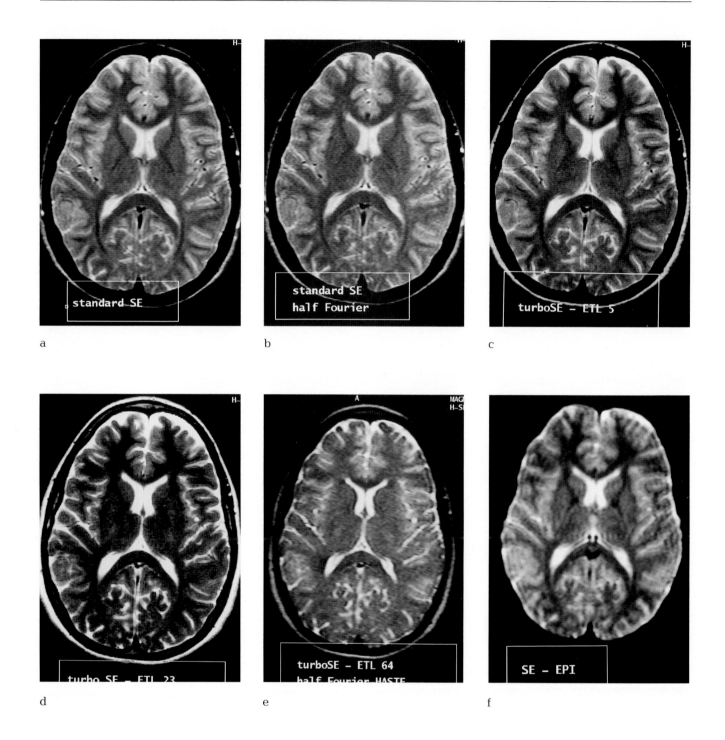

a

b

c

d

e

f

Figure 2.20

Comparison of acquisition times for various T_2-weighted MR imaging techniques. (All images are acquired with 128 × 256 matrix and 5 mm slice thickness.) (a) Conventional spin echo (acquisition time 5 min 24 s). (b) Half Fourier conventional spin echo (acquisition time 3 min 4 s). (c) Turbo spin echo with ETL = 5 (acquisition time 2 min 24 s). (d) Turbo spin echo with ETL = 23 (acquisition time 53 s). (e) HASTE (turbo spin echo with ETL = 64, half Fourier) (acquisition time .92 s). (f) SE-EPI (acquisition time 220 ms).

the repetition time *TR*, the number of phase encode steps N_p and the number of excitations N_{ex}:

$$t_{acq} = TR \, N_p N_{ex} \tag{11}$$

The number of echoes in a spin echo acquisition is the product of the number of phase encode steps N_p and the number of excitations N_{ex}.

A new parameter *T*, the total readout time, is the product of the echo sampling time (EST) (Fig. 2.2) and the number of echoes[8]

$$T = \text{EST} \times N_p N_{ex} \tag{12}$$

By Eqn (9) the signal-to-noise ratio is proportional to the square root of the number of echoes:

$$\text{S/N} \propto V \sqrt{N_p N_{ex}} \tag{8}$$

Rearranging Eqn 12,

$$N_p N_{ex} = \frac{T}{\text{EST}} \tag{13}$$

By combining Eqns (9) and (13), it can be seen that the signal-to-noise ratio is also proportional to the square root of the total readout time, i.e.

$$\text{S/N} \propto \sqrt{T} \tag{14}$$

(this equation will have greater relevance in the discussion of EPI that follows).

To scan faster using spin echo, either *TR*, N_p or N_{ex} can be reduced. By Eqn (11), with a decrease in *TR*, N_p or N_{ex}, there will be a linear decrease in scan time. Unfortunately, *TR* affects more than the acquisition time; therefore a decrease in *TR* is also associated with a decrease in the amount of T_2 or proton density contrast, the number of slices and the signal-to-noise ratio. Decreasing N_p for a fixed field of view results in decreased spatial resolution along the phase encode axis. Reduction in either N_p or N_{ex} also leads to a reduction in signal-to-noise ratio in proportion to the square root of these quantities (as shown in Eqn (9)). In general, halving the acquisition time results in a 40% ($\sqrt{2}$) decrease in signal-to-noise ratio.

Another way to scan faster without this loss of S/N is to use gradient echo techniques[9] (Fig. 2.17). Since these techniques have a lower flip angle, they require a much shorter *TR* to return to near-equilibrium magnetization. As discussed above, ultrafast gradient echo techniques such as TurboFLASH and Fast-SPGR are able to acquire images in less than a second, although contrast is typically less than that seen in a conventional spin echo. This poor contrast necessitates the use of additional 'magnetization preparation' pulses—with an increase in scan time of 30–40%.

Yet another (much more efficient) way to scan faster (without the egregious loss of S/N) is to cover multiple lines of *k*-space during each *TR* interval or 'shot' (Fig. 2.20). This is the basis for fast or turbo spin echo (FSE or TSE), gradient spin echo (GRASE) (Fig. 2.21), multishot echo planar imaging (EPI) (Fig. 2.22), and single shot EPI (Figs 2.21 and 2.22). With increasing *k*-space coverage per shot, the acquisition time is decreased in direct proportion. Unlike single line *k*-space trajectory techniques (e.g. conventional spin echo), FSE and GRASE techniques suffer only a minimal signal-to-noise penalty with faster scanning. In fact, if it were not for T_2 decay, there would be no loss of signal-to-noise ratio at all compared with conventional *k*-space trajectories. With ultrafast techniques such as single shot EPI, S/N is reduced primarily because of the higher bandwidths used.

k-space

FSE and GRASE are discussed along with an introduction to *k*-space in Chapter 1. Actually, these techniques are only part of a spectrum extending from conventional spin echo (CSE) to single shot EPI (Figs 2.20–2.22). In CSE, a single line of *k*-space is filled for each 90° pulse and each *TR*. In FSE, multiple lines of *k*-space are filled, depending on the ETL. In HASTE (half Fourier turbo spin echo), the ETL is 128, covering one-half of *k*-space (half Fourier). This 'RF-EPI' is extremely fast, producing images in less than 1 s (Fig. 2.20). In GRASE, some of the spin echoes in an FSE technique are replaced by gradient echoes.[10] Contrast in GRASE techniques reflects the effective *TE* and the ratio of gradient to spin echoes. In multishot EPI, all of the spin echoes are replaced by gradient echoes—but *k*-space is still segmented into multiple shots, each filling ETL lines in *k*-space. The relationship between the number of shots N_s, the ETL, and the total number of k_y lines in *k*-space (N_p) is

$$N_s \times \text{ETL} = N_p \tag{15}$$

In single shot EPI, all lines of *k*-space are filled by multiple gradient reversals, producing multiple gradient echoes in a single acquisition during a single T_2^* decay, i.e. $N_s = 1$ and ETL $= N_p$.

In view of the importance of *k*-space in the description of these techniques, it is useful to amplify on some of the introductory comments made in Chapter 1. As noted there, *k*-space represents the raw data matrix prior to reverse Fourier transformation into an image. The axes of *k*-space are k_x (horizontal) and k_y (vertical) (Fig. 2.23). The

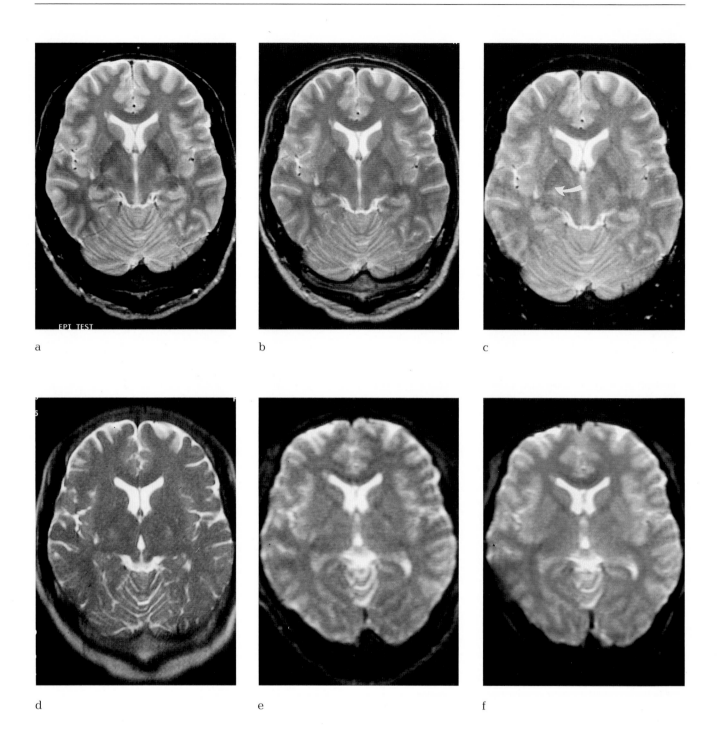

Figure 2.21

Spectrum of fast T_2-weighted imaging including
GRASE and HASTE. (a) Conventional T_2-weighted
spin echo: (b) Fast spin echo (ETL = 5). (c) GRASE
(ETL = 9, 2:1 gradient echo; spin echo). Note the subtly
greater definition of the medial border of the right
globus pallidus in GRASE compared with FSE (arrow),
although it is still somewhat less conspicuous than on
conventional spin echo (a). (d) HASTE (half Fourier
turbo spin echo with ETL = 128) shows very little
definition of basal ganglia. (e) Single shot SE-EPI
shows little sensitivity to magnetic susceptibility
effects. (f) Single shot FID-EPI appears very similar to
SE-EPI. S/N is somewhat better than in (e) owing to
shorter TE. CSF is bright despite the 90° pulse, since
TR is effectively infinite (i.e. no saturation effects).

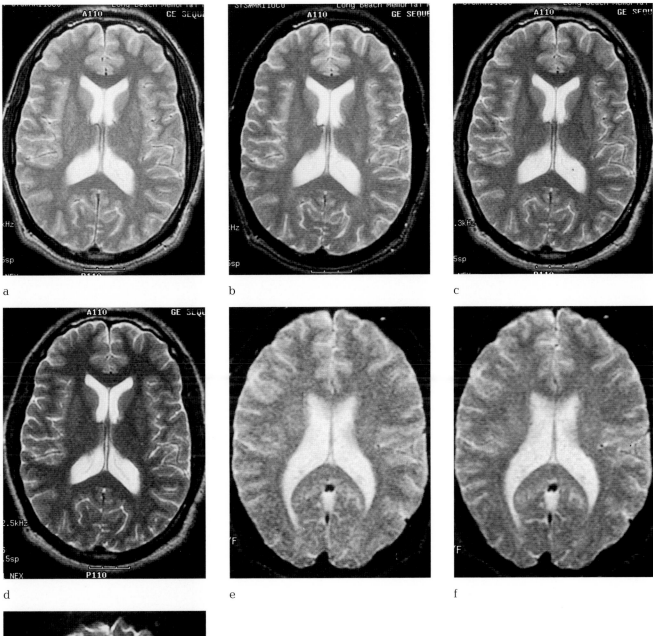

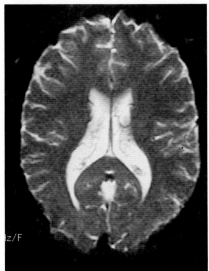

Figure 2.22

T_2-weighted imaging of the brain: spectrum of fast scanning techniques. (a) Conventional T_2-weighted spin echo. (b) 8-echo train fast spin echo. (Note somewhat brighter subcutaneous fat than in (a).) (c) 32-echo-train fast spin echo. (d) 64-echo-train fast spin echo. (Note the decreasing signal intensity from brain compared with CSF. This is due to an increasing magnetization transfer effect resulting from the increasing echo-train length.) (e) 32-shot EPI (ETL = 8). (f) 8-shot EPI (ETL = 32). (g) Single shot EPI (ETL = 256). (Note the 30° positive angulation (relative to canthomeatal line) for all EPI sequences (e)–(g) compared with 0° angulation for spin echo and fast spin echo sequences (a)–(d). Note the decreasing signal-to-noise ratio as the number of shots is decreased in (e)–(g), which is due in part to the necessity for higher and higher bandwidths.)

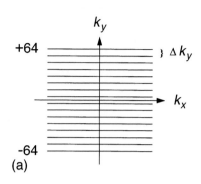

(a)

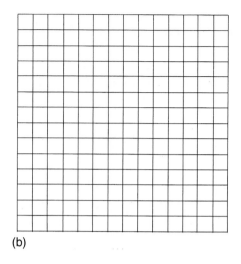

(b)

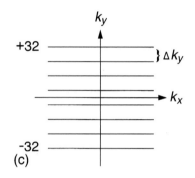

(c)

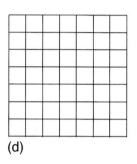

(d)

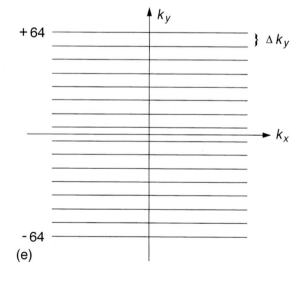

(e)

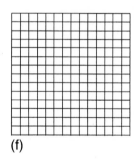

(f)

Figure 2.23

Comparison of image area in k-space and (x, y)-space. (a,b) A small phase increment Δk_y in k-space (a) results in a large field of view in (x, y)-space (b). The 128 lines in k-space result in a low-resolution image in (x, y)-space (b). (c,d) The line spacing Δk_y in k-space has been doubled (c), halving the field of view in (x, y)-space (d). Since the number of k-space lines has been halved, the overall area of the image in k-space is unchanged (d). The resulting halving of both the FOV and the number of matrix elements in (x, y)-space leaves the spatial resolution unchanged. (e,f) By keeping the phase increment Δk_y doubled in k-space (e), the FOV remains small in (x, y)-space (f). By increasing the number of Fourier lines to 128 in k-space (e), the spatial resolution is doubled in (x, y)-space (f).

units of measurement along these axes are in spatial frequencies (cycles/mm). For 1 mm spatial resolution, the span of spatial frequencies from the bottom to the top of *k*-space must be 1 cycle/mm. Thus the maximum k_y values are ±0.5 cycles/mm (at the periphery) and 0 cycles/mm in the center.

The k_x data results from the readout of a single echo. The number of points along k_x is the same as the number of points used to digitize the echo (e.g. 256). The spacing Δk_x between the points along k_x reflects the strength of the readout gradient and the time for which it is activated. To be more specific, the spacing (in cycles/mm) is such that two points at the periphery of the FOV describe the highest (Nyquist) frequency (±BW).

The total number of lines k_y is the same as the number of phase encode projections N_p. The spacing Δk_y between these lines depends on the phase encode gradient *increment* (in mT/m) and the time (in ms) for which the phase encode gradient is applied. (In practice, the time for which the phase encode gradient is applied remains the same for each of the phase encode steps—only the gradient strength is changed. This is the distinguishing characteristic of the 'spin warp' technique.) The spacing Δk_y determines the FOV along the phase encode (y) axis. The larger the spacing, the smaller the FOV. Thus at a given matrix size, the greater the spacing between points along k_x or the wider the separation of lines k_y (smaller FOV), the larger the area of the *k*-space trajectory. By definition:

$$k_x = \gamma G_x \Delta t \qquad (16)$$

$$k_y = \gamma G_y t_y \qquad (17)$$

where k_x and k_y are spatial frequencies (in cycles/mm), γ is the gyromagnetic ratio (42.57 mHz/T for hydrogen), G_x and G_y are the gradient strengths (in mT/m, incremental or fixed), Δt is the dwell time and t_y is the time for which the phase encode gradient is applied.

From the above discussion, it can be seen that *k*-space (the raw data matrix) has physical dimensions. The incremental phase (or frequency) gain is the spacing between points k_y or k_x. The greater the spacing Δk, the smaller the FOV (along either axis). The number of k_y lines in *k*-space corresponds to the matrix size and, with the spacing Δk (FOV), determines the spatial resolution. This is illustrated in Fig. 2.23. In Fig. 2.23(a), Δk_y and Δk_x are small, so the FOV in Fig. 2.23(b) is large. For a 128² matrix, spatial resolution is relatively poor. In Fig. 2.23(c), Δk_y and Δk_x are large, so the FOV in Fig. 2.23(d) is small. For a 64² matrix, spatial resolution is still poor. In Fig. 2.23(e) the spacing

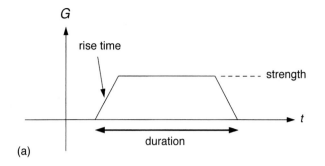

(a)

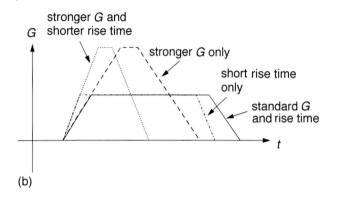

(b)

Figure 2.24

Gradient performance parameters. (a) Gradient performance can be characterized by the maximum strength (in mT/m) and the rise time (in ms or μs). The gradient strength (in mT/m) divided by the rise time (in ms) is known as the slew rate. (b) This illustrates the effect of change in gradient strength and rise times. The area under the gradient versus time curve determines the incremental phase advance, which in turn determines the FOV (larger areas corresponding to smaller FOVs). High-performance gradients allow greater areas under the curve in less total time.

Δk_x and Δk_y are again large, so the FOV in Fig. 2.23(f) is small. Since there are now 128 Fourier lines, spatial resolution is doubled. Notice that physical dimension of the *k*-space trajectory in Fig. 2.23(c) is twice that of Figs 2.23(a,c). As a general rule, the larger the area covered by *k*-space, the better the spatial resolution—since a larger area could be produced by large Δk spacing (small FOV) or by many lines (large matrix). Regardless of how high spatial resolution is achieved, at a given bandwidth, high resolution requires strong gradients.

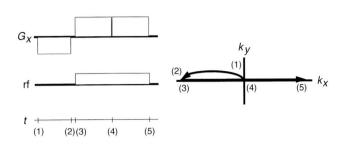

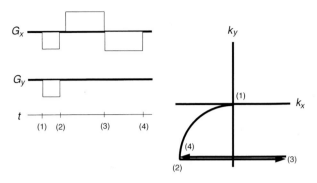

Figure 2.25

One-dimensional k-space trajectory. Prior to gradient activation, we begin in the center of k-space (1). With activation of a negative G_x at time (1), we move to the left along k_x to arrive at (2). At time (3) the positive G_x is activated, moving the k-space trajectory to the right. At time (4), the area under the positive lobe equals the area under the negative lobe, and we have returned to the center of k-space (4). Continued readout and application of the positive G_x gradient moves us to the right edge of k-space (5). As we move from (3) to (5), the rf channel (A/D converter) is opened and 128 points are sampled, corresponding to the readout of a single spin echo.

Figure 2.26

Two-dimensional k-space trajectory. In this example, negative G_x and G_y lobes are activated simultaneously. The negative G_x lobe moves us to the left of the origin in k-space and the negative G_y lobe moves us down in k-space. At the end of the application of both gradients, we are at (2) in the lower left-hand corner of k-space. Subsequent activation of a positive G_x moves us to the right (3), during which time 128 points could be sampled during a spin echo readout. When the next negative G_x lobe is applied, we move to the left in k-space, allowing readout of an additional 128 points for a second spin echo.

The physical equivalent of the k-space trajectory is the pulse sequence diagram (PSD) (Fig. 2.11). Gradient performance is characterized by three parameters: strength, rise time and duration (Fig. 2.24a). (Another gradient parameter, namely slew rate, is the maximum gradient strength divided by the minimum rise time.) Activation of the phase encode gradient leads to a certain amount of marginal phase accumulation at a particular point. This depends on the integral of the gradient over time—or, stated differently, the area under the gradient versus time curve. Whether this is accomplished by the gradient pulse in Fig. 2.24(a) or by any of those in Fig. 2.24(b) is inconsequential, since only the area under the curve is important. The advantage of high-performance gradients—with their greater strength and shorter rise times—is that the same area can be generated in less time. In Fig. 2.24(b), the dot–dash lines demonstrate that shorter rise times (at the same maximum gradient strength) shorten the duration of the gradient pulse compared with standard rise times shown in Fig. 2.24(a) (which is the same as the solid line in Fig.

2.24b). The dashed line shows the effect of stronger gradients at the old (slower) rise times. The dotted line in Fig. 2.24(b) shows the effect of faster rise times *and* stronger gradients—with marked reduction in the time the gradients are applied. This is the essence of the benefit from high-performance gradients. However it is achieved, the area under the gradient-versus-time curve determines the k-space trajectory and the FOV.

The simplest example of demonstrating the use of k-space is the concept of encoding along a single dimension (1D), e.g. readout (Fig. 2.25).[12] Typically, data sampling is coordinated with this k-space trajectory, and a series of equally spaced samples is taken, shown as sample points 1, ..., 128 below the k_x line. At the beginning, no gradient events have occurred and the k_x position is at the origin. A typical readout from a gradient echo sequence begins with activation of a negative lobe of the readout gradient G_x. (A momentary lull or zero gradient amplitude does not affect the k_x positioning.) This negative lobe acts to dephase spins along the readout axis, or move the position of k_x off-center to the left. A positive lobe acts to rephase spins or move the k_x 'trajectory' to the right. As it passes through zero, spins are maximally rephased and an echo is produced.

In this example, a Fourier transform of these 128 points yields a 1D projection of the object. Spacing these same 128 samples further apart and extending the two endpoints (either through higher gradient amplitudes or longer sampling duration) produce higher spatial resolution along this axis. If the number of samples is doubled to 256 with the same two endpoints maintained, the net effect to double the range of frequencies or bandwidth. If the readout gradient is the same and the dwell time is halved, the result is a doubling of the BW and the FOV.

This same analysis can be extended to two dimensions of k-space. In Fig. 2.26, the negative first lobe of G_x shifts the k-space position to the left (as in the example above). The simultaneous negative lobe G_y shifts the k-space position downward to the left lower corner. If there were no later G_y gradient application, filling of k-space would not progress upward along k_y. As in the example above, the next positive lobe of the x-gradient causes a rightward trajectory along k_x, during which the first echo is acquired. If there were a second negative lobe, the position in k-space would move leftward, and a second echo would be produced.

The second pass would merely repeat the first, albeit in the opposite direction. (In practice the phase encode would be activated to move upward along k_x.) In discussing this effect, we say that the second echo is 'time-reversed', or filled in 'backwardly', from the first. (As discussed below, this may have the effect of introducing '$N/2$ ghosts' into the image if eddy current-induced phase errors are uncorrected of if the gradient timing is slightly off.)

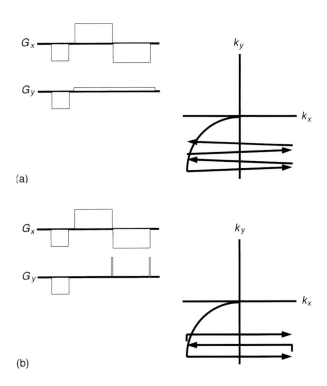

Figure 2.27

EPI k-space trajectory. (a) In the original description of EPI, initial negative G_x and G_y lobes move us to the lower left-hand corner of k-space. The G_x gradient is subsequently alternated positive and negative 128 times as the G_y gradient is left continuously 'on'. This produces a ramped trajectory in k-space, with changes in direction as G_x is reversed. (b) In the blipped version of EPI, the phase encode gradient G_y is 'blipped' very briefly to add a stepwise phase increment, resulting in a more Cartesian trajectory through k-space (which is easier to Fourier-transform).

Echo planar imaging

It is easy to extrapolate from this simple example to other methods to fill k-space via a series of gradient echoes. This initial concept for fast imaging filled k-space following a single rf pulse, i.e. in a single measurement or 'shot'. This was dubbed 'echo planar imaging' (EPI) by Sir Peter Mansfield in 1977 because an entire 2D raw data set (i.e. a 'plane' of data) could be filled during a single echo.[13] In order to do this, the readout gradient must be reversed rapidly from maximum positive to maximum negative 128 times during a single T_2^* decay (which is on the order of 100 ms). Each lobe of the readout gradient above or below the baseline corresponds to a separate k_y line of k-space and thus determines the number of phase encode steps N_p. The area under the G_x lobe determines the FOV, larger areas corresponding to smaller fields of view.[14] Thus single shot EPI places tremendous demands on the gradients in terms of maximum strength and minimum rise time. During each G_x reversal, a gradient echo is produced and is read out rapidly (*very* rapidly). (While the echo sampling time for the usual 256^2, $\pm 16\,\text{kHz}$ technique is 8 ms, 256 points must now be sampled in a *fraction* of a millisecond.) As we shall see below, this also places tremendous demands on the A/D converter.

In the original EPI method, the phase encode gradient was kept on continuously during the acquisition, resulting in a zigzag coverage of k-space (Fig. 2.27a). This led to some difficulties during Fourier transformation compared with the usual 'Cartesian' k-space trajectories.

To rectify this situation, the phase encode gradient was subsequently applied briefly when the readout gradient was zero, i.e. when the k-space position was at either end of the k_x axis. This method was referred to as 'blipped' phase encoding, since the duration of the phase encoding pulse was minimal (typically $<200\,\mu\text{s}$). The technique was called blipped EPI, and the k-space trajectory (Fig. 2.27b) was much more amenable to Fourier transformation.[15] In the following discussion, EPI implies 'blipped EPI', unless otherwise stated.

Even with blipped EPI, phase errors may result from the multiple positive and negative passes through k-space (i.e. alternating polarity of the readout gradient). If gradient-induced eddy currents build up or if there is a slight but systematic mismatch in the timing of the odd and even echoes, a complete replica or ghost of the main image will appear along the phase encode axis. Since ghosts are derived from half the data (even or odd passes), they are called '$N/2$ ghosts' (Fig. 2.28).

The gradient requirements to perform single shot EPI can be estimated from a few basic assumptions. First, the signal needs to be collected before it has significantly decayed owing to T_2 (or, in a real magnet, $T_2{}^*$) processes (Fig. 2.29a). As k-space is traversed from the bottom to the top, T_2 decay leads to blurring (called T_2 blurring). In order to keep the blurring to less than one pixel, the total readout time T must be kept to one or two T_2 values. Actually, for the blurring to be one pixel in width it can be shown that[16]

$$T < \pi T_2/2 \qquad (18)$$

Thus for a tissue with a $T_2 = 60$ ms, T would be 94 ms. (For total readout times greater than shown in Eqn (18), the pixel dimension becomes greater than that predicted from the FOV divided by the number of matrix elements.)

In EPI, each gradient reversal leads to a gradient echo and a new line in k-space. The number of k_y lines (N_p) together with the total readout time T determines the maximum time available to

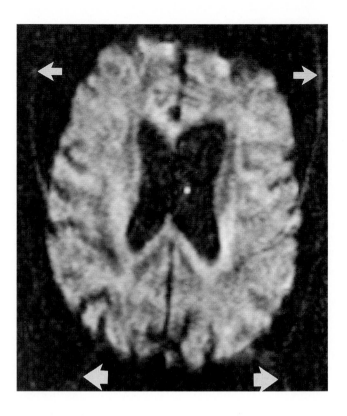

Figure 2.28

EPI artifacts. This EPI diffusion image has both chemical shift artifact (small arrows) and $N/2$ artifact (large arrows). The chemical shift artifact is approximately one-sixth of the FOV, while the $N/2$ artifact is approximately one-half of the FOV.

sample *each* echo, the so-called echo sampling period (ESP) (Fig. 2.29b):[14]

$$\text{ESP} = T/N_p \qquad (19)$$

In our example, if $T = 94$ ms and $N_p = 128$ then ESP = 700 µs.

During the ESP, the gradient must rise and fall and—if there is time—plateau in between (Fig. 1.30a). If the rise time is too long, the gradient may not even have time to achieve its full strength before it is time to begin falling (Fig. 2.30b). This defines the criterion for the minimum slew rate SR_{min} required to achieve the maximum gradient strength G_{max} in time ESP/2 (Fig. 2.30c):

$$\text{SR}_{\text{min}} = \frac{G_{\text{max}}}{\text{ESP}/2} \qquad (20)$$

Thus 25 mT/m gradients and an ESP of 700 µs (minimum rise time of 350 µs) would require a minimum SR of 71 mT/m per ms. A slew rate lower than this would not allow us to use the full

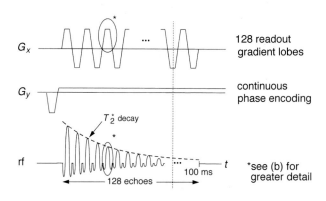

a

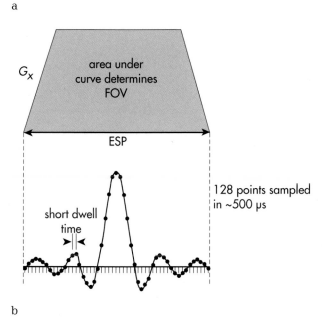

b

Figure 2.29

EPI readout. (a) During a single T_2^* decay (below), 128 echoes are formed from 128 reversals of the readout gradient G_x. During this time, the phase encode gradient is either continuously on (as shown here) or blipped in between each readout gradient reversal. The G_x gradient lobe and one of the gradient echoes (✱) are shown in greater detail in (b), where it can be seen that the G_x lobe demonstrates a trapezoidal waveform. The area under the curve determines the FOV, larger areas leading to smaller FOVs. The G_x gradient lobe can also have a sinusoidal (quarter-wave) ramp. During the time for which the gradient lobe G_x is applied, a gradient echo is formed (below) and digitized by the A/D converter. In order to have 128 readout projections, this signal must be sampled 128 times during the echo sampling period ESP. This necessitates extremely short dwell times, resulting in extremely high bandwidths for single shot EPI.

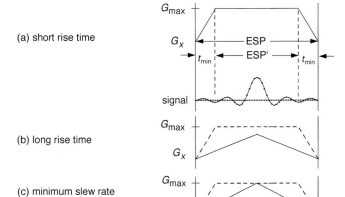

Figure 2.30

EPI readout gradient. (a) With a short rise time, the gradient is able to plateau at its maximum value prior to falling. The shorter the rise time and the stronger the gradient, the greater the area under the curve and the smaller the FOV. If the system is only capable of sampling on the plateau then this time is limited to ESP'. (b,c) In these situations, there would be no opportunity to sample the echo with long rise times (b) or if only the minimum slew rate is available to achieve G_{max} prior to falling (c). The signal shown in (a) assumes that it can be sampled during ramp up and ramp down, as well as on the plateau during the full time ESP.

strength of the gradients. While the *minimum* rise time required to reach G_{max} is ESP/2, there are several additional concerns that further lower the minimum rise time in practice. Some systems can *only* sample the data on the plateau, not on the ramps (e.g. during time ESP' in Fig. 2.30a). In Figs 2.30(b,c) where the gradient only has time to be ramped up and down without plateauing, the actual sampling time might have been zero. Obviously systems that are able to sample as the gradient goes up and down (i.e. to perform 'ramp sampling'), have an advantage compared with systems that cannot.

The shorter the sampling time, the higher the bandwidth. High bandwidths pose two potential problems. Since noise is proportional to the square root of bandwidth, the shorter the sampling time, the higher the bandwidth, the greater the noise and the lower the S/N (Fig. 2.31). In addition, higher bandwidths place additional demands on

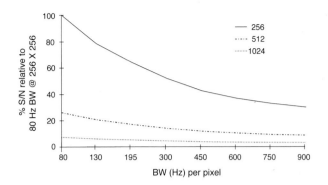

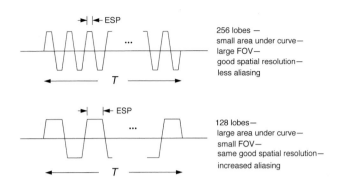

Figure 2.31

S/N versus matrix size and BW. S/N drops
precipitously with increasing matrix and increasing
bandwidth.

Figure 2.32

EPI spatial resolution. The top figure demonstrates 256
reversals of the readout gradient, producing 256 lobes
and 256 phase encode lines. With such rapid gradient
reversal, there is little area under the curve; therefore
the FOV is relatively large. Alternatively, the readout
gradient can be reversed 128 times, producing 128
lobes and 128 phase encode lines with a greater area
under the curve, leading to a smaller FOV. Although
the spatial resolution is comparable in the two cases,
there is a greater chance of aliasing in the latter
scenario.

the analog-to-digital converter (ADC). Conventional ADCs may not be able to sample quickly
enough to achieve the BWs required for EPI. The
maximum sampling speed is reflected in the
maximum achievable bandwidth of the ADC. For
an ESP of 700 µs with ramp sampling, the dwell
time for 256 readout projections would be 700/256
µs = 2.7 µs. This corresponds to a bandwidth of
$(1/2.7) \times 10^6$ Hz = 370 kHz = ±185 kHz. If the ADC
cannot sample this quickly, the BW is reduced,
leading to a smaller FOV and potential aliasing. In
order to prevent wraparound, we can modify Eqn
(5):

$$BW_{min} > \gamma G \times FOV/2$$

For $G = 25$ mT/m and FOV = 40 cm ($\gamma = 42.57$
mHz/T),

$$BW_{min} > ±210 \text{ kHz}$$

In general, single shot EPI techniques require
ADCs with total bandwidths on the order of MHz
rather than the kHz maximum total bandwidths
used for CSE.[14] Sampling on the rise—whether it
is a partial sine wave or a linear ramp—eases the
burden on the gradients considerably.[14] It has the
advantage of allowing the entire ESP to be used
for sampling—not just the plateaus. This results in
lower bandwidths, less noise and decreased
demands on the ADC.

As discussed above, the area under the gradient-versus-time curve determines the distance Δk
between points in k-space, i.e.

$$\Delta k_x = \int_0^{\Delta t} \gamma G_x \, dt \qquad (21)$$

and

$$\Delta k_y = \int_0^{t_y} \gamma G_x \, dt \qquad (22)$$

The greater the spacing Δk, the smaller the field
of view. Thus, the greater the area under the
curve, the smaller the FOV (Fig. 2.29b).

The area under the curve for a trapezoidal gradient pulse is determined by the maximum gradient
strength G_{max}, the minimum rise time t_{min} and the
ESP (Fig. 2.30a):

$$area = G_{max} (ESP - 2t_{min}) + G_{max} \, t_{min}$$

$$= G_{max} (ESP - 2t_{min}) \qquad (23)$$

Thus the shorter the minimum rise time and the
stronger the gradient, the greater the area (Fig.
2.24b).

As shown in Fig. 2.32, there is a tradeoff between the two determinants of spatial resolution in EPI: matrix size and field of view. If half the matrix elements were acquired during a given total readout time T, the ESP could double. This would potentially double the area under the curve, halving the FOV (Fig. 2.32, lower). Since the matrix has also been halved, this would leave spatial resolution unchanged—but would increase the chance of aliasing. If twice the matrix elements (N_p) during a given T were acquired, ESP would be halved, potentially halving the area under the curve *if* the gradients could keep up (Fig. 2.32, upper). Half the area translates to twice the FOV, again maintaining spatial resolution. This has the advantage of a lower chance of aliasing but it puts greater demands on the gradients in terms of rise time and slew rate. In the end, the only way to have high spatial resolution (which requires *both* a large number of matrix elements *and* a small FOV) is to use high-performance gradients.

One of the problems with single shot EPI is that any phase errors tend to propagate all the way through k-space. (This is not a problem for conventional spin echo, where the TR is long compared to T_2 so that the signal—and no phase errors—remain at the end of the cycle.) The usual phase error in a conventional spin echo image arises from motion from line to line over the TR interval. By comparison, there is little opportunity for involuntary or even physiologic motion during a typical 100 ms single shot EPI acquisition. Instead, protons resonating at frequencies different from the main Larmor frequency tend to build up phase errors, which increase over time. Since the temporal progression is mapped along the phase encode axis, these errors are mismapped along the phase encode axis. Fat protons, for example, resonate at a frequency 220 Hz below water. This will result in the phase of fat protons lagging behind the phase of water protons. Since position along the phase encode axis is based on the phase of water protons, fat signal will be mismapped, producing chemical shift artifact (Fig. 2.28). For conventional spin echo, the chemical shift artifact is along the readout axis and is predicted from the bandwidth per pixel, which is in turn derived from the echo sampling time as shown in Eqn (3). In EPI, chemical shift artifact is along the phase encode axis, because it has a much lower BW than along the readout axis.

At this point, it is useful to distinguish the total BW from the BW per pixel along the phase encode and readout axes in EPI. As shown in Eqns (2) and (3), the total and per pixel BWs along the readout gradient are:

$$BW_{tot} = \frac{N_x}{EST} \quad (2)$$

$$BW_{per\ pixel} = \frac{1}{EST} \quad (3)$$

For the phase encode direction, $BW_{per\ pixel}$ is determined by the total echo sampling time T (since there is no phase correction once sampling has started in EPI). Thus

$$BW_{phase,\ per\ pixel} = \frac{1}{T} \quad (24)$$

For $T = 100$ ms, for example,

$$BW_{phase} = 10\ Hz/pixel$$

The total BW in phase is derived from the time it takes to sample one line in k_y, which is also the echo sampling period ESP:

$$BW_{phase,\ total} = \frac{N_p}{T} = \frac{1}{ESP} \quad (25)$$

$BW_{per\ pixel}$ in the read direction is the total time an echo is read out, i.e. ESP (again):

$$BW_{read\ per\ pixel} = \frac{1}{ESP} \quad (26)$$

The total BW in read is the dwell time or the sampling interval. This is the ESP divided by the total number of readout projections:

$$BW_{read,\ total} = \frac{N_x}{ESP} \quad (27)$$

These bandwidth formulas are summarized in Table 2.2, along with a typical numerical example.

Table 2.2

	BW		
	Read	*Phase*	
Per pixel	1/ESP	1/T	Formula
Total	N_x/ESP	1/ESP	

Example[a]	BW	
	Read	*Phase*
Per pixel	1 kHz	10 Hz
Total	100 kHz	1 kHz

[a] For $T = 100$ ms, $N_p = 100$, $N_x = 100$, ESP = 1 ms.

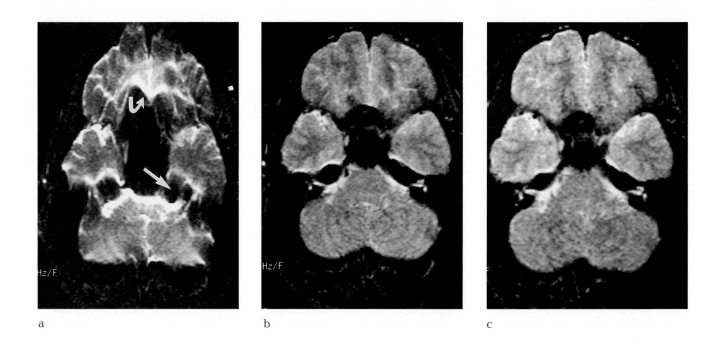

a   b   c

Figure 2.33

EPI susceptibility effects. (a) Single shot EPI demonstrates marked distortion of the skull base due to differences in diamagnetic susceptibility between air and tissue. (b) 8 shot EPI sequence markedly reduces the geometric distortion due to differences in diamagnetic susceptibility. Persistent distortion is noted along the anterior margin of the temporal bones (straight arrow) and above the sphenoid sinus (curved arrow). (c) 32-shot EPI results in minor diminution in degree of susceptibility-induced distortion although the image quality is generally inferior because of artifacts introduced in the interleaving of the 32 shots.

For a 220 Hz chemical shift between fat and water and $T = 100$ ms (i.e. $BW_{phase} = 10$ Hz/pixel), there would be a 220/10 = 20 pixel chemical shift along the phase encode axis. The fat image would then be shifted 20/100 or one-fifth of the FOV (Fig. 2.28a). For this reason, a spectroscopic fat saturation ('FatSat') pulse must be applied prior to a single shot EPI acquisition.

Intrinsic nonuniformities in B_0 and diamagnetic susceptibility effects result in variable resonance frequencies and growing phase errors as well. For example, the chemical shift associated with the diamagnetic susceptibility differences between air in the sinuses and tissue is estimated at 1 ppm, or about one-third of the chemical shift between fat and water. Over the course of a single shot EPI readout, the phase errors that build up, lead to several centimeters of spatial mismapping.[17] Thus one of the persistent technical difficulties with EPI is distortion at the base of the brain, particularly where air in the sinuses is in close proximity with brain (Fig. 2.33a). (For this reason, most axial EPI sequences are now angled +30° to the canthomeatal line to avoid the paranasal sinuses (Fig. 2.22).)

By dividing the EPI readout into multiple shots N_s, phase errors have less time to build up, with subsequent decrease in the diamagnetic susceptibility artifacts (Fig. 2.33b) This is called multishot EPI[11] or—since k-space is segmented into multiple acquisitions—segmented EPI.[18] (As noted above, $N_p = N_s \times ETL$.) For an eight-shot EPI acquisition at the same BW as the comparable single shot technique, there would be one-eighth the phase encode error. Unfortunately, multishot techniques also take a lot longer than single shot techniques; therefore they are more susceptible to motion artifacts and new artifacts arising from the potential misregistration of the multiple shots.[19]

While multishot EPI may not be as fast as single shot EPI, it does have certain advantages compared with FSE. For about half the time it takes to acquire an 8ETL FSE sequence, a 16-shot (16ETL) multishot EPI sequence has contrast much closer to conventional spin echo, i.e. greater sensitivity to magnetic susceptibility artifacts such as

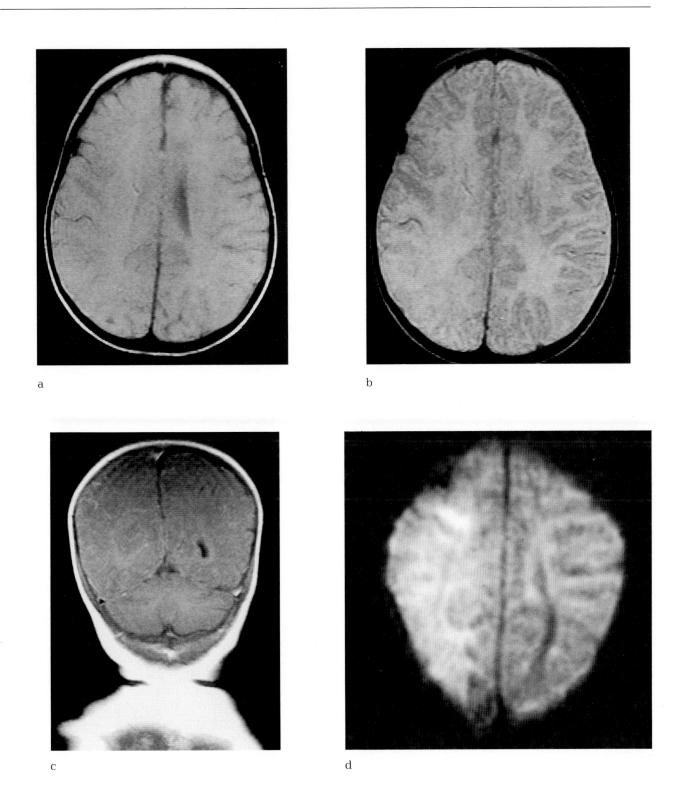

a

b

c

d

Figure 2.34

Non-accidental trauma. (a) Proton-density-weighted image demonstrates subtle effacement of sulci in the right hemisphere. (b) T_2-weighted image demonstrates subtle loss of gray/white differentiation. (c) Gadolinium-enhanced T_1-weighted image shows sulcal effacement and subtle vascular stasis on the right. (d) EPI–diffusion image demonstrates high signal intensity in the territory of the right middle cerebral artery. While the conventional spin echo imaging was suggestive of diffuse brain edema secondary to a contusion, the EPI diffusion image showing vascular territory hyperintensity is much more suggestive of infarction, which would suggest strangulation, strengthening the case for child abuse.

hemorrhage.[14] Because each echo in FSE is produced by a 180° rf pulse (which takes time and increases the specific absorption rate, SAR), the total time per slice and the total rf heating are greater than for a multishot EPI[19] (which only uses gradient reversal to produce echoes). For this reason, more slices can be acquired per *TR* interval with multishot EPI than with FSE (or GRASE either, for that matter). Unfortunately, even at a large number of shots, some diamagnetic susceptibility artifact remains at the skull base. (This is the tradeoff for faster imaging.)

Contrast in single shot and multishot EPI depends on the 'root' sequence from which it is derived (i.e. the succession of 90° and 180° rf pulses), rather than on the composite gradient or spin echoes.[14] In this context, it is useful to separate the 'root sequence' from the 'signal'. For example, a single 90° rf pulse produces an FID *signal*. A 180°–90°–180° combination is an IR *root* with a spin echo signal. (A 90°–180° is a spin echo root *and* a spin echo signal.) For echo train techniques covering multiple lines in *k*-space, the 'signal' for each rf excitation (or *TR*) is more accurately termed a readout module (ETL echoes long). Thus FSE is a $90°–(180°)_{ETL}$, i.e. a 90° rf pulse followed by ETL 180° rf pulses. IR-FSE is a $180°–90°–(180°)_{ETL}$, i.e. a 180° followed by a FSE readout module, ETL echoes long.

In the same way, EPI can be considered a readout module—whether as a single or multishot technique. For example, a 90°–180°–EPI would be a spin echo root with an EPI readout module, i.e. SE-EPI (Fig. 2.21e). An rf pulse (less than 90°) followed by an EPI readout module would be a GRE-EPI, i.e. an EPI sequence with gradient echo contrast (Fig. 2.21f). Similarly, diffusion gradients can be added for EPI-diffusion imaging (Fig. 2.34).[20,21] Unlike FSE, where echoes acquired with weaker values of the phase encode gradient (in the center of *k*-space) determine contrast ('effective *TE*'), all the echoes in EPI are acquired with the *same* value of the phase encode gradient. Thus contrast on SE-EPI is determined from the temporal rephasing of the 180° RF pulse; in GRE-EPI, it is determined by the time between the negative phase encode gradient prepulse and the EPI readout module. Contrast in a T_2-weighted EPI is very much like a T_2-weighted conventional spin echo; i.e. signal is determined by T_2 decay, and flowing blood appears dark. Contrast in a GRE-EPI sequence is $T_2{}^*$-weighted—which means it is perfect for performing first-pass 'perfusion' sequences with gadolinium (Fig. 2.34) or dysprosium.[21] (As with other low-flip-angle, conventional gradient echo images, flowing blood is bright—

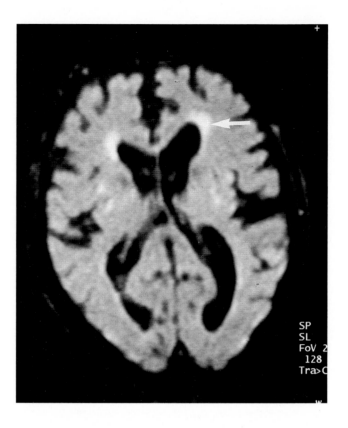

Figure 2.35

IR-SE-EPI. Using a *TI* of 3000 ms and an effectively infinite *TR*, this single shot EPI-FLAIR image demonstrates effective nulling of CSF with good T_2-weighting, showing bright interstitial edema (arrow).

which will be useful for EPI-MR angiography sequences.) Should T_1 contrast be desired in an EPI sequence, a 180° prepulse can be applied, i.e. an inversion–recovery root, IR-EPI (Fig. 2.35).

The combination of EPI–diffusion imaging and EPI–perfusion imaging appears to be particularly promising for the evaluation and management of acute stroke.[22] In EPI–perfusion imaging, the transient drop in signal intensity as the gadolinium bolus passes provides indirect evidence of the state of perfusion of the tissue. From this data, relative cerebral blood volume (rCBV) and mean transit time (MTT) maps can be generated (see Chapter 3). (Actually, the sensitivity to perfusion in vessels of a particular size depends on the specific EPI sequence used. Performing EPI perfusion imaging with a spin echo technique (SE-EPI) provides sensitivity to the microcirculation alone, while a GRE-EPI sequence provides sensitivity to both the microcirculation and the capillary circulation.]

With decreasing perfusion from normal, the EPI perfusion study is the first to become positive. As the blood supply drops below about 20 ml/min per 100 g of brain tissue, reversible ischemic changes begin.[23] As the ATP levels fall, the sodium potassium pump fails and the cells become nonfunctional and begin to swell. This is known as 'cytotoxic edema'. It is associated with decreased water diffusion and high signal on EPI diffusion images. Cytotoxic edema is reversible. If blood supply is re-established (e.g. through thrombolysis), these cells can return to normal. On the other hand, if the ischemia is sufficiently severe or prolonged, the cells may go on to irreversible infarction. Infarction leads to cell rupture, vasogenic edema, and high signal on conventional T_2-weighted images. Early on in this process, there is still a population of swollen, cytotoxic cells. Thus early infarcts are also positive on EPI diffusion images. Therefore a positive EPI diffusion study does not guarantee that irreversible infarction has not already occurred. In practice, it is uncommon that a positive EPI–diffusion study is ultimately associated with a totally normal MRI examination. Thus EPI–perfusion imaging is the most sensitive test for ischemia, followed by EPI–diffusion imaging and then conventional T_2-weighted spin echo imaging.

At the time of the initial presentation, if the perfusion and diffusion defects are matched, the infarct is unlikely to worsen.[22] A diffusion defect smaller than the perfusion defect defines an 'ischemic penumbra' that is at risk for extension of the infarct. Unless the brain recruits collateral blood supply or interventional procedures (e.g. thrombolytics) are instituted, the completed infarct is more likely to be the size of the perfusion defect than the diffusion defect. It has recently[22] been suggested that this mismatch between the size of the abnormalities on EPI perfusion and diffusion imaging be used as the criterion for institution of thrombolysis rather than the 3–6 h duration of symptoms.

The only downside to EPI at the moment appears to be physiologic peripheral nerve stimulation.[24] This tingling sensation in the skin occurs where the change in gradient field is greatest at the edges of the coil. It depends on dB/dt, rise time, G_{max} and patient body habitus.[25]

References

1. Wood ML, Fourier Imaging. In: *Magnetic Resonance Imaging*, 2nd edn (ed DD Stark, WG Bradley) 21–66. Mosby-Year Book, St Louis, 1992.

2. Bradley WG, Kortman KE, Crues JV, Central nervous system high-resolution magnetic resonance imaging: effect of increasing spatial resolution on resolving power. *Radiology* 1985; **156**: 93–8.

3. Bradley WG, Rogers L, Chen F-Y, Ramirez G, Correlation of high resolution MRI with pathology to determine Gleason grading of prostate cancer. *Radiology* 1995; **197(P)**: 253.

4. Bradley WG, Flow Phenomena. In: *Magnetic Resonance Imaging*, 2nd edn (ed DD Stark, WG Bradley) 253–98. Mosby-Year Book, St Louis, 1992.

5. Le Bihan D, Turner R, Diffusion and Perfusion. In: *Magnetic Resonance Imaging*, 2nd edn (ed DD Stark, WG Bradley) 335–71. Mosby-Year Book, St Louis, 1992.

6. Moseley ME, Cohen Y, Mintorovitch J, et al. Early detection of regional cerebral ischemia in cats: comparison of diffusion- and T2-weighted MRI and spectroscopy. *Magn Reson Med* 1990; **14**: 330–46.

7. LeBihan D, Delannoy J, Levin RL. Temperature mapping with MR imaging of molecular diffusion: application to hyperthermia. *Radiology* 1989; **171**: 853–7.

8. Weber DM, Echo Planar Imaging, monograph, GE Medical Systems, Milwaukee, WI, 1993.

9. Frahm J, Gyngell ML, Hanicke W, Rapid Scan Techniques. In: *Magnetic Resonance Imaging*, 2nd edn (ed DD Stark, WG Bradley) 165–218. Mosby-Year Book, St Louis, 1992.

10. Oshio K, Feinberg DA. GRASE (gradient- and spin-echo) imaging: a novel fast MRI technique. *Magn Reson Med* 1991; **20**: 344–9.

11. Butts, Riederer SJ, Ehman RL, Thompson RM, Jack CR, Interleaved echo planar imaging on a standard MRI system. *Mag Res in Med* 1994; **31(1)**: 67–72.

12. Twieg DB. The k-trajectory formulation of the NMR imaging process with applications in analysis and synthesis of imaging methods *Med Phys* 1983; **10**: 610–21.

13. Mansfield P, Multi-planar image formation using NMR spin echoes. *J. Phys Chem* 1977; **10**: L55.

14. Mansfield P, Pykett IL. Biological and medical imaging by NMR. *J Magn Reson* 1978; **29**: 355–73.

15. Edelman RR, Wielopolski R, Schmitt F. Echo-planar imaging. *Radiology* 1994; **192**: 600–12.

16. Farzaneh, et al, Analysis of T2 limitations and off-resonance effect on spatial resolution and artifacts in echo-planar imaging. *Mag Res in Med* 1990; **14**: 123–39.

17. Jezzard P, Balban RS, Correction for geometric distortion in echo planar images from Bo field variations. *Mag Res in Med* 1995; **31(1)**: 65–73.

18. Butts K, Riederer SJ, Ehman RL, et al. Interleaved echo planar imaging on a standard MRI system. *Magn Reson Med* 1994; **31**: 67–82.

19. Siewert B, Patel MR, Mueller MF, Gaa J, Darby, et al, Brain lesions in patients with multiple sclerosis: detection with echo-planar imaging. *Radiology* 1995; **196(3)**: 765–71.

20. DeLaPaz RL, Echo-planar imaging. *Radiographics* 1994; **14(5)**: 1045–58.

21. Dardzinski BJ, Sotak CH, Fisher M, Hasegawa Y, Li L, Minematsu K, Apparent diffusion coefficient mapping of experimental focal cerebral ischemia using diffusion-weighted echo-planar imaging. *Mag Res in Med* 1993; **30(3)**: 318–25.

22. Kucharczyk J, Vexler ZS, Roberts TP, Asgari HS, et al, Echo-planar perfusion-sensitive MR imaging of acute cerebral ischemia. *Radiology* 1993; **188(3)**: 711–17.

23. Sorensen AG, Buonanno FS, Gonzolez RG, Schwamm LH, et al, Hyperacute stroke: Evaluation with combined multisection diffusion-weighted and hemodynamically weighted echo-planar imaging. *Radiology* 1996; **199**: 391–401.

24. Jacobs BC, Brant-Zawadzki M, Ischemia. S In: *Magnetic Resonance Imaging*, 2nd edn (ed DD Stark, WG Bradley) 636–69. Mosby-Year Book, St Louis, 1992.

25. Mansfield P, Harvey PR, Limits to neural stimulation in echo-planar imaging. *Mag Res in Med* 1993; **29**: 746–58.

3

Echo planar imaging: technology and techniques

Robert M Weisskoff and Mark S Cohen

Introduction

Magnetic resonance imaging (MRI) has proven to be an extremely sensitive and increasingly specific modality for in vivo diagnostic scanning. Yet, for all its efficacy, MRI remains costly and MRI scan times, which are long compared with physiological motion and patient tolerance, limit its use in certain situations. In this chapter, we describe the use of echo planar imaging (EPI), an emerging technology that, by dramatically reducing scan times, expands the limits of conventional MRI. While conventional MR methods build images from repeated radiofrequency (rf) excitations and sampling of the MR data, EPI methods can form complete images from a single rf excitation. Though considerable progress has been made over the past few years on gradient echo and faster spin echo methods that speed encoding, applications are emerging for which the ultimate temporal resolution (as little as $\frac{1}{30}$ s) provided by EPI is beneficial or necessary. This chapter introduces EPI, discussing both the principles of its implementation and its emerging applications.

Motivation

Of the commonly available diagnostic imaging examinations (e.g. ultrasound, fluoroscopy and X-ray CT), magnetic resonance is often the slowest. In most cases, the longer scan time of MRI are justified by the increased soft tissue contrast available with MR. However, there are at least three drawbacks of these lengthy times: motion artifacts, limited applications and increased cost.

Motion can have a particularly devastating effect on MR images. Because of the Fourier encoding process used in MRI, local motion can have global effects on the MR image and its contrast.[1,2] Thus respiration, pulsation, peristalsis and other movements that occur during the exam can result in substantial distortion of the MR image.

For certain cyclical motions like cardiac pulsation and respiration, it is possible to synchronize the MR data acquisition with the source of the motion itself, by such means as ECG triggering, respiratory gating or respiratory-ordered phase encoding. Though these methods can be remarkably effective, they also make scan setup more complex and can result in contrast distortion. In cardiac triggered scans, for example, irregular heartbeat translates into variable TR and thus variable T_1 contrast.[3]

In addition to involuntary physiological motions, artifacts from 'voluntary' patient motion reduce the diagnostic yield of MR scans substantially, particularly for those exams, such as cervical and lumbar spine, where pain is the primary symptom. This problem is exacerbated in hospital-based centers that often serve a high proportion of non-ambulatory patients. Because of claustrophobia, as many as 15% of patients refuse MR scans, or are not sufficiently cooperative to produce diagnostic images. It is likely that the claustrophobia is aggravated by long examination times. While techniques to minimize motion artifacts continue to evolve, motion remains one of the primary corrupters of clinical image quality.

In addition to corruption by motion, the relatively low speed of conventional MR limits the range of its application. Despite its high intrinsic tissue contrast and proven sensitivity to a wide variety of pathological conditions, the majority of clinical MRI is still limited to the central nervous system. Of the many factors that account for this, the limitations of MRI in the presence of motion weigh heavily, even though the medical indications for sensitive diagnostic procedures in the abdomen and thorax offer potential areas of growth for MRI.

Beyond these applications, recent discoveries of physiological contrast in MR such as diffusion imaging in stroke, susceptibility contrast in the brain and heart, BOLD and flow imaging of activation in the brain, fundamentally require high speed and/or motion artifact-free images to exploit this contrast clinically. These techniques have the potential to extend dramatically the types of exam that can be performed in the MR scanner, from purer anatomic scans to those that include a functional component.

Finally, with multiple forces focused on decreasing the cost of MR scans, there is pressure to decrease the duration of the MR exam. In the USA, for example, third party reimbursement for MR scans has dropped by nearly half in the last five years, and all indications are that this trend will continue. While the duration of the scan is not necessarily the primary driver of these costs, increasing the range of indications and decreasing the duration of the individual exams is one scenario for the continued fiscal success of MRI. EPI is a potentially important tool in evolving this scenario.

Organization

This chapter is organized in three basic parts. In the first, we describe the basics of EPI: how to think about it, and how its implementation differs from conventional MRI. In the second, we give some examples of the current clinical applications of EPI. These applications include 'standard' MR imaging done quickly (e.g. rapid intracranial imaging in uncooperative patients and T_2 imaging of the liver), as well as new applications that are helped by ultrahigh-speed imaging (e.g. blood volume mapping and diffusion imaging of acute stroke). In the final section, we describe specific artifacts of EPI and set EPI in context with other high-speed imaging techniques.

Echo planar imaging basics

In this section, we describe EPI as an imaging technique. We first review the common description of the MR imaging process, called the k-space formalism, and then describe conventional and fast imaging techniques in terms of that formalism. This formalism will be helpful both in this section and below, when we describe image artifacts specific to EPI. We then describe the contrast behavior of EPI, again comparing it with conventional imaging. Finally, we introduce some of the technical aspects of EPI implementations, in order to give a flavor of its differences from conventional imaging requirements.

k-space

As described in Chapter 2, one of the most efficient ways to describe the MR image formation process is through a notation that reflects the mathematics of the image formation. The phase- or frequency-encoding gradient in MRI gives protons a location-specific resonance frequency, and thus encodes the spatial location of the object into frequencies. Ultimately, it is the spatial frequencies that are encoded by MR. The Fourier transform decodes these frequencies back into locations in the reconstruction computer. The encoding process can be described entirely by describing the history of these encoding gradients in a particularly simple way. The sum of their past history (i.e. their integral) up to a given point in time describes which particularly spatial frequency is being encoded at that moment:

This k-space method is a useful formalism proposed by a number of investigators and developed by Twieg[4,5] and Ljunggren[6] for describing and manipulating the MR raw data collected in the Fourier-encoded scanning methods commonly used in MR imaging. The distance from the origin of k-space, and thus the spatial frequency information acquired at any given time, depends solely upon the history of the applied gradients:

$$\boldsymbol{k}(t) = \gamma \int_0^t \boldsymbol{G}(t') \, dt',$$

where $\boldsymbol{k}$ is the k-space displacement, a 2D vector for 2D imaging, γ is the gyromagnetic ratio and $\boldsymbol{G}$ is the vector of the phase- and frequency-encoding gradients at a given time. Usually, one

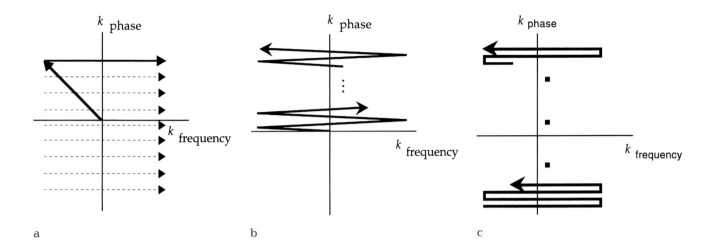

Figure 3.1

k-space trajectories. (a) The typical, conventional spin warp imaging k-space trajectory. It is rectilinear, and each horizontal line starts afresh with a new excitation. (b) The original EPI with a constant phase-encoding gradient without pre-encoding. The trajectory zig-zags (constant velocity in the phase-encoding direction), and does not necessarily cover k-space uniformly. (c) The current EPI trajectory used in most applications. By using blipped phase-encoding pulses at the zero-crossings of the readout gradient, rectilinear k-space coverage is re-established.

axis of k-space describes the phase and the other the frequency of the MR signal.

Signals corresponding to low spatial frequencies (i.e. the general shape of the object) are concentrated near the origin of k-space. Information about higher spatial frequencies (e.g. edges and smaller objects) is spread further from the origin. Thus, leaving the gradients on for a longer time or increasing their amplitude results in better encoding smaller features of the sample. Where the integral of the applied gradients is zero (i.e. where the signal is undisturbed by the gradients) the MR signal is usually at its greatest. For this reason, each time the MR signal crosses either axis in k-space, it is said to form a 'gradient echo'.

Every location in k-space corresponds to a combination of the integrals of the applied gradients. Since these integrals evolve over time, the position of the MR signal on the k-space plane can be thought of as a trajectory. If the time spent in spatial encoding is short compared with other temporal factors (such as T_2-related signal decay or patient motion) then the appearance of the final image is independent of the specific k-space trajectory. On the other hand, if k-space is not completely and/or evenly sampled, various artifacts may appear in the final image.[4]

Fast imaging and k-space

In a conventionally acquired MR image, the k-space trajectory is a simple raster. The phase encoding pulse 'moves' the trajectory to a given location vertically, and then the frequency-encoding gradient moves across k-space horizontally (Fig. 3.1a). The excitation is repeated N times, changing the phase-encoding gradient each time so that a different starting vertical position can be accessed with each excitation. From the k-space point of view, all that is required to make an image is that enough of k-space be sampled that reconstruction is possible. Conventional imaging fills one line every TR. With $TR = 500$ ms, filling 256 lines takes about 2 min; with $TR = 2000$ ms, filling 256 lines takes about 8 min. One way to make fast images is simply to fill up k-space faster by decreasing TR. Shortening TR is the key to the 'FLASH'-like pulse sequences (see Chapter 2). Another way to decrease scan time is to acquire more than one line of k-space with every excitation. Fast spin echo (RARE-like sequences) sequences do exactly this, using multiple 180° pulses to produce additional spin echoes, each of which has a unique phase-encoding associated with it (see Chapter 1). A fast spin echo sequence

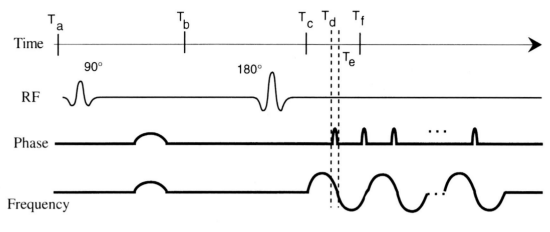

a

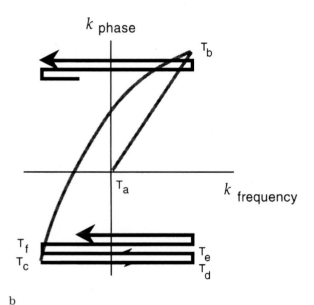

b

Figure 3.2

EPI pulse sequence. (a) Pulse sequence for a prototypical EPI spin echo acquisition. The rf pulses and slice selection are the same as for conventional spin warp imaging, while the oscillating readout gradient and blipped phase-encoding gradient encode the imaging data from the single rf excitation.
(b) The detailed k-space trajectory for this sequence. The sequence starts at T_a, pre-encoding translates the acquisition to one corner of k-space at T_b, and refocusing reflects this point across the center of k-space to T_c. The first frequency-encoding half-lobe translates the trajectory horizontally to T_d, at which time a phase-encoding blip translates vertically at T_e. The negative half-lobe moves the trajectory back across k-space horizontally to T_f. The pattern then continues until k-space coverage is complete.

that encodes eight echoes (an echo train length of eight) will fill up k-space eight times faster. The goal of single-shot imaging is to fill all of k-space in a single rf excitation.

In 1977, Peter Mansfield[7,8] proposed the technique known as echo planar imaging or EPI. With this method, the complete 2D encoding process is completed during the free induction decay following a single excitation pulse. In the original implementation, a small gradient was applied along the phase-encoding axis while rapidly alternating pulses were applied with the frequency-encoding gradient (Fig. 3.1b). Because of the resulting 'zig-zag' k-space trajectory, and because only half of k-space was covered in these early implementations, images produced from a single excitation were not useful, but nevertheless were tremendously promising and exciting. The problems resulting from the

sampling of only one half of k-space become increasingly severe as the field strength is increased. In 1987 Mansfield's group[9] introduced the FLEET (fast low-angle excitation echo planar technique) and BEST (blipped echo planar single-pulse technique) methods that solve the reconstruction problems by acquiring two images, one for the positive and one for the negative halves of the k-phase. Using these techniques and variants, Mansfield was able by 1987 to collect complete MR images in as little as 100 ms. These techniques have progressed to produce high-quality images of the head[10] and body[11] using the MBEST technology on their 0.5 T research system.

At approximately the same time, the 'Instascan' method was introduced in 1986 by Pykett and Rzedzian.[12-15] Like echo planar imaging, it utilizes rapidly oscillating gradients to spatially encode the

MR signal. Instascan was developed between 1983 and 1986 to overcome the problems resulting from the larger, 2.0 T, static fields that were being used in imaging. In the original Instascan presentation, all of the spatial encoding was performed under the rf-elicited Hahn spin echo. Second, pre-encoding pulses were applied along the phase- and frequency-encoding axes; as a consequence, k-space is scanned symmetrically from $-k$ to $+k$ values. Finally, rather than leaving the phase-encoding gradient on continuously during acquisition, one gradient was pulsed briefly between each frequency-encoding period. Like MBEST, the result is a rectilinear, rather than a zig-zag, k-space trajectory (Fig. 3.1c)—almost identical to the trajectory used in conventional imaging, though acquired in a small fraction of the total scan time.

The distinctions between these early methods have become sufficiently blurred over time that it is simpler to describe all single-shot, oscillating gradient imaging techniques as 'echo planar' techniques. In addition, to avoid continued explosion of acronyms, for the remainder of this chapter, we shall simply call the data acquisition method 'EPI', and use the conventional acronyms for the rf pulse sequences that give it contrast. Thus a 90° pulse (or α pulse) with no refocusing will be called 'gradient echo EPI', a 90–180° sequence 'spin echo EPI', and a 180° inversion preparatory pulse before a spin echo sequence 'inversion recovery EPI'.

We now consider in greater detail the k-space trajectory for spin echo EPI. This pulse sequence is shown in Fig. 3.2(a). As in conventional MRI, spatial information is encoded by the use of two gradient sets along orthogonal axes. The effects of the oscillating frequency-encoding gradient and blipped phase-encoding gradient are shown in their k-space representations in Fig. 3.2(b). Because the phase- and frequency-encoding gradients are used alternately, rather than simultaneously, the trajectories along the frequency axis of k-space are flat, rather than tilted, and trace out a 'rasterlike' pattern. The raw data space is therefore covered more homogeneously, and the image reconstruction process is similar to that of conventional imaging, except that every other line of k-space is scanned in the opposite direction. The displacement in k-space along the frequency axis is determined by the duration and amplitude of the frequency-encoding gradient pulses, while the total displacement along the k-phase axis is determined by the duration and amplitude of the phase-encoding gradient pulses *and* by the total number of scan lines.

Contrast behavior

One of the simplest ways of thinking about EPI is to consider it simply as an accelerated acquisition that one can combine with any conventional pulse sequence (see Fig. 3.3). While this simplification ignores certain artifacts that will be discussed

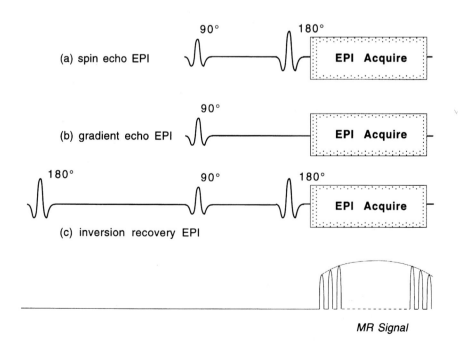

Figure 3.3

EPI acquisition/conventional rf. EPI is simply a way of acquiring the imaging data very quickly. As such, it can be thought of as an acquisition block that can be placed in any MRI pulse sequence. Thus spin echo (a), gradient echo (b) and inversion recovery (c) imaging are compatible with EPI.

below, it provides a useful model for understanding the contrast of EPI images. For example, spin echo EPI has contrast behavior like that of conventional spin echo images (Fig. 3.4). Unlike the gradient echo methods (FLASH, GRASS etc), it is possible to use relatively long echo times to obtain true T_2 weighting, since a spin echo is indeed created by the rf pulses. Furthermore, because the technique uses only a single excitation pulse, it is possible to obtain 'infinite TR' images: scans whose contrast is independent of T_1. Since a common—though by no means universal—property of biological tissues is the tendency for disease to be associated with simultaneous increases in both T_1 and T_2, T_1 contamination of T_2 images has a tendency to wash out some of the inherent T_2 contrast possible in the system. That is, in conventional spin echo images, the T_1 increase causes a signal loss while the T_2 increase results in a relative contrast gain. As a consequence, lesion conspicuity is often compromised by residual T_1 contrast in T_2-weighted scans. Spin echo EPI therefore offers the advantage of significantly improved diagnostic contrast behavior.

In addition, T_1 contrast can be added in exactly the same manner as it is conventionally. That is, it is possible to introduce a 'TR' period, though in this case TR represents the time between complete images rather than lines of k-space. In fact, the standard basis set of MR images, namely spin-density-, T_2- and T_1-weighted scans, can be acquired with only two excitatory RF pulses. After the first 90° pulse, double echo EPI acquisitions with short and long TE are acquired, yielding the proton-density and T_2-weighted contrasts respectively, with an effective TR of infinity. A second 90° pulse is applied half a second or so later, and a short TE Instascan image is acquired. This image will have T_1 contrast like that of a 500 ms TR conventional image. The overall imaging time will therefore be only half a second. Note therefore that, paradoxically, in EPI the 'long-TR' (T_2-weighted) scans require less *actual* scan time than the short-TR (T_1-weighted) scans.

T_1 contrast may also be added by spin inversion. Preceding the EPI spin echo sequence with a 180° rf pulse produces inversion recovery (IR) contrast (Fig. 3.3c). Such images have roughly twice the T_1 sensitivity of short-TR (partial saturation) scans, and are therefore useful in making highly T_1-weighted images (Fig. 3.5). In addition, unlike conventional imaging, for which the contrast per unit time is actually better with saturation recovery, the total scan times are sufficiently short with EPI that net contrast can be optimized with little impact on total scan time.

The same applications that have been proposed for IR in conventional imaging work equally well with EPI, with the added advantage that long TRs between k-space lines (which typically drive conventional IR acquisitions beyond 12 min) have negligible impact on total examination time. Thus, choosing an inversion time (TI, the time between the first 180° pulse and the 90° nutation pulse) corresponding to the time at which the magnetization of fat is at a minimum (about 170 ms at 1.5 T) produces nearly complete fat suppression,

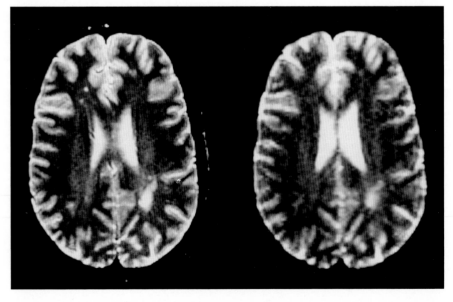

a   b

Figure 3.4

Conventional/EPI image. Spin echo EPI images have T_2 contrast comparable to that of their conventional analogs, as demonstrated in this image pair: (a) conventional 256 × 256, 20 cm FOV, TE = 80 ms, TR = 2500 ms, spin echo image (time 10.5 min) of a patient demonstrating a white matter lesion due to AIDS; (b) single-shot EPI image, 128 × 128, 20 cm FOV, TE = 80 ms, TR = infinite (time 0.1 s).

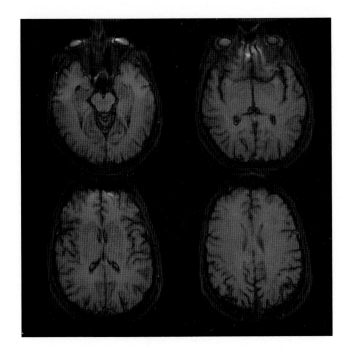

Figure 3.5

EPI inversion recovery contrast. Inversion recovery can be particularly useful for generating excellent gray/white contrast while simultaneously suppressing fluid (FLAIR), but is time-consuming and prone to motion artifacts using conventional techniques. Using EPI, these long *TI* (≈1200 ms) and long *TR* (≈5000 ms) images are acquired in the same examination time as conventional EPI spin echo images.

creating the Instant analog to 'STIR' imaging.[16–18] Preconditioning with an inversion pulse in high-speed FLASH imaging has also been utilized to advantage (see below), but the resulting contrast behavior is different from that seen in conventional MRI.

Gradient strategies and *k*-space coverage

Performing all of the MR spatial encoding in only a few milliseconds requires strong and rapidly switched gradients. As can be seen from the *k*-space description, the spatial resolution in standard Fourier reconstructions along any axis is determined by the maximum displacement of the *k*-space trajectory along the corresponding axis. This position is, in turn, determined by the integral of the applied gradient. In order to use brief gradient pulses, large gradient amplitudes must be applied to give the same overall integral. The large amplitudes require high current capability, and the rise time requirements place severe voltage demands on the gradient power sources. For example, if we consider a standard trapezoidal read gradient with rise time τ, flat-top amplitude *G* and duration *T*, we see that the resolution, Δx is given by

$$\Delta x = \frac{1}{\gamma GT}$$

The current into the gradient coil (with inductance *L*) required to achieve this resolution is proportional to *G*, and the peak voltage is proportional to *G*/τ. Thus, for a fixed readout period, the amplifier power (which is proportional to voltage × current) is proportional to $(1/\Delta x)^2$. In addition, if we want to maintain the same resolution, but shorten the readout time, we find that the power scales as $(1/T)^3$. That is, shortening the readout increases the peak current proportionally, but increases the required voltage quadratically: one factor for the increased peak current and one factor for the decreased rise time to achieve that peak. Thus merely halving the readout time costs a factor of eight in amplifier power.

Because it is so costly to shorten this readout time, strategies for decreasing the echo time are particularly important for EPI imaging. Figure 3.6 illustrates one common strategy, adapting the partial *k*-space reconstructions used to decrease overall imaging time in conventional MRI. As shown in Fig. 3.6(a), the minimum echo time is driven by the need to cover *k*-space before the spin echo occurs. By acquiring less than half of *k*-space before the spin echo, and using partial Fourier reconstruction techniques (see e.g. MacFall et al[19]), less time between the 180° pulse and the spin echo is required. Note that this reconstruction technique is completely analogous to partial-NEX imaging in conventional MRI; that is, *k*-space is only partially filled in the phase-encoding direction (Fig. 3.6b). However, the *application* is analogous to that of partial echo imaging in conventional MRI to minimize echo time. Since the phase-encoding direction is the 'long time' direction in EPI, several other analogies also exist between phase encoding in EPI and frequency encoding in conventional MRI. These analogies will be discussed further in the section on artifacts.

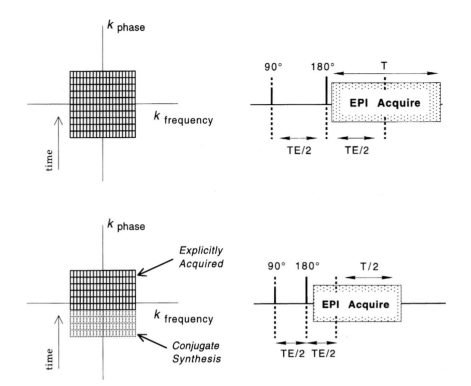

Figure 3.6

Partial Fourier techniques to control *TE*. The relatively long readout period used in EPI can limit the minimum echo time for spin and gradient echo images. As seen on the pulse sequence in (a), for an EPI acquisition time *T*, the minimum echo time would be >*T* for a full *k*-space reconstruction. However, by acquiring fewer lines of *k*-space before the spin echo (b) than after, this minimum echo time can be shortened considerably.

We have just seen that partial Fourier reconstruction in the phase-encoding direction in EPI can be used to control *TE*. In addition, partial Fourier acquisitions in the frequency-encoding direction are also useful in order to increase the achievable spatial resolution. As shown in Fig. 3.7, offsetting the block of *k*-space along the frequency-encoding direction and using conjugate synthesis techniques allows a near doubling of the effective spatial resolution without increasing the total single-shot readout time.[20] Because *k*-space is only complex-conjugate symmetric, at least half of the data must be acquired for these reconstructions, so decreases in echo time and increases in spatial resolution cannot be combined simultaneously.

Finally, if we relax the restriction that all the EPI data must be acquired in a single excitation, significant increases in resolution, or decreases in amplifier power requirements, can be achieved. For example, by acquiring two blocks of data on separate excitations, the resolution may be doubled in either the frequency- or phase-encoding direction.[14] The 'mosaicking' together of two *k*-space tiles is illustrated in Fig. 3.8. Alternatively, *k*-space can be tiled in multiple excitations, either by encoding multiple lines under a single spin echo (interleaved EPI[21]) or by using multiple

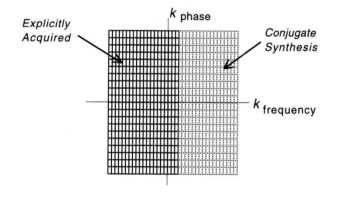

Figure 3.7

Partial Fourier techniques to improve resolution. By offsetting the *k*-space data in the frequency-encoding direction, and using partial Fourier reconstruction in this direction, the resolution in the frequency-encoding direction can be nearly doubled compared to full *k*-space reconstruction. This technique is particularly useful for brain T_2 studies, for which partial *k*-space in the phase-encoding direction is not required to shorten *TE*.

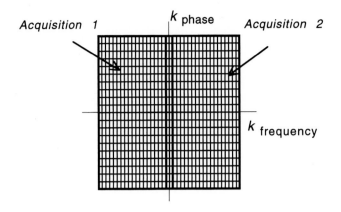

Figure 3.8

Mosaic. By relaxing the 'one-excitation one-image' constraint, EPI encodes can be used to acquire higher-resolution images by using multiple excitations. In this technique, alternate excitations acquire alternate halves of k-space, which are then pieced together like a mosaic tile in order to reconstruct the higher-resolution images.

180° pulses as well (GRASE[22]). With interleaved imaging, there is a continuum of possible trade-offs between total image acquisition time, spatial resolution, degree of motion artifacts, etc. However, in the rest of this chapter, we shall focus on single-shot, or at most double-shot, imaging and its applications.

Hardware issues and present implementations

Echo planar imaging is one of the most demanding applications for an MR scanner. EPI scanning is improved by modifying nearly every subsystem of the scanner: gradient amplifiers and coils, receiver, data acquisition and computer systems are all involved. While a complete discussion of these modifications is beyond the scope of this chapter, we shall summarize here some of the more common changes.

As discussed above, to maintain spatial resolution in the readout direction requires large-amplitude, rapidly switched gradient waveforms. In addition, resolution in the phase-encoding direction also requires rapidly switched gradients in the *frequency*-encoding direction, because extent in k-space in the phase-encoding direction depends on the number of phase-encoded lines (see Fig. 3.6) that can be achieved under the spin echo or FID. Since these echoes last on the order of T_2^* ($\approx$20–100 ms in most organs), acquiring 64–128 lines in this brief time requires rapid oscillations of the frequency-encoding gradients. Thus achieving reasonable resolution in these short times has required a rethinking of MRI gradient amplifiers and gradient systems. For example, to achieve 3 mm resolution with a 500 µs trapezoid with 100 µs ramps (i.e. 300 µs flat-top) required about 2.5 G/cm gradients. With typical whole body gradient coils, the peak current would be about 250 A, or twice the output of typical amplifiers on conventional high-end MR scanners. More importantly, ramping up to this 250 A in 100 µs required 2500 V, about 10 times the normal voltage output of conventional MR systems. Thus the net result is that single-shot EPI with conventional amplifiers would require nearly 20 times the power of current systems. (As an aside, trying to achieve 'conventional' resolution—1 mm—in a single shot in the same total readout time currently used for conventional imaging—10 ms—would require about 5000 times the power of a current scanner, or roughly the output of a small power station!)

One solution to this power problem is to modify the type of power amplifier used to perform encoding. A simple modification is to use a capacitor across the coil to make the encoding device a resonant system. Such a system stores the energy required for encoding and spreads it out through the encoding cycle. Thus, since the inductive load of the coil guarantees that high voltage (quick gradient ramp up) and high current (high amplitude at peak) are not required at the same instant in time, a resonant L–C circuit that is precharged to the necessary voltage can be used to perform encoding. Such techniques (see e.g. Rzedzian[15]) have found application in a number of vendors' EPI systems.

Another technique to allow EPI with conventional amplifiers is to change the gradient coils themselves. Since the power required also scales as the gradient coil size to the fifth power, reducing the size of the gradient coil (see e.g. Wong et al[23]) can also allow EPI, albeit for a more limited range of applications. At least one vendor currently supplies an EPI-compatible head gradient coil attachment, and a number of others have proposed products that are expected to enter the marketplace in the next few years.

In addition to gradient amplifier changes, the gradient coils themselves have required modification for EPI. Because eddy-current artifacts are potentially severe in EPI (see below), shielded gradient coils seem a requirement for EPI. In addition, the higher current and faster switching times usually put dramatic mechanical stress on the gradient coils themselves, so body gradient coils completely potted in fiberglass epoxy or concrete have become the norm. (One pleasant side benefit of these coils has been their reduced acoustic noise in conventional scanning!)

Not only must the gradients be rapid and powerful, but the image data must be collected very rapidly, requiring a wide receiver bandwidth, and fast analog-to-digital converters that must sample at rates as high as 1 MHz, roughly 30 times faster than conventional MRI. The entire receiver chain, from the body rf coil to the audio filters, must accept the increased bandwidth.

In EPI, the alternating left–right trajectory through k-space requires a few additional steps in image reconstruction, the details of which are beyond the scope of this chapter (the interested reader may wish to consult the literature for more details[24–27]). In addition, high-speed imaging is usually helped by high-speed reconstructions and large data storage on the computer system. It is easy (and becoming increasingly common) to acquire as many as 2000 EPI images in just a few minutes. Even though the individual images are not always used for functional applications, they must be reconstructed and stored for processing. Such large numbers of images and large data sets (300 MBytes/hour) were not envisioned in the software architecture of most conventional MR systems' databases, and are all being rethought for EPI applications.

EPI applications

In this section, we outline some of the emerging clinical applications of EPI. These applications depend either on EPI's ability to obtain T_2-weighted images even in the presence of motion or on EPI's ability to acquire images densely in time. Most of the early inventors and developers of EPI techniques would have been surprised at the time if they had known the direction EPI has most recently taken. A quick look at the medical literature from 1991 to 1995 shows that of the nearly 200 references to EPI, more than half describe its use for functional imaging of the brain, an application unimagined in EPI's early days. It appears that the most clinically exciting applications of EPI are not those that simply reduce overall scan time, but rather those that extend the applications of the MR scanner beyond the range accessible to normal diagnostic radiology devices.

Brain imaging

Brain imaging provides a good example of the trends in EPI. Ultrafast imaging allows 'guaranteed' freedom from motion artifacts in very short periods of time. In addition, however, it allows new uses of the MR scanner, accessing image contrast that is difficult or impossible to obtain with conventional imaging techniques. After discussing rapid cranial imaging, we therefore discuss at length EPI imaging of brain blood hemodynamics, diffusion imaging and imaging of neuronal activation.

Rapid cranial imaging

In general clinical practice, examinations of the central nervous system make up typically 40–70% of the patient load. If EPI affords a reduction in examination time for these patients, while maintaining uncompromised diagnostic image quality, it will have important beneficial impacts on both scan costs and patient acceptance of the MRI procedure. To this end, considerable attention has been paid to improving the image quality of cranial images with spin echo EPI.[20,28] While the comparative sensitivity of EPI and conventional MRI in the detection of disease is still under investigation, preliminary studies (see e.g. Fig. 3.4) are encouraging, and confirm that the overall contrast behavior follows that of conventional acquisitions, even in the presence of gross patient motion (see e.g. Fig. 3.9). Using suitable instant imaging protocols, the total examination time for complete brain studies will be well under one minute for a typical head screening. The insensitivity of ultrafast imaging to patient motion should all but completely eliminate scan failures in uncooperative subjects. Thus, while EPI imaging may not replace conventional T_2 imaging as a method for speeding up clinical protocols, it may be added on with minimal time to assure some diagnostic quality scans for nearly all patients.

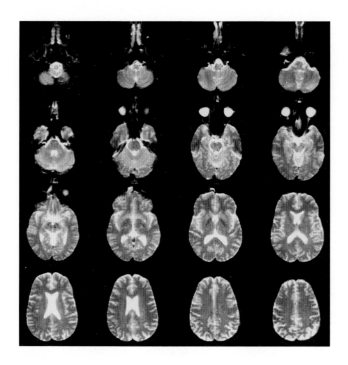 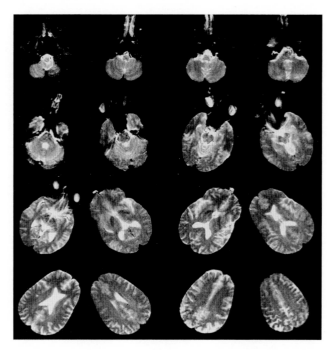

Figure 3.9

T_2-weighted studies and gross motion. Single-shot brain EPI images are uncontaminated by even the grossest of head motion, as demonstrated in this multislice image. Using the partial Fourier technique in the frequency-encoding direction (Fig. 3.7), this 16-slice set was acquired in 4 s while the patient was moving his head back and forth in the magnet. (TE = 80 ms, 128 × 128, 20 cm FOV.)

Physiological imaging and cerebral blood volume (CBV) mapping

Functional studies of the brain (in PET, for example) are attracting increased interest in the diagnosis of important diseases such as Alzheimer's-type dementia and in assessing the viability of tissue that may display no signal intensity changes on standard MRI or CT. Although this dementia cannot yet be treated, the presence of a definitive diagnostic study may, as in multiple sclerosis, reduce substantially the number of otherwise unnecessary additional diagnostic procedures. Many significant lesions (e.g. acutely ischemic regions) are frequently invisible with even the best anatomic studies, yet functional scans such as SPECT and PET can reveal them. Several functional MRI methods are discussed below: dynamic analysis of contrast agent distribution, designed to produce quantitative determination of regional perfusion, and diffusion imaging, which produces changes that depend on cerebral ischemia.

The first functional method we describe involves the observation of cerebral blood flow, by tracking the distribution of injected contrast agents dynamically. As a result of their large magnetic susceptibilities, paramagnetic lanthanide chelates, such as gadolinium diethylene triamine pentaacetic acid (Gd-DTPA) or dysprosium-DTPA (Dy-DTPA), when in high concentration in the bloodstream, produce large magnetic field gradients across vascular boundaries. When field echo methods are used for imaging, these induced gradients act to reduce T_2^* relaxation times. As a consequence, the signal recovered in gradient echo imaging methods is reduced in the vicinity of the blood vessels when the concentration of contrast agent is high. The T_2 relaxation time is also reduced by locally high concentrations of paramagnetic contrast, though the mechanism is somewhat different, depending on the diffusion of protons in the field gradients produces by the intravascular agent.

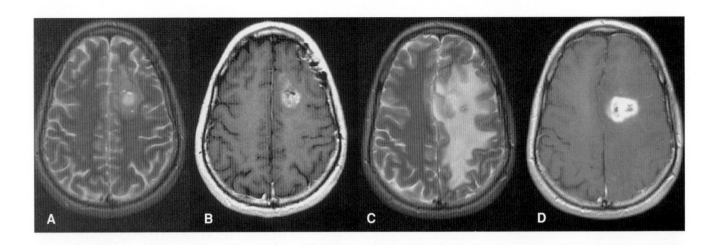

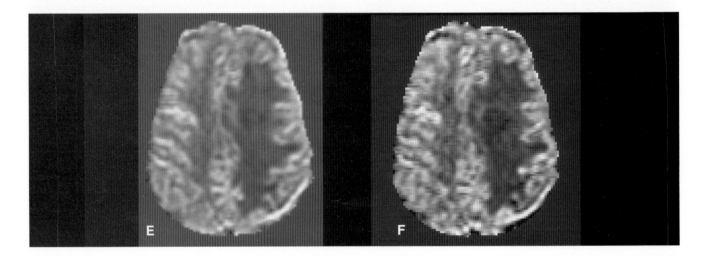

a

Figure 3.10

Blood volume mapping. (a) Radiation necrosis. Radiation necrosis versus recurrence in a 42-year-old male 1 year post X-ray therapy for Grade III/IV astrocytoma. A and B: November 1993 T_2-weighted and post-Gd T_1-weighted images respectively. C and D: T_2-weighted and post-Gd T_1-weighted images six months later, showing increased T_2 signal abnormality, increased enhancement and greater mass effect. E: Gd-based rCBV map shows no areas of rCBV greater than contralateral (normal) white matter. F: rCBV mapping with dysprosium (Dy-DTPA-BMA, Nycomed) also demonstrates no areas of rCBV greater than contralateral (normal) white matter. (Dysprosium has essentially no T_1 effect, and therefore the integrity of the blood–brain barrier is less of an issue than with Gd-based rCBV maps.) These images therefore suggest radiation necrosis rather than tumor. Biopsy showed radiation necrosis with no tumor.

The T_2 relaxation effect of Dy-DTPA was noted by Villringer et al[29] in rat brain, and has been expanded into a robust imaging technique. In this technique, a clinically acceptable dose of contrast agent (typically 0.2 mmol/kg antecubital i.v.) is rapidly injected, and spin echo or gradient echo EPI takes place, typically acquiring 8–12 slices every 1–1.5 s. While the agent remains compartmentalized in the vasculature, protons everywhere in the brain are affected by the magnetic field inhomogeneities caused by the intravascular agent. Thus, even though the blood volume is less than 5%, it is possible to decrease the MR signal by 50% or more with agents. The biophysics of these agents is particularly interesting. For example, spin echo (T_2) and gradient

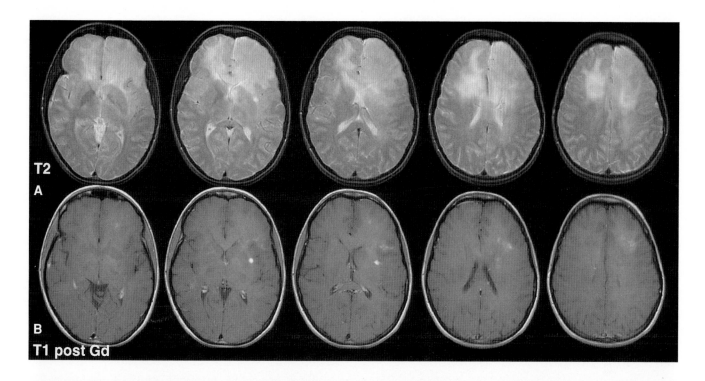

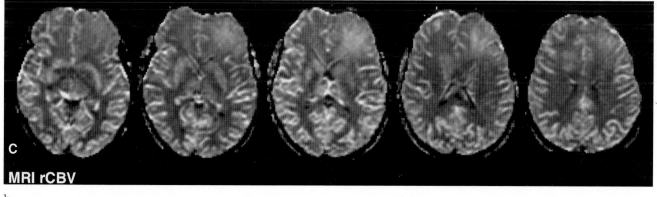

b

Figure 3.10 *continued*

(b) Tumor degeneration. Radiation effect versus tumor degeneration. 29-year-old female 4 years s/p X-ray therapy for left frontal astrocytoma. A: Conventional T_2-weighted images show diffuse increased signal intensity consistent with radiation effect or recurrent tumor. B: Post-Gd T_1-weighted images show diffuse mild enhancement. C: Relative CBV maps show a large area of increased rCBV, suggesting high capillary count tissue and therefore malignancy rather than radiation effect. Biopsy showed anaplastic astrocytoma. Note the infiltrative pattern of high rCBV, consistent with the known infiltrative patterns of gliomas.

echo (T_2*) images are sensitive to differently sized vessels in which the agent is compartmentalized (see e.g. Weisskoff et al[30] and Boxerman et al[31]), so that while gradient echo images are preferentially sensitive to larger (venule and bigger) vessels, spin echo images are preferentially sensitive to capillary-sized vessels. By integrating this signal change (see e.g. Rosen et al[32]) or, more precisely, the change in the effective relaxivity ΔR_2, over time a voxel-by-voxel map of the regional cerebral blood volume (rCBV) is produced.

CBV maps based on spin echo imaging show strong correlation with [18F]fluorodeoxyglucose PET studies of metabolism in tumors. That is, tumors that have high microscopic blood volume also have high metabolism.[33] It is reasonable to assume that this correlation results from the underlying relation between microvessel angiogenesis and growth in cancers.[34] Thus the MR scanner has the ability to acquire both high-resolution anatomic and functional images that are inherently coregistered, and which can be acquired in a single exam. Examples of CBV maps are shown in Figs 3.10(a,b). The FLASH method has also been used[35] to evaluate contrast agent dynamics, but these studies are limited in a number of ways: because of the briefness of the first-pass effect, FLASH studies tend to be limited to one or at most two slices. In addition, current FLASH studies are T_2*- (macroscopic blood volume) rather than T_2- (microscopic blood volume) weighted, and thus may not have the same correlation with underlying pathology.

Diffusion imaging and stroke

Like functional imaging, diffusion imaging offers a new tool for MRI in patients. By using large, bipolar gradient pulses, MR images can be made sensitive to the random diffusion of water molecules in tissues. Brownian motion is a biologically common and generally familiar phenomenon. Water molecules in most tissues are never at rest, and constantly undergo a random dance through the biological medium. Their walk can take them through the intra- and extracellular spaces, inside and out of red blood cells, etc. Often the physio-chemical environment profoundly affects the path these molecules take. For example, the environments in the interstitial space and in the intracellular space in the brain are quite different, and there is non-infinite permeability to water through cell membranes. Changes in any of these compartments can affect the net diffusivity of the water, which, in turn, can be measured with MRI.

Diffusion is a random process, and can be described in many ways. For our purposes, the simplest analogy might be to the blurring of a spot of ink. The diffusion coefficient D helps to describe how spread out the drop becomes after some period of time. In general, along some direction, the width of the blur depends on the square root of time T and the diffusion coefficient:

$$x_{\mathrm{rms}} = \sqrt{2DT},$$

where 'rms' stands for root mean square, which is just a fancy way to describe the average width. (The average displacement is zero: there is no net transport of water—it just blurs out.) In many materials (like a glass of water, or the gray matter in the brain) diffusion is isotropic; that is, water randomly walks equally in all directions. However, more generally, diffusion can be different in different directions. For example, in a stalk of celery, water diffuses much more easily along the stalk than perpendicularly to it. So the diffusion coefficient in the parallel direction is considerably higher than the coefficient in the perpendicular direction. Many tissues in the body show similar diffusion anisotropy: white matter fiber tracts in the brain, myofiber architecture in the heart and other muscles show large diffusion anisotropy. To completely describe anisotropic diffusion, then, actually requires six numbers: three to describe the amount of diffusion in each of the three main directions, and three to describe the orientation of these primary directions in absolute space. (Technically, homogenous diffusion is thus described by a tensor, or a 3 × 3 symmetric matrix.) While biological systems are anything but homogenous, the general mobility of water is great enough that, on the timescale and dimensions of most MR imaging, this matrix completely describes the waters' diffusion. Thus, while the intra- and extracellular spaces have quite different water diffusivities, the measured diffusion coefficient (see below) tends to be a weighted average of these values, because the water actually spends a good fraction of its random walk in both regions in any given experiment. While diffusion is relatively easy in the extracellular space (i.e. D is high) and more encumbered in the intracellular space (i.e. D is low), the net apparent diffusion constant is somewhere between these. It is also a fair summary at this time that the exact relationship between these compartmental diffusivities, the permeability between the compartments, and the geometries of the compartments is not yet fully understood.

While water diffusion is actually already incorporated in a number of MR parameters, such as T_1 and T_2, diffusion can also be measured independently. The most common method, originally proposed for spectroscopy in the 1960s, is the 'pulsed gradient method' (PGM) or Stejskal–Tanner method.[36] This method has been adapted for imaging by many investigators (see e.g. LeBihan et al[37]). The PGM involves strong motion-encoding of the MR sequence. That is, PGM is the exact opposite of flow compensation for MRI: its goal is to enhance the signal loss due to water motion. The utility of the PGM method is that the signal loss is a relatively simple function of the strength of the gradient G, its duration δ, the spacing Δ between the beginning of one pulse and

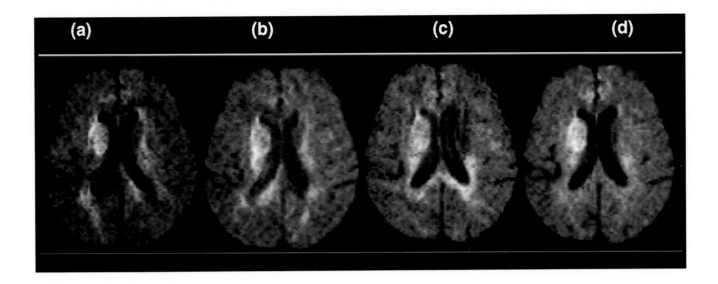

Figure 3.11

Diffusion anisotropy. White matter in the brain is anisotropic, allowing more rapid diffusion along the fibers than against them. This can be shown by comparing images with diffusion weighting in three orthogonal directions, (a)–(c), which show hyperintensity in the white matter when the diffusion encoding is perpendicular to the fibers. However, by combining information from three orthogonal directions, an orientation-independent image can be made, (d), which more readily shows ischemia-induced changes without artifacts from (normal) white matter anisotropy.

the beginning of the next, and the diffusion coefficient D:

$$S(G) = \exp\left[-D\gamma^2 G^2\delta^2(\Delta - \frac{1}{3}\delta)\right]S_0,$$

where S_0 is the signal in the absence of the pulsed gradients, and thus includes normal T_1 and T_2 weighting terms. Thus by changing G, or δ, one may measure the diffusion coefficient D. Commonly in the literature, the constants to the right of D are clumped together, and called b,

$$b = \gamma^2 G^2\delta^2(\Delta - \frac{1}{3}\delta),$$

and thus the signal loss caused by the diffusion gradient is $\exp(-bD)$. Biologically, typical values of D lie in the range $(0.3-2.0) \times 10^{-5}$ cm^2/s, and thus b values on the order of 10^5 s/cm^2 are required to cause substantial (and thus detectable) signal loss. Such large values of b typically require a 1 G/cm gradient for 30–50 ms. D measured in this case is the diffusion coefficient along the direction of the applied gradient. To measure D in an isotropic medium, only one pair of measurements is required: one with and one without the large gradient present. However, in an anisotropic medium, six different measurements are required to fully parameterize the diffusion, though as few as four can be used when certain simplifying assumptions are allowed. This anisotropy is shown in the brain in Fig. 3.11. While gray matter shows diffusional signal losses that are the same in all three directions, white matter shows a much more profound directional dependence to the diffusional loss. Only when the diffusion gradient is applied along the direction of the fibers is there substantial signal loss.

One difficulty with this measurement process is that the large b value creates huge potential for motion artifact from gross patient motion. For example, if $G = 1$ G/cm, $\delta = 40$ ms and $\Delta = 50$ ms, unsteady velocities as low as 0.1 mm/s will corrupt these images. (Such unsteady motion could come both from inadvertent patient motion as well as from intrinsic motions of the brain itself!) As a result, most efforts to image diffusion have either used some type of modified conventional acquisition (e.g. navigator pulses)[38, 39] or single-shot (echo planar) imaging.[40] Navigated acquisitions attempt to measure and correct the displacement artifacts, while echo planar imaging seeks to eliminate the artifact altogether by acquiring the data in a single excitation, eliminating view-to-view artifact entirely.

While MRI measurement of diffusion was originally proposed as a method for quantifying perfusion,[41] there are a number of difficulties, both technical and theoretical, with this idea.[42] The more recent excitement regarding the measurement of diffusion in cerebral ischemia originated with the observation by Moseley et al[43] in cats that there is a profound change in measured diffusion very early in the natural history of experimentally induced focal ischemia. That is, well before there were observable changes on T_2-weighted scans, the diffusion coefficient was seen to drop in the ischemic regions. A number of groups have reproduced this work in animal models, and the currently favored hypothesis explaining these changes is that cell swelling occurs very quickly after ischemic insult. This swelling decreases the extracellular volume, and thus the fraction of the 'easy' (high-D) part of the protons' walk is decreased, forcing them to spend more time in the turgid intracellular space. As a result, the net apparent diffusion is smaller after the cells have swollen.

This change in diffusion has now been well documented in humans as well.[44] Diffusion changes appear to be detectable at the earliest time post-ischemia that any patient can be placed in the scanner, and diffusion-weighted images (DWI) show local decreases in D (increases in signal intensity on diffusion-weighted scans) of as much as 50%. If the ischemia does not resolve, and the tissue becomes infarcted, the diffusion changes can linger for several days or even weeks. However, the infarcted region is also visible as a T_2 abnormality (T_2-bright) at this and later stages. This increased T_2 is presumably due to increases in free water in the tissue caused by edema, though here too there is some controversy regarding the exact nature of the MR-visible changes. There have been some experiments that attempt to age strokes on the basis of their DWI appearances. This work is still in its infancy, and may ultimately be hindered by population heterogeneity—both patient-to-patient as well as region-to-region variations within the brain. Nevertheless, the observation of profound changes in D with ischemia, and the possibility that these changes are reversible when ischemia is reversed, makes DWI an exciting technology for monitoring the evolving treatment of cerebral ischemia, especially when coupled with the hemodynamic imaging described above.

Figure 3.12 illustrates the combination of diffusion and hemodynamic imaging using EPI in evaluating acute cerebral ischemia. Figure 3.12(a) demonstrates the profound reduction of diffusional signal loss (hyperintensity on diffusion-weighted scans) in this trace-diffusion-weighted image. Figure 3.12(b) shows rCBV and rCBF maps of the same patient, demonstrating a larger territory that is at risk owing to its perturbed hemodynamics. EPI is fast enough to allow this type of evaluation even in the setting of acute management: these images represent part of a 15 min imaging protocol that can be performed on an emergency basis even in a busy, in-patient setting.

Imaging of neuronal activation

While not necessarily a 'clinical' application yet, imaging neurological function by MRI has become a burgeoning research application. As has been observed using a variety of techniques (see e.g. Kwong et al,[45] Ogawa et al[46] and Bandettini et al[47]), both T_1- and T_2*-weighted images subtly change their contrast to reflect local changes in blood flow and (presumably) oxygenation in response to neuronal activation. Ultrahigh-speed imaging has been particularly vital for imaging these changes, especially at clinical field strengths (i.e. 2.0 T and below), because it decouples motion artifacts from contrast changes. That is, while patient motion complicates the statistical analysis of signal changes over time,[48] patient motion during the conventional MR encoding process spreads motion artifacts throughout the image,[2] thus compromising the intrinsic contrast of the study. In addition, the dense data acquisition in EPI allows for complete brain coverage, as opposed to the few slices available through fast gradient echo techniques, or the ability to image single slices very densely in time to detect subtle temporal changes in activation.

Typically, 3–5% signal changes have been observed robustly with primary motor and sensory changes using gradient echo EPI studies, with somewhat smaller signal changes observed in higher-order, cognitive tasks. While the implications for fundamental brain science are particularly profound,[49] the clinical opportunity to be able to produce both anatomic and functional images in the same scanning session is also tremendous.

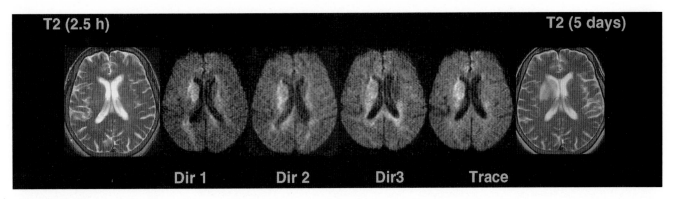

a

Figure 3.12

Stroke. (a) Diffusion-weighted imaging and white matter anisotropy. White matter anisotropy and DWI artifacts. This patient was imaged 2.5 h after the onset of left hemiparesis and hemineglect. T_2 fast spin echo images (FSE) are normal. Diffusion-weighted images (DWI) show clear hyperintense signal in the right basal ganglia on any one direction sampling, but also demonstrate hyperintensities in the white matter that degrade the diagnostic quality of the study. Combining three directions into a single, summary image (the trace of the diffusion tensor, or an 'isotropic' diffusion-weighted image) reduces these artifacts and matches well the five day follow-up MRI that documents the infarct.

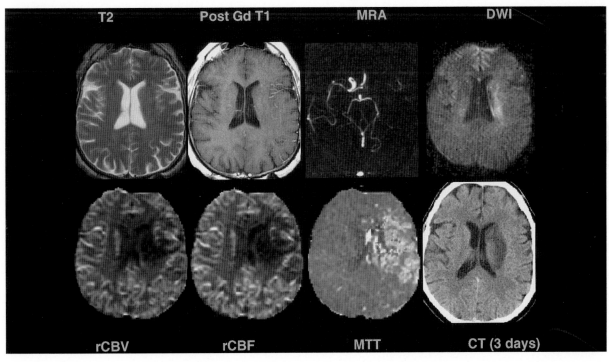

b

(b) Hemodynamic mapping. This patient was imaged 2 h after the onset of right hemiplegia and aphasia. The T_2-weighted images are normal; post contrast T_1-weighted images show intravascular enhancement but no parenchymal damage. The MRA documents absence of flow in the left MCA. There is only a small DWI abnormality, with a much larger rCBV, rCBF and MTT abnormality. Based on this mismatch, the patient was treated with hypervolemia and hypertensive therapy; this caused his aphasia to resolve (his symptoms became blood-pressure dependent). Follow-up imaging documents the infarct extended in to the region of abnormal rCBF despite initial normal DWI, but may have been smaller than it could have been owing to the hypertensive therapy.

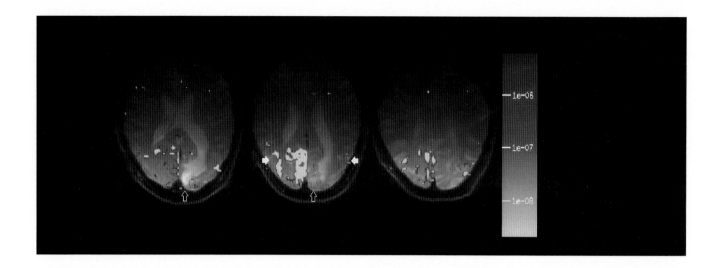

Figure 3.13

Hemianopia. A small area of tissue is affected by stroke, located in the primary visual cortex (indicated by open arrows). Activation mapping demonstrates that on the unaffected side there is a large area of activation, consistent with both primary, secondary and higher centers of visual processing. However, on the affected side there is absence of activation not only in the affected primary visual cortex but also in the expected areas of activation outside the primary visual cortex, in regions known to correspond to higher centers of vision (indicated by solid arrows). Hence a stroke in one area is demonstrated to affect distant cortex. Underlying gray-scale image: T_2-weighted oblique axial spin echo image. Functional overlay: t-test p-value, ranging from $p = 10^{-5}$ to $p = 10^{-9}$. The test was applied to 90 images acquired during full-field stimulation with LED goggles alternating with darkness. (Courtesy of Dr AG Sorensen.)

Two examples are shown in Figs 3.13 and 3.14. In the first, patients with chronic stroke that presented with hemianopia were given full-field visual task studies. In normals, the complete primary visual cortex (area V1) is affected in gradient echo EPI images. However, as shown in Fig. 3.13, because of the retinotopic mapping of the primary visual cortex, visual field deficits map directly into signal change deficits in the affected regions of the visual cortex fMRI image. Thus it is possible to determine by imaging at what stage along the processing pathway an anatomic lesion may be having a functional effect.

The second example demonstrates that imaging tasks have the potential to replace more invasive tests that currently assess functionality. This case illustrates an fMRI version of the Wada test (see e.g. Charles et al[50]) used to determine laterality of language functions before cortirectomy or other brain surgeries. In the invasive study, intracarotid injection of depressants is used to determine which hemisphere has greater control of language functions. By performing the language functions within the scanner, however, noninvasive EPI fMRI can be used to detect which hemisphere is more activated by the language tasks. Figure 3.14 demonstrates the laterality observed in a robust eloquent task, focusing on the differences between verb generation (from visually presented language cues) and passive fixation. While not a neuroscientifically simple task, it does appear to activate robustly lateralized regions that are related to language.

Body imaging

Tomographic imaging of the abdomen, while still dominated by X-ray CT in many cases, is finding increasing MR applications. While improved breathholding schemes,[51] respiratory compensation[52] and phased-array receiver coil techniques[53] continue to improve conventional T_1-weighted imaging in the body, EPI is an extremely effective technique to acquire artifact-free T_2-weighted images. As in the brain, T_2 contrast is often more

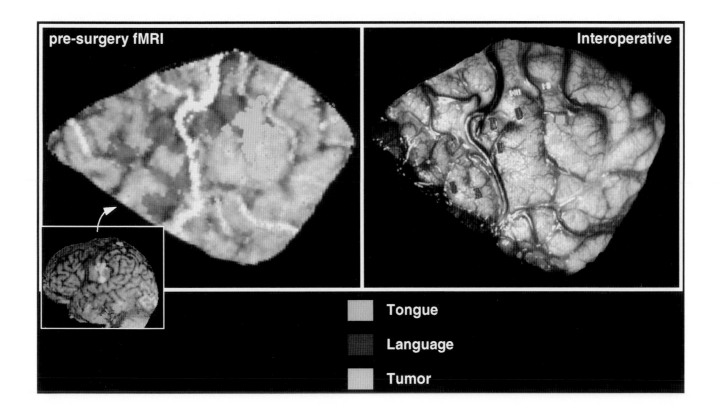

Figure 3.14

Functional imaging with EPI: Wada test. Comparison between fMRI and cortical stimulation mapping of language function and sensorimotor function (tongue) in a 21-year-old patient with a dominant hemisphere rolandic tumor producing seizures. fMRI and Wada test were in accord in predicting left dominance, which was confirmed by obtaining speech arrest during stimulation in areas with green flags on the right. (Courtesy of Dr R Benson.)

effective at demonstrating lesion–parenchymal contrast.

Simple breathhold, multislice T_2 imaging of the liver has demonstrated liver lesions, both benign and malignant, as bright lesions against the dark, short T_2 normal parenchyma (Fig. 3.15). Because of the absence of motion artifacts, focal lesions are easily detected[54] on these T_2-weighted scans. In addition, there is some evidence that hemangiomas can be distinguished from metastases by using very long (>100 ms) echo times: only hemangiomas continue to be visible on these heavily T_2-weighted scans.

Imaging of the pancreas, especially of pancreatitis, also appear efficacious with T_2-weighted EPI scans in a single breathhold,[55] with good delineation of pancreatic margins and ducts uncontaminated by respiratory and GI tract motion (Fig. 3.16).

As in the brain, functional imaging of the abdominal organs using a bolus of contrast material (both Gd-based chelates and iron oxide agents) is also possible with EPI. Dynamic imaging of the liver is possible, and shows promise for distinguishing tissue perfused by the portal and hepatic circulations.[56] Dynamic imaging of the kidney, both to quantify kidney physiology[57] and to detect renal artery stenosis, have shown promising preliminary results. In addition, the EPI-STAR technique[58] without contrast agents has shown excellent promise for showing arterial and parenchymal flow in the kidneys.

In addition to these T_2-weighted studies, diffusion-weighted EPI (see above) is also possible in the abdomen.[59] By using cardiac gating to eliminate occasional motion artifacts, diffusion images in the kidney or liver may provide additional clinical information about the status of these tissues.

The ability of EPI to freeze anatomic motion has also been used to extend non-ionizing radiation

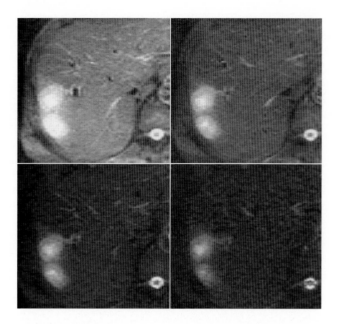

Figure 3.15

Liver. EPI allows motion-artifact-free, T_2-weighted images of the liver, as well as multiple *TE* acquisitions in a single breathhold to improve lesion characterization. These images (*TE* = 25, 50, 75 and 100 ms; *TR* = 3000 ms; 128 × 128, 40 × 20 cm FOV) demonstrate a colon cancer metastasized to the liver. These images show both the central necrosis as well as a peripheral reaction zone typical of these lesions. (Images courtesy of Drs P Hahn and S Saini.)

imaging studies to cases that might only be studies by X-ray CT, but for which the radiation hazards are a counter indication. Examples of these uses include prolonged monitoring of the GI tract[60] and imaging of the developing fetus.[61] For further discussion of these applications, see the recent review of EPI imaging in the abdomen by Muller and Edelman.[62]

Cardiac imaging

One of the earliest clinical application of EPI was for imaging the beating heart,[63] demonstrating that EPI could indeed freeze cardiac motion. As we describe below, there are a number of different ways to use EPI to visualize the heart and its dynamics, and EPI cardiac applications have grown to include single-breathhold quantification of cardiac ejection fraction, assessment of cardiac hemodynamics (relative perfusion) with and without contrast agents, quantification of the internal dynamics of the myocardium (strain imaging), and the use of diffusion to visualize myocardial fiber orientation in the beating heart.

Anatomic imaging

Since single-shot EPI can be used to acquire a single image in a short time compared with the

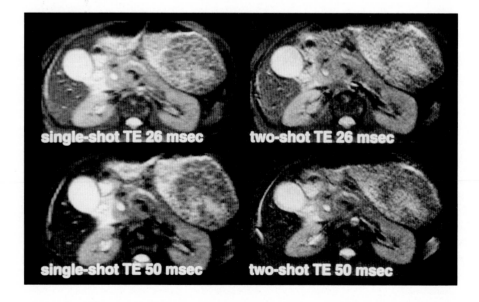

Figure 3.16

Pancreas. Absence of respiratory artifact, good T_2 contrast and robust fat suppression allow good visualization of the pancreas, pancreatic masses and enlarged ducts. In this example, the inflamed duct is easily visualized as hyperintense even on the shorter-*TE* images. These images also show the use of mosaic (Fig. 3.8) imaging in the abdomen to improve spatial resolution. (Images courtesy of Drs P Hahn and S Saini.)

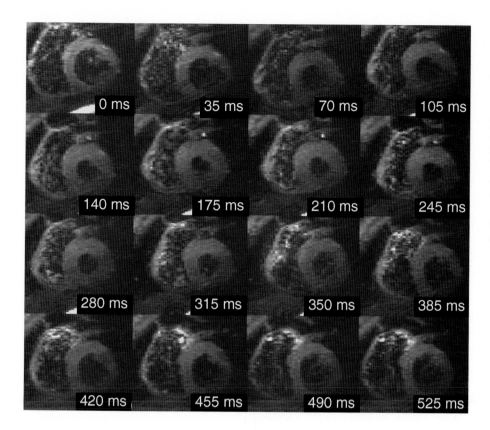

0 ms	35 ms	70 ms	105 ms
140 ms	175 ms	210 ms	245 ms
280 ms	315 ms	350 ms	385 ms
420 ms	455 ms	490 ms	525 ms

Figure 3.17

Black blood EPI heart. Spin echo EPI images of the heart typically show the myocardium bright against dark blood. By progressively delaying the image acquisition after R-wave, cine images of the beating heart can be produced. These images were acquired with 128 × 128, 40 × 20 cm FOV, TE = 30 ms, TR = 2 × RR, using a 5 × 11 surface coil on the anterior chest wall.

cardiac cycle, it is possible to construct multislice movies of the beating heart using several techniques.[17] Using spin echo imaging (without or with dephasing gradient to spoil the ventricular blood signal),[64] black blood images can be acquired (Fig. 3.17). By gating this acquisition, and varying the time of the acquisition relative to R-wave, images throughout the cardiac cycle are routinely acquired. A cine view can then be constructed across multiple heartbeats that reflects average cardiac behavior through the cardiac cycle. Since the image acquisition takes so little time (50–100 ms), it is also possible to image multiple slices in each R–R interval and, by permuting the slice order between R–R periods, obtain multislice, multiphase images in a single breathhold.

One particularly efficient means of quantifying cardiac function using this technique is to obtain only two phases of the cardiac cycle in each R–R interval: one at end-diastole (ED) and one at end-systole (ES). By again permuting the order of the slices, it is possible to create ES and ED images of N slices in just N heartbeats, leaving $N/2$ heartbeats between each slice's repetition. This relatively long duration between re-excitation allows for good T_1 recovery (i.e. high signal), and yet allows eight slices to be obtained in a relatively easy eight-heartbeat breathhold. Using this technique, Hunter[65] was able to show the ejection fraction could be calculated from this single breathhold with accuracy comparable to that of a much longer, conventional cine MR acquisition.

'Real time'

Alternatively, short-TR (<100 ms) gradient echo EPI has been used to make ungated 'real-time' movies of the beating heart, even in patients with severe arrhythmias that make gated imaging impossible. The bright blood, real-time movies have also been used to image visualize valve leaflets[66] and valvular insufficiency. When imaging at speeds greater than 10 images per second, these movies reflect not just the average disturbances than can also be seen in conventional MR cine views, but also the non-reproducible disordered flow in any given cardiac contraction.[67] While the flow properties of EPI are somewhat complex

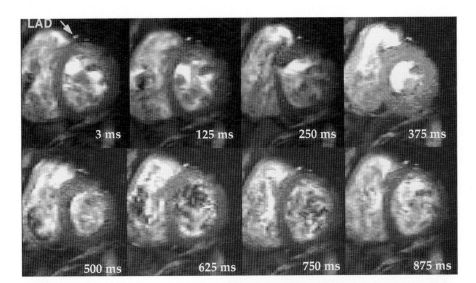

Figure 3.18

EPI coronary. Gradient echo EPI images of the heart typically show the myocardium darker against bright blood. Simple flow compensation in the slice-selection direction allows clear visualization of the left coronary artery. (Images courtesy of Dr B Poncelet.)

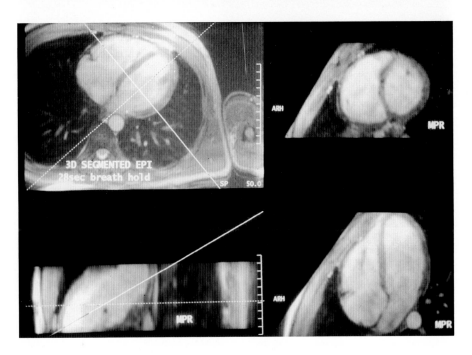

Figure 3.19

Interleaved EPI heart. Gradient echo EPI can also be interleaved across heartbeats in order to generate 3D images of the heart in a single breathhold. Such data acquisition allows post-acquisition visualization of the heart in both short- and long-axis views. (Images courtesy of Dr R Edelman.)

because of evolution during the echo train,[68,69] its ability to visualize complex flows has been documented,[70] but remains relatively unexploited in clinical studies. What has been exploited, however, is the relative ease of quantitative, cine velocity measurements in the great and pulmonary vessels using EPI.[71]

In addition to measuring myocardial dynamics, EPI has been used to visualize and quantify flow in the coronary vasculature. Both single-shot techniques (Fig. 3.18) and, more recently, multi-shot EPI (Fig. 3.19) have successfully delineated the coronary arteries, and have even been used to measure velocity in these arteries.[72] These studies

have been used to demonstrate the ability of EPI to perform stress–coronary flow studies in the scanner, and have shown reduced coronary velocity reserve (with dipyridamole stress) in patients.

Functional imaging

In addition to imaging the myocardial and coronary anatomy, EPI can also be used to aid functional assessment of myocardial hemodynamics. In direct analogy to the brain studies described

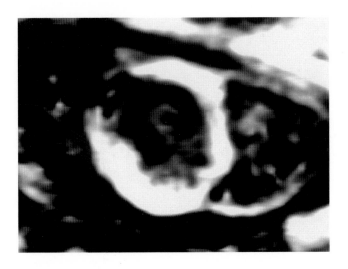

Figure 3.20

Contrast agents and myocardial perfusion. Clinically available MR contrast agents are highly extracted on their first pass through the coronary circulation. The changes in this extraction due to pharmacological stress may allow evaluation of myocardial ischemia and infarction. This image shows the uptake (peak change in transverse relaxivity) 1 min post-antecubital injection of 0.2 mmol/kg of Dy-DTPA on a spin echo EPI image ($TE = 35$, $TR = 2 \times$ RR, 128×128 on 40×20 cm FOV). The region that shows absence of uptake corresponds to an ischemic segment identified by PET.

above, dynamic studies with EPI both with and without contrast agents have been used to characterize the perfusion of the myocardium.

Contrast agents
A number of studies have successfully shown that EPI can efficiently track a peripheral venous injection of contrast material,[73,74] and, unlike fast conventional MR techniques (see e.g. Atkinson et al[74]), can evaluate the changes in multiple slices from a single injection. While rapid, but incomplete, extravasation makes the direct physiological interpretation of these studies difficult using clinically available contrast media, they nonetheless show a characteristically delayed and blunted uptake in regions of focal disease. With the clinical advent of true intravascular agents, quantification will become more tractable[76] in terms of blood volume and blood flow, but clinical usefulness may be established even from the less physiologically

well-defined delayed 'uptake' of the agent. Figure 3.20 shows a typical 'uptake' map, achievable with currently approved contrast media, showing focally reduced uptake in segments corresponding to a PET-defined perfusion deficit.

$T_2{}^*$ changes without contrast
As in the brain, the changing oxygenation of the blood can produce myocardial signal changes in T_2- and $T_2{}^*$-weighted studies. These changes have been measured both at 4.0 T[77] and at 1.5 T using EPI. In these studies, a potent vasodilator (e.g. dipyridamole or adenosine) is infused during gradient echo EPI imaging. Because flow changes much more than contractile function under this pharmacological stress, the oxygen extraction decreases owing to the increased delivery of oxygen to the tissue. As a result, venous blood become more oxygenated, and tissue $T_2{}^*$ is increased, and thus $T_2{}^*$-weighted images show a signal increase. In pathological segments, this change is not observed, either because the resting oxygen extraction is already very low (no function), or because there is insufficient flow reserve so that vasodilatory stress increase the flow much less in the affected segment. Figure 3.21 illustrates one example of this technique.

Imaging myocardial contraction
EPI is also an efficient imaging technique for measuring local myocardial contractile function. In analogy to conventional MR techniques, there are two primary classes of tools to image this contraction: 'tagging' and 'phase contrast'. In tagging methods,[78,79] stripes of magnetization are laid down, and proceed to distort as the heart beats. EPI allows excellent contrast in the tagged methods because of the lack of beat-to-beat variability in the tag/tissue contrast.[80] In phase-contrast methods, just as in phase-contrast angiography, velocity encoding pulses are used to encode the velocity of the tissue into phase of the image. The phase then can be integrated to estimate myocardial strain[81] or used directly to estimate strain rate.[82] Strain or strain rate can be used to produce images that show focal changes corresponding to myocardial contractile dysfunction. In these applications, EPI is used to speed up the acquisitions, and make them less sensitive to cardiac arrhythmia. Figure 3.22 illustrates the power of these techniques to image the internal motion of the myocardium, demonstrating a

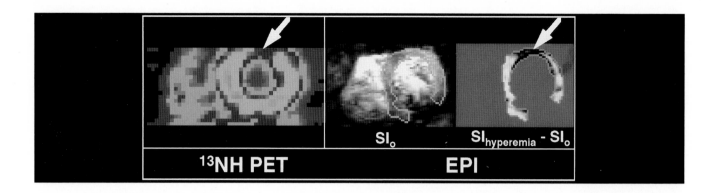

Figure 3.21

T_2^* in heart during stress. Endogenous deoxyhemoglobin can also provide useful contrast in the myocardium, as demonstrated here. This gradient echo EPI image ($TR = 10 \times RR$, $TE = 29$ ms, 128×128 on 40×20 cm FOV) shows the signal change in the myocardium 5 min after administration of a dipyridamole challenge. The normal myocardium increases its signal intensity as the increased blood flow tends to increase the average oxygenation of the venous blood. The anterior segment of the heart demonstrates no such change, implying either that flow reserve is impaired or that resting oxygen extraction is abnormally low. Either conclusion is consistent with the abnormality visualized by PET in the same segment.

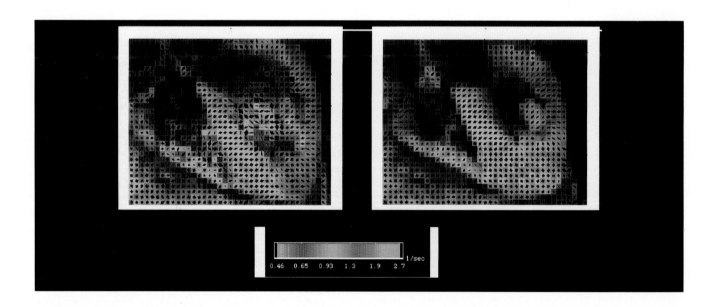

Figure 3.22

Transmural contractility measurement. Velocity-induced phase shifts can be used to quantify the internal motion of the myocardium, eliminating cardiac rotation and translation. This image of a patient with hypertrophic cardiomyopathy demonstrates that focal contractile abnormalities can be identified by using simple algebraic combinations of the strain rate tensor, in this case the natural logarithm of its second characteristic polynomial. A septal defect is clearly seen on this image, which was not observed on echo. (Image courtesy of Drs V Wedeen and G Beache.)

contractile dysfunction near the apex of this patient with hypertrophic cardiomyopathy. This dysfunction was not visible on ultrasound in this patient.

Imaging myocardial fibers

Finally, EPI has recently demonstrated its potential to image not just myocardial motion, but also the underlying myocardial fibers. Just like white matter in the brain, myocardial fibers show anisotropic diffusion, with diffusion being easiest along the fibers. Cardiac pulsation make the measurement of diffusion even more complex, but EPI appears to allow its unambiguous measurement nonetheless.[83,84] Figure 3.23 is an intersecting long- and short-axis view of the heart, with anisotropic diffusion shown as a octahedron, pointing in the direction of the myocardial fibers. In addition to mapping this structure, diffusion imaging in the heart may play a potentially greater role if ischemia has the same effect in the myocardium that it does in the brain.

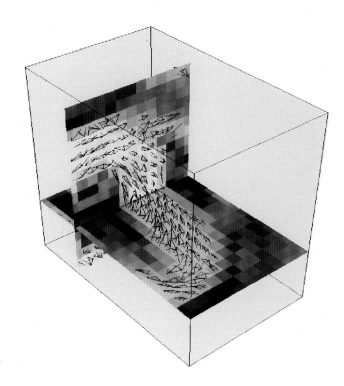

Figure 3.23

Cardiac fibers. Diffusion anisotropy is visible in the heart as well as in brain white matter (Fig. 3.11), and can be used to track the myocardial fibers. This image shows an intersecting long- and short-axis image, with the diffusion anisotropy displayed as a pyramid. The connection of the fibers between the planes is easily visualized. (Image courtesy of Drs V Wedeen and T Reese)

EPI limitations and alternatives

In this section, we discuss some of the artifacts and other drawbacks specific to EPI. In general, EPI produces artifacts similar to any low-bandwidth conventional technique: increased chemical shift artifacts, increased distortion due to magnetic susceptibility artifacts, and increased blurring. In addition, the rapid, oscillating gradients that define EPI are louder than conventional gradients, and have, in some cases, produced a demonstrable biological effect: peripheral nerve stimulation. After discussing these effects, we put EPI in context compared with other current and emerging ultrafast imaging techniques.

EPI limitations

Chemical shift

The primary chemical shift artifact in MR images arise from the subtle differences in the effective resonance frequencies of water, fat and (in implant work) silicone protons. Chemical shift artifacts occur in conventional MR images when the frequency differences between pixels due to spatial encoding are smaller than the intrinsic differences in resonance frequencies between chemical species. The result is spatial displacement of fatty structures (and silicone implants) compared with aqueous tissues. Conventionally, these artifacts are in the frequency-encoding direction, because it is the read gradient that generates a frequency difference between pixels. There are no artifacts in the phase-encoding direction, because the phase 'clock' is restarted with each excitation.

EPI, on the other hand, acquires each line of 128 raw data points in less than 1 ms, so that the nominal bandwidth per pixel is greater than 1 kHz.

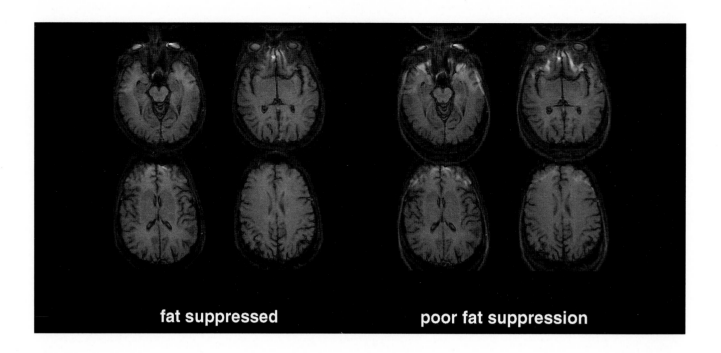

Figure 3.24

Chemical shift artifact. The long, continuous EPI readout creates narrow bandwidth in the phase-encoding direction. In the absence of fat suppression, the chemical shift artifact associated with the proton moieties is quite large, as shown on this spin echo (TE = 80 ms) EPI brain image.

Because this bandwidth is much greater than the nominal fat/water shift of 220 Hz at 1.5 T, chemical shift along the frequency-encoding axis is invisible in EPI images. However, in EPI, artifacts can be generated along the phase-encoding axis. Following the k-space diagram of Fig. 3.2(b), consider acquiring an EPI image with a 500 µs read period. The time between successive raw data points along the phase-encoding direction (the columns of data as represented in Fig. 3.2b) is 0.5 ms, so that 64 lines with a total readout duration of 32 ms produces an effective bandwidth per pixel of only 30 Hz. (This is the same bandwidth per pixel that might be acquired in a conventional image along the frequency-encoding axis with a 256-point image using a 4 kHz bandwidth.) As a result, the fat/water shift artifacts in uncorrected EPI images can be quite severe, extending for approximately eight pixels (at 1.5 T) in the phase-encoding direction, or a spatial shift of about one-eighth of the image. An example of such an artifact is shown in a brain image in Fig. 3.24. Similar considerations require correction of images from other long-readout single- and few-shot imaging methods such as spiral imaging.[85]

Because of this potential for large chemical shift artifacts, a variety of solutions have been implemented to eliminate such artifacts in EPI by suppression of either lipid or fat signals. These techniques are exactly analogous to those used in conventional imaging to saturate one chemical species, and are now used routinely in nearly all EPI acquisitions.

Artifacts

The unique data sampling characteristics of EPI techniques can lead to artifacts different than those seen in conventional imaging. Several major classes are important: spatial distortion from T_2^* (or T_2) decay, and from off-resonance effects; ghosting from inadequate control of gradient waveforms or sampling; and large chemical shift effects. Other artifacts, such as contrast aberrations from T_2 decay during sampling, or positional shifts secondary to velocity, are more subtle and may not noticeably affect the image appearance.

The T_2 decay, susceptibility-based distortion and chemical shift artifacts all arise from the same ultimate source: phase and amplitude changes during the long, continuous EPI readout. Amplitude changes (i.e. T_2 and T_2^* decay) cause blurring, and frequency changes cause spatial distortion. A more complete discussion of these effects can be found in Farzaneh et al.[86] In general, spatial distortion artifacts become significant when the total time for spatial encoding is comparable to T_2^*. Whereas short relaxation times result in line broadening in spectroscopy, in imaging the consequence will be a widening of the point spread function, that is, a blurring of the image features.

Since the effective bandwidth in EPI is quite low (see the discussion of chemical shift above) along the phase-encoding axis, small deviations in resonance frequency result in relatively large displacements in the image. For example, local deviations in magnetic susceptibility can cause these frequency variations. In the brain, the air sinuses typically cause shift of about a 1 ppm (60 Hz at 1.5 T) in the resonance frequency; with the 32 ms read period example used above, this shift produces as much as a two-pixel local distortion. In the brain, these potential distortions are particularly important in two cases. First, in patients who have recently undergone surgery, there are typically increased susceptibility effects near the site of surgery. Since this site can be the area of interest for the referring physician, EPI imaging can be artifactual. Second, some imaging applications such as surgical or radiation planning require good absolute positional accuracy, which can be compromised in EPI compared with conventional imaging.

However, at least for moderate susceptibility effects, this distortion can be corrected because its magnitude can be easily measured. A number of investigators[87–89] have presented methods for correction of these artifacts in both EPI and conventional imaging. EPI is particularly beneficial for these corrections, since it allows the acquisition of the correction data so rapidly. In addition, an increasing number of techniques have become available for automated shimming[90–93] to improve the baseline homogeneity. These techniques are particularly important in the abdomen and heart, for which the wide variability of patients' body habitus produces a wide variability of field uniformity.

N/2 ghosts

Another unique artifact on EPI scans is the N/2 or Nyquist ghost. These are ghost images that appear

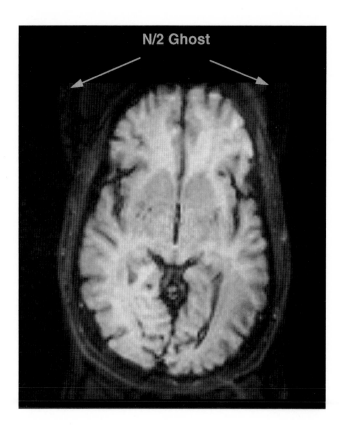

Figure 3.25

N/2 ghost. Any mismatch between the even and odd lines of k-space produces an N/2 ghost in the resulting EPI image, demonstrated here. Careful hardware alignment and/or software correction schemes are used to eliminate this artifact.

half an image away in the phase-encoding direction. Such ghosts appear because the even and odd lines of k-space are traversed in the opposite directions in the raster trajectory. Anything that is systematically different between these even and odd lines will lead to these artifacts. They can be due to hardware timing adjustment, eddy currents, and even very rapid flow. While there are pulse sequence modifications that can eliminate these effects (see e.g. Feinberg et al[94]), it is far more common to use either hardware or software calibrations to reduce such artifacts. As a general rule, these artifacts tend to be somewhat worse in the body than in the head, and tend to become somewhat more troublesome as the spatial resolution is increased. An example of an uncorrected N/2 ghost is shown in Fig. 3.25.

Acoustic noise

The large, rapidly switched, gradient fields of the present implementation of EPI produce relatively loud (90–110 dB) sound bursts, predominantly at the switching frequency of the gradients. Commercially available earplugs (e.g. E-A-R, from Cabot Corporation, Indianapolis, IN) offer as much as 40 dB of acoustic attenuation at this frequency, so that there has thus far been no issue of patient acceptance. In addition, the increasing use of acoustically driven headphones providing patient entertainment often provide sufficient acoustic attenuation as well. As discussed above, the increased robustness of most whole body EPI gradient coils, which is required for purely mechanical reasons to offset increased stress due to the high currents and voltages of EPI encoding, has led to decreased acoustic noise on the conventional scans.

Safety issues

The primary source for concern with EPI has been due to reports of apparent nerve stimulation in the scanner.[95–97] Electrical currents induced in the body by time-varying magnetic fields seem to be the cause of these effects. Reilly[98,99] has reviewed the available data on excitatory thresholds for magnetic stimulation of the peripheral nerves and heart, and has modeled these excitable systems in order to predict threshold behavior. According to these data, while the electrical thresholds for cardiac and peripheral stimulation are similar, the rate constants characterizing the excitable tissues of the heart are generally much longer than those seen in neural tissues. As a consequence, the predicted thresholds, measured in dB/dt (the rate of change of the magnetic field), for cardiac stimulation are much greater in the heart than in the peripheral nerves at the frequencies used for EPI. Furthermore, the relatively small area subtended by the heart suggests that larger time-varying magnetic fields will be required for cardiac stimulation than for peripheral nerves. This assertion is supported by animal work[100] in which extra systoles have been generated by magnetic stimulation in dogs, but at much higher rates of magnetic field change, up to 3000 T/s. In addition, recent work has suggested that there may be opportunities to reduce stimulation by modifying the gradient waveforms,[101] though it is unclear whether these methods will have a practical impact on the current clinical market. Ultimately,

the practical acceptance of single-shot imaging clearly requires sufficient experience with the method to indicate its overall safety.

Other possible biohazards, such as rf heating, have been a concern in conventional imaging sequences. Since the spatial-encoding scheme is all that is altered in EPI, its rf heating properties are exactly the same as in conventional sequences, except that rf power is typically deposited for a shorter period of time, thus depositing relatively less total energy.

Practical aspects and alternative techniques

SNR versus resolution

Ultimately the goal of achieving EPI's temporal resolution and reduced imaging time results in a set of tradeoffs. Since MRI is a technique that exploits extremely small signals, achievable signal-to-noise ratio is often a limiting factor in image quality. It is a convenient metaphor to consider SNR as a limited currency that can be used to purchase contrast resolution, temporal resolution, or spatial resolution—the major determinants of image quality. Owing to the elimination of T_1-related signal changes and absence of motion artifacts, EPI images have a general advantage of improved SNR and T_2 contrast behavior for the time they are acquired. In EPI, spatial resolution is traded for temporal and contrast improvements. In many organ systems, the loss in 'useful' spatial resolution is much ameliorated because of the decreased motional distortion as described above.

In most reported experiences, single excitation EPI images generally have adequate SNR for voxel volumes of about 15 mm³ in the brain using a quadrature head coil with echo times as long as 75 ms. This is equivalent to a 7 mm slice thickness and a 1.5 mm × 1.5 mm in-plane resolution. When smaller voxel volumes are required, for thinner slices or for better in-plane resolution, single-shot techniques do not necessarily have enough SNR, and the tradeoffs between multiple excitation EPI and other fast but more conventional imaging techniques such as interleaved spirals or fast spin echo become possible (see below).

The abdominal organs tend to present more of a challenge, both because their T_2 values are shorter than those of the central nervous system, and because the raw SNR achievable in these organs using body or large surface coils is poorer. At present, most scanners produce acceptable image quality for voxel volumes of 30 mm³ and greater. As in any MRI technology, SNR in EPI is determined both by measurement parameters, such as TR, TE, TI and slice thickness, and by T_1, T_2, proton density and motion of the patient's body tissues. The final image quality therefore depends upon a careful match of measurement parameters to the clinical application. The image contrast behavior in EPI is much like that in conventional MRI, making predictions of contrast and SNR a straightforward task.

EPI and other fast techniques

At its conception, EPI was by far the fastest MR imaging technique described, with many orders of magnitude of speed separating it from conventional techniques. In the intervening two decades, a number of alternative techniques have filled the gaps in between (and even a bit beyond) conventional and EPI acquisition times. While a complete comparison between these techniques is well beyond our intended scope, we conclude with some general comparisons of technical requirements, achievable SNR and contrast issues among these techniques. We limit the discussion to EPI, fast gradient echo imaging, spiral scanning, RARE (fast spin echo) and BURST imaging.

Essentially, any 'fast' technique must, by its nature, scan through k-space very quickly. As described above, EPI achieves this trajectory by switching the gradients rapidly. Fast gradient echo techniques (see e.g. Haase et al[102] and Haase[103]) fill k-space more rapidly decreasing by TR dramatically. Spiral MRI (see e.g. Meyer et al[85]), like EPI, uses a planar trajectory, but uses a spiral rather than raster filling of k-space. RARE imaging[104] uses multiple 180° pulses to refocus the original excitation multiple lines, to fill multiple lines of k-space. BURST imaging[105,106] uses multiple, hard rf pulses and a relatively slow readout gradient to produce multiple encoded echoes in the same TR period. The current, voltage, power, stimulation threshold and raw SNR for these techniques are compared in Table 3.1. There are a number of interesting features that can be seen from this table. First, for comparable imaging time, all the techniques require fairly similar power needs, and produce fairly similar SNR

Table 3.1 Summary of requirements for fast imaging sequences. Throughout the abbreviations are: Δx = resolution, γ = gyromagnetic ratio, N is number of phase encode lines, T_{acq} is the duration of the entire image encoding. The 'G' column gives the peak amplitude of the gradient (or, alternatively, the peak current in the gradient coil) required to achieve a given resolution. 'Risetime' refers to the typical risetime required within any frequency encoded line, 'V_{peak}' is the peak voltage across the coil required, Peak 'i-V' is the product of voltage and current, which would be the peak power required in a linear amplifier (this can be much smaller in an energy storage device, such as a resonant power system). M_o refers to the magnetization available for imaging.

	G (I_{peak})	Risetime	V_{peak}	Peak i-V	M_o
EPI	$\dfrac{N}{\gamma\Delta x T_{acq}}$	$0.1\dfrac{T_{acq}}{N}$	$\dfrac{10N^2}{\gamma\Delta x T_{acq}^2}$	$\dfrac{10N^{3\,*}}{\Delta x^2 T_{acq}^3}$	1
FLASH	$\dfrac{N}{\gamma\Delta x T_{acq}}$	$0.1\dfrac{T_{acq}}{N}$	$\dfrac{10N^2}{\gamma\Delta x T_{acq}^2}$	$\dfrac{10N^3}{\Delta x^2 T_{acq}^3}$	$\sqrt{\dfrac{T_{acq}}{2NT_1}}$
BURST	$\dfrac{N}{\gamma\Delta x T_{acq}}$	$0.1T_{acq}$	$\dfrac{10N}{\gamma\Delta x T_{acq}^2}$	$\dfrac{10N^2}{\Delta x^2 T_{acq}^3}$	$\sqrt{\dfrac{1}{N}}$
Spiral	$\dfrac{\pi}{4}\dfrac{N}{\gamma\Delta x T_{acq}}$	$*$	$\dfrac{2.8N^2}{\gamma\Delta x T_{acq}^2}$	$\dfrac{2.2N^3}{\Delta x^2 T_{acq}^3}$	1

(BURST imaging is the exception, requiring considerably lower power, but producing lower SNR). They differ much more in their contrast behavior and their image artifacts. To determine SNR in this chart, we have used the observation that, to first order, the SNR of nearly all MR imaging sequences can be written very simply as

$$SNR \sim f(M)VT^{1/2}$$

where $f(M)$ describes the available magnetization for imaging (TE, TR, flip angle etc) due to the rf preparation, V is the voxel volume and T is the time spent encoding. (There are a number of potential subtleties, especially when k-space is not sampled uniformly, but these tend to make only small changes in this equation.)

Spirals

Because spirals have such nice flow properties,[107] they are an excellent sequence for interleaving multiple acquisitions, and such interleaves are accessible with more existing scanner's gradient hardware. They are also more efficient by about $\pi/4$ because the spiral covers only enough k-space to make a cylindrically symmetric point-spread function. This efficiency impacts both hardware costs as well as peripheral nerve stimulation limits, as shown in Table 3.1. While these terms are only of order unity, they are nontrivial from an engineering point of view. In addition, like EPI, the contrast and temporal resolutions are not coupled, and conventional spin echo contrast is easily achieved. Spirals, too, face a number of technical challenges. As a single-shot technique, they require high-power amplifiers on two axes (as opposed to one for EPI), and the susceptibility and chemical shift artifacts that lead to shifts in the phase-encoding direction lead to significant cylindrical blurring in spirals, which must be measured and compensated for in order to achieve optimal image quality.[108]

Turbo FLASH

Because of their nearly universal accessibility, very fast FLASH-like sequences have been used extensively for fast imaging applications. Because they have very short readout periods, they have very few of the artifacts described above for EPI or spirals. However, one must pay a large cost in either SNR or volume coverage compared with EPI because of the inefficiency in the magnetization

preparation in FLASH (i.e. throwing away the transverse magnetization). As a concrete example, consider a dynamic imaging application that seeks to image the brain once every 3 s at 128×64 resolution. We could acquire 15 EPI slices (one slice every 200 ms) with a 64 ms readout period per slice, and a 90° flip angle for all slices. If we use regular FLASH imaging to acquire just one slice with the same resolution in this time ($TR = 50$ ms, 4 ms acquisition of conventional readout per readout, total encoding time 256 ms, flip 20°) Using our SNR equation, the relative SNR of the FLASH/EPI is $0.15 \times 1 \times (256/64)^{1/2} = 0.3$; that is, the increased encoding time does not make up for the decreased magnetization. (We could make up for this by decreasing the bandwidth of the FLASH sequence dramatically, say from 16 kHz to 2 kHz, making each FLASH read 32 ms long. The SNRs would then be comparable, but so would the artifacts!) In addition, if we wanted to image 15 slices with the FLASH technique (which is not actually possible with conventional gradients, but is possible with the kinds of gradients available for EPI), we could do this by decreasing the time between slices to 3 ms (with TR still 50 ms), and reading out each for 1 ms. In this case, the SNR ratio falls even farther, to 0.15.

In addition, since the rf pulses are the source of most image contrast, fast gradient echo techniques must intertwine temporal and contrast resolutions. However, a number of techniques that use preparation pulses to achieve T_1 and even T_2 contrast have proven feasible and, as demonstrated in Chapter 2, have a number of clinical applications. Nevertheless, these techniques further limit the temporal efficiency of these sequences. As a result, their most potent use has not been in the ultrafast (<3 s) domain, but rather in filling the gap between ultrafast and conventional imaging.

BURST

First suggested in an abstract by Hennig, but recently reinvented by a number of groups, there is an entirely different method of filling k-space that requires neither short TR nor quickly switched gradients. By using multiple, short rf pulses in the presence of slowly varying gradients, and reading these pulses back out again by rewinding these gradients, BURST allows for ultrafast imaging without any kind of high-performance waveform. Like FLASH techniques, however, it suffers SNR penalties because of small available magnetization for imaging. Compared with EPI, optimized BURST techniques seem limited for comparable resolution and readout times to SNRs lower by a factor of $N^{1/2}$, where N is the number of phase-encoding steps. While recent work has provided 3D images with presentable SNR in as little as 2 s, the image quality and contrast still are at too preliminary a stage to assess the ultimate clinical usefulness of this class of techniques.

Conclusions

We have presented in this chapter both a technical introduction to EPI and some samples of its current clinical and near-clinical applications. Commercially available EPI can provide diagnostically valuable images in as little as 50–100 ms, and, more importantly, its ability to simply make scans more quickly is becoming valuable by creating a new range of applications in the MRI scanner. These include functional and physiological imaging of the brain in cancer and stroke, as well as cardiac and abdominal MRI. While eliminating nearly all motion artifacts, EPI is subject to a number of other, unique, artifacts, including chemical shift and susceptibility artifacts in the phase-encoding direction and $N/2$ ghosting. While implementation of EPI on conventional scanners does require hardware modifications, it ultimately offers a number of potentially useful advantages over other ultrafast techniques. Its potential as both a clinical and basic clinical research tool continues to grow as the number of EPI-equipped scanners increases, and, if its past is any predictor of its future, ultrafast imaging will be used for an even wider variety of examinations in the future.

References

1. Ehman RL, McNamara MT, Brasch RC et al, Influence of physiologic motion on the appearance of tissue in MR images. *Radiology* 1986; **159**: 777–82.

2. Henkelman RM, Bronskill MJ, Artifacts in magnetic resonance imaging. In: *Reviews of Magnetic Resonance in Medicine* (ed JC Gore) 1–126. Pergamon Press, New York: 1987.

3. Rogers WJ, Shapiro E, Effect of RR interval variation on image quality in gated, two-dimensional, Fourier MR imaging. *Radiology* 1993; **186**: 883–7.

4. Twieg DB, The *k*-trajectory formulation of the NMR imaging process with applications in analysis and synthesis of imaging methods. *Med Phys* 1983; **10**: 610–21.

5. Twieg DB, Acquisition and accuracy in rapid NMR imaging methods. *Magn Reson Med* 1985; **2**: 437–52.

6. Ljunggren S, A simple graphical representation of Fourier-based imaging methods. *J Magn Reson* 1983; **54**: 338–43.

7. Mansfield P, Pykett IL, Biological and medical imaging by NMR. *J Magn Reson* 1978; **29**: 355–73.

8. Mansfield P, Maudsley A, Planar spin imaging by NMR. *J Magn Reson* 1977; **27**: 101–19.

9. Chapman B, Turner R, Ordidge R et al, Real time movie imaging from a single cardiac cycle by NMR. *Magn Reson Med* 1987; **5**: 546–54.

10. Ordidge R, Coxon R, Howseman A et al, Snapshot head imaging at 0.5 T using the echo planar technique. *Magn Reson Med* 1988; **8**: 110–15.

11. Stehling M, Howseman A, Ordidge R et al, Whole-body echo-planar MR imaging at 0.5 T. *Radiology* 1989; **170**: 257–63.

12. Rzedzian RR, Pykett IL, An instant technique for real-time MR imaging. *Radiology* 1986; **161**(P): 333.

13. Pykett IL, Rzedzian RR, Instant images of the body by magnetic resonance. *Magn Reson Med* 1987; **5**: 563–71.

14. Rzedzian R, High speed, high resolution spin echo imaging by Mosaic scan and MESH. *Soc Magn Reson Med* 1987; **51**.

15. Rzedzian RR, A method for instant whole-body MR imaging at 2.0 Tesla and system design considerations in its implementation. *Proc 6th Ann Mtg Soc Magn Reson Med, New York, 1987.*

16. Bydder G, Young I, MR imaging: clinical use of the inversion recovery sequence. *Comput Assist Tomogr* 1984; **9**: 659–75.

17. Cohen MS, Weisskoff RM, Ultra-fast imaging. *Magn Reson Imaging* 1991; **9**: 1–37.

18. Ordidge R, Gibbs P, Chapman B et al, High-speed multislice T_1 mapping using inversion-recovery echo-planar imaging. *Magn Reson Med* 1990; **16**: 238–45.

19. MacFall J, Pelc N, Vavrek R, Correction of spatially dependent phase shifts for partial Fourier imaging. *Magn Reson Imaging* 1988; **6**: 143–55.

20. Weisskoff RM, Dalcanton JJ, Cohen MS, High-resolution 64 msec instant images of the head. *Magn Reson Imaging* 1990; **8** (supp 1): 93.

21. Butts KS. Jr, Ehman R, Thompson R, Jack C, Interleaved echo planar imaging on a standard MRI system. *Magn Reson Med* 1994; **31**: 67–72.

22. Oshio K, Feinberg D, GRASE (Gradient- and SpinEcho) imaging: a novel fast MRI technique. *Magn Reson Med* 1991; **20**: 344–9.

23. Wong E-C, Jesmanowicz A, Hyde J, High-resolution, short echo time MR imaging of the fingers and wrist with a local gradient coil. *Radiology* 1991; **181**: 393–7.

24. Tropper M, Image reconstruction for the NMR echo-planar technique and for a proposed adaptation to allow data acquisition. *J Magn Reson* 1981; **42**: 193–202.

25. Bruder H, Fischer H, Reinfelder H, Schmitt F, Image reconstruction for echo planar imaging with nonequidistant *k*-space sampling. *Magn Reson Med* 1990; **23**: 311–23.

26. Hyder F, Rothman D, Blamire A, Image reconstruction of sequentially sampled echo-planar data. *Magn Reson Imaging* 1995; **13**: 97–103.

27. Zakhor A, Weisskoff R, Rzedzian R, Optimal sampling and reconstruction of MRI signals resulting from sinusoidal gradients. *IEEE Trans Sig Process* 1991; **39**: 2056–65.

28. Weisskoff RM, Rzedzian RR, High-resolution instant images in the brain. *Radiology* 1989; **173**: 1272.

29. Villringer A, Rosen BR, Belliveau JW et al, Dynamic imaging with lanthanide chelates in normal brain: contrast due to magnetic susceptibility effects. *Magn Reson Med* 1988; **6**: 164–74.

30. Weisskoff R, Zuo C, Boxerman J, Rosen B, Microscopic susceptibility variation and transverse relaxation: theory and experiment. *Magn Reson Med* 1994; **31**: 601–10.

31. Boxerman J, Hamberg L, Rosen B, Weisskoff R, MR contrast due to intravascular magnetic susceptibility perturbers. *Magn Reson Med* 1995; **34**: 555–66.

32. Rosen BR, Belliveau JW, Aronen HJ et al, Susceptibility contrast imaging of cerebral blood volume: human experience. *Magn Reson Med* 1991; **22**: 293–9.

33. Aronen H, Gazit I, Louis D et al, Cerebral blood volume maps of gliomas: Comparison with tumor grade and histologic findings. *Radiology* 1994; **191**: 41–51.

34. Folkman J, What is the evidence that tumors are angiogenesis dependent? *J Natl Cancer Inst* 1990; **82**: 4–6.

35. Edelman RR, Mattle HP, Atkinson DJ et al, Cerebral blood flow: assessment with dynamic contrast-enhanced $T2^*$-weighted MR imaging at 1.5 T. *Radiology* 1990; **176**: 211–20.

36. Stejskal E, Tanner J, Spin-diffusion measurements: spin echoes in the presence of a time dependent field gradient. 1965; **42**: 288–92.

37. LeBihan D, Breton E, Lallemand D et al, Separation of diffusion and perfusion in intravoxel incoherent motion MR imaging. *Radiology* 1988; **168**: 497–505.

38. de Crespigny A, Marks M, Enzmann D, Moseley M, Navigated diffusion imaging of normal and ischemic human brain. *Magn Reson Med* 1995; **33**: 720–8.

39. Ordidge R, Helpern J, Qing Z, Knight RVN, Correction of motional artifacts in diffusion-weighted MR images using navigator echoes. *Magn Reson Imaging* 1994; **12**: 455–60.

40. Turner R, LeBihan D, Single-shot diffusion imaging at 2.0 tesla. *J Magn Reson* 1990; **86**: 445–52.

41. Le Bihan D, Breton E, Lallemand D et al, MR imaging of intravoxel incoherent motions: application to diffusion and perfusion in neurologic disorders. *Radiology* 1986; **161**: 401–7.

42. Henkelman RM, Does IVIM measure classical perfusion? *Magn Reson Med* 1990; **16**: 470–5.

43. Moseley M, Cohen Y, Mintorovitch J et al, Early detection of regional cerebral ischemia in cats: comparison of diffusion and *T*2 weighted MRI and spectroscopy. *Magn Reson Med* 1990; **14**: 330–46.

44. Warach S, Gaa J, Siewert B et al, Acute human stroke studied by whole brain echo planar diffusion-weighted magnetic resonance imaging. *Ann Neurol* 1995; **37**: 231–41.

45. Kwong KK, Belliveau JW, Chesler DA et al, Dynamic magnetic resonance imaging of human brain activity during primary sensory stimulation. *Proc Natl Acad Sci USA* 1992; **89**: 5675–9.

46. Ogawa S, Tank DW, Menon R et al, Intrinsic signal changes accompanying sensory stimulation: functional brain mapping with magnetic resonance imaging. *Proc Natl Acad Sci USA* 1992; **89**: 5951–5.

47. Bandettini PA, Wong EC, Hinks RS et al, Time course EPI of human brain function during task activation. *Magn Reson Med* 1992; **25**: 390–7.

48. Woods RP, Cherry SR, Mazziotta JC, Rapid automated algorithm for aligning and reslicing PET images. *J Comput Assist Tomogr* 1992; **16**: 620–33.

49. Cohen M, Functional magnetic resonance imaging of the human brain. *Epilepsia* 1992; **33**(supp 3): 2.

50. Charles P, Abou-Khalil R, Abou-Khalil B et al, MRI asymmetries and language dominance. *Neurology* 1994; **44**: 2050–4.

51. Naganawa S, Jenner G, Cooper T et al, Rapid MR imaging of the liver: comparison of twelve techniques for single breath-hold whole volume acquisition. *Rad Med* 1994; **12**: 255–61.

52. Fredrickson J, Wegmuller H, Herfkens R, Pelc N, Simultaneous temporal resolution of cardiac and respiratory motion in MR imaging. *Radiology* 1995; **195**: 169–75.

53. Campeau N, Johnson C, Femlee J et al, MR imaging of the abdomen with a phased-array multicoil: prospective clinical evaluation. *Radiology* 1995; **195**: 769–76.

54. Reimer P, Ladebeck R, Rummeny E et al, Initial feasibility studies using single-shot EPI for the detection of focal liver lesions. *Magn Reson Med* 1994; **32**: 733–7.

55. Reimer P, Saini S, Hahn P et al, Techniques for high-resolution echo-planar MR imaging of the pancreas. *Radiology* 1992; **182**: 175–9.

56. Reimer P, Saini S, Kwong K et al, Dynamic gadolinium-enhanced echo-planar MR imaging of the liver: effect of pulse sequence and dose on enhancement. *J Magn Reson Imaging* 1994; **4**: 331–5.

57. Wolf G, Hoop B, Cannillo J et al, Measurement of renal transit of gadopentetate dimeglumine with echo-planar MR imaging. *J Magn Reson Imaging* 1994; **4**: 365–72.

58. Wielopolski P, Adamis M, Prasad P et al, Breath-hold 3D STAR MR angiography of the renal arteries using segmented echo planar imaging. *Magn Reson Med* 1995; **33**: 432–8.

59. Muller M, Prasad P, Siewert B et al, Abdominal diffusion mapping with use of a whole-body echo-planar system. *Radiology* 1994; **190**: 475–8.

60. Evans D, Lamont G, Stehling M et al, Prolonged monitoring of the upper gastrointestinal tract using echo planar magnetic resonance imaging. *Gut* 1993; **34**: 848–52.

61. Baker P, Johnson I, Gowland P et al, Measurement of fetal liver, brain and placental volumes with echo-planar magnetic resonance imaging. *Br J Obstr Gyn* 1995; **102**: 35–9.

62. Muller M, Edelman R, Echo planar imaging of the abdomen. *Top Magn Reson Imaging* 1995; **7**: 112–19.

63. Rzedzian RR, Pykett IL, Instant images of the human heart using a new, whole-body MR imaging system. *AJR* 1987; **149**: 245–50.

64. Edelman R, Wielopolski P, Schmitt F, Echo-planar MR imaging. *Radiology* 1994; **192**: 600–12.

65. Hunter G, Hamberg L, Weisskoff R et al, Measurement of stroke volume and cardiac output within a single breath hold with echo-planary MR imaging. *J Magn Reson Imaging* 1994; **4**: 51–6.

66. Davis C, McKinnon G, Debatin J et al, Single-shot versus interleaved echo-planar MR imaging: application to visualization of

cardiac valve leaflets. *J Magn Reson Imaging* 1995; **5**: 107–12.

67. Weisskoff R, Crawley A, Wedeen V, Flow sensitivity and flow compensation in instant imaging. *Proc 9th Ann Mtg Soc Magn Reson Med New York, 1990*, 398.

68. Duerk J, Simonetti O, Theoretical aspects of motion sensitivity and compensation in echo-planar imaging. *J Magn Reson Imag* 1991; **1**: 643–50.

69. Butts R, Riederer S, Analysis of flow effects in echo-planar imaging. *J Magn Reson Imag* 1992; **2**: 285–93.

70. Wedeen V, Crawley A, Weisskoff R et al, Real time MR imaging of structured fluid flow. *Proc 9th Ann Mtg Soc Magn Reson Med, New York, 1990*, 164.

71. Firmin D, Klipstein R, Hounsfield G et al, Echo-planar high-resolution flow velocity mapping. *Magn Reson Med* 1989; **12**: 316–27.

72. Poncelet B, Weisskoff R, Wedeen V et al, Time of flight ouantification of coronary flow with echo-planar MRI. *Magn Reson Med* 1993; **30**: 447–57.

73. Edelman R, Li W, Contrast-enhanced echo-planar MR imaging of myocardial perfusion: preliminary study in humans. *Radiology* 1994; **190**: 771–7.

74. Saeed M, Wendland M, Yu K et al, Identification of myocardial reperfusion with echo planar magnetic resonance imaging. Discrimination between occlusive and reperfused infarctions. *Circulation* 1994; **90**: 1492–501.

75. Atkinson D, Burstein D, Edelman R, First-pass cardiac perfusion: evaluation with ultra-fast MR imaging. *Radiology* 1990; **174**: 757.

76. Wilke N, Kroll K, Merkle H et al, Regional myocardial blood volume and flow: first-pass MR imaging with polylysine–Gd–DTPA. *J Magn Reson Imaging* 1995; **5**: 227–37.

77. Balaban R, Taylor J, Turner R, Effect of cardiac flow on gradient recalled echo images of the canine heart. *NMR Biomed* 1994; **7**: 89–95.

78. McVeigh E, Zerhouni E, Noninvasive measurement of transmural gradients in myocardial strain with MR imaging. *Radiology* 1991; **180**: 677–83.

79. Axel L, Dougherty L, MR imaging of motion with spatial modulation of magnetization. *Radiology* 1989; **171**: 841–5.

80. Tang C, McVeigh E, Zerhouni E, Multi-shot EPI for improvement of myocardial tag contrast: comparison with segmented SPGR. *Magn Reson Med* 1995; **33**: 443–7.

81. Pelc L, Sayre J, Yun K et al, Evaluation of myocardial motion tracking with cine-phase contrast magnetic resonance imaging. *Invest Radiol* 1994; **29**: 1038–42.

82. Wedeen V, Magnetic resonance imaging of myocardial kinematics. Technique to detect, localize, and quantify the strain rates of the active human myocardium. *Magn Reson Med* 1992; **27**: 52–67.

83. Reese T, Weisskoff R, Smith R et al, Imaging myocardial fiber architecture in vivo with magnetic resonance. *Magn Reson Med* 1995; in press.

84. Edelman R, Gaa J, Wedeen V et al, In vivo measurement of water diffuson in the human heart. *Magn Reson Med* 1994; **32**: 423–8.

85. Meyer C, Hu B, Nishimura D, Macovski A, Fast spiral coronary artery imaging. *Magn Reson Med* 1992; **28**: 202–13.

86. Farzaneh F, Riederer SJ, Pelc NJ, Analysis of *T*2 limitations and off-resonance effects on spatial resolution and artifacts in echo-planar imaging. *Magn Reson Med* 1990; **14**: 123–39.

87. Bruder H, Fischer H, Schmitt F, Reinfelder H, Reconstruction procedures for echo planar imaging. *Proc 8th Ann Mtg Soc Magn Reson Med, Amsterdam, 1990*, 359.

88. Weisskoff R, Davis T, Correcting gross distortion on echo planar images. *Proc 11th Ann Mtg Soc Magn Reson Med, Berlin, 1992*.

89. Sumanaweera T, Glover G, Binford T, Adler J. MR susceptibility misregistration correction. *IEEE Trans Med Imaging* 1993; **12**: 251–9.

90. Prammer M, Haselgrove J, Shinnar M, Leigh J, A new approach to automatic shimming. *J Magn Reson* 1988; **77**: 40–52.

91. Gruetter R, Boesch C, Fast, noniterative shimming of spatially localized signals, in vivo analysis of the magnetic field along axes. *J Magn Reson* 1992; **96**: 323–34.

92. Scheider E, Glover G, Rapid in vivo proton shimming. *Magn Reson Med* 1991; **18**: 335–47.

93. Reese T, Davis T, Weisskoff R, Automated shimming at 1.5 T using echo-planar image frequency maps. *J Magn Reson Imaging* 1996; in press.

94. Feinberg D, Turner R, Jakab P, von Kiennlin M, Echo planar imaging with asymmetric gradient modulation and inner volume excitation. *Magn Reson Med* 1990; **13**: 162–9.

95. Cohen MS, Weisskoff RM, Rzedzian RR, Kantor HL, Sensory stimulation by time-varying magnetic fields. *Magn Reson Med* 1990; **14**: 409–14.

96. Budinger T, Fischer H, Hentchel D et al, Physiological effects of fast oscillating magnetic field gradients. *J Comput Aided Tomogr* 1991; **15**: 909–14.

97. Harvey P, Mansfield P, Sensory stimulation due to switched gradients. 1992.

98. Reilly J, Peripheral nerve stimulation and cardiac excitation by time-varying magnetic fields: a comparison of thresholds. The Office of Science and Technology, Center for Devices and Radiological Health, US Food and Drug Administration, 1990.

99. Reilly J, Peripheral nerve stimulation by induced electric currents: exposure to time-varying magnetic fields. *Med Biol Engng Comput* 1989; **27**: 101–10.

100. Bourland J, Mouchawar G, Nyehuis J et al, Transchest magnetic (eddy-current) stimulation of the dog heart. *Med Biol Engng Comput* 1990; **28**: 196–8.

101. Harvey P, Mansfield P, Avoiding peripheral nerve stimulation: gradient waveform criteria for optimum resolution in echo-planar imaging. *Magn Reson Med* 1994; **32**: 236–41.

102. Haase A, Frahm J, Matthaei K, FLASH imaging: rapid NMR imaging using low flip angles. *J Magn Reson* 1986; **67**: 258–66.

103. Haase A, Snapshot FLASH MRI. Applications to *T*1, *T*2, and chemical shift imaging. *Magn Reson Med* 1990; **13**: 77–89.

104. Hennig J, Nauerth A, Freidberg H, RARE imaging: a fast imaging method for clinical MR. *Magn Reson Med* 1986; **3**: 823–33.

105. Lowe I, Wysong R, DANTE ultrafast imaging sequence. *J Magn Reson* 1993; **101**: 106–9.

106. Duyn J, van Gelderen P, Barker P et al, 3D bolus tracking with frequency-shifted BURST MRI. *J Comput Assist Tomogr* 1994; **18**: 680–7.

107. Meyer C, Hu B, Nishimura D, Macovski A. Fast spiral coronary artery imaging. *Magn Reson Med* 1992; **28**: 202–13.

108. Noll D, Pauly J, Meyer C et al, Deblurring for non-2D Fourier transform magnetic resonance imaging. *Magn Reson Med* 1992; **25**: 319–33.

4

Clinical use of diffusion-weighted imaging

Joseph V Hajnal and Graeme M Bydder

Introduction

Translational molecular diffusion is a process in which molecules move along random paths, colliding with and moving past each other. In a homogeneous fluid of infinite extent diffusion may be a truly random phenomenon, but the extent to which water molecules diffuse in tissues is affected not just by the properties of the cytosol itself but also by the presence of cellular structures, which provide barriers to free movement. Diffusion in these circumstances is said to be restricted. In tissues that have a highly organized but asymmetric structure, diffusion may be more restricted in one direction than in another. An important example of this is myelinated white matter, where diffusion of water molecules across fibers is much more restricted than that along fibers. Diffusion that has strong directional dependence of this type is said to be anisotropic.

In the presence of a spatially varying magnetic field, random motion of protons in diffusing water molecules results in irreversible dephasing of the magnetic resonance signal, producing a reduction in its amplitude. Since spatially varying magnetic fields are used for slice selection and spatial encoding in all magnetic resonance (MR) images, diffusion of water molecules results in a reduction in signal intensity in all images, although the effect is normally quite small. By deliberately applying large magnetic field gradients in particular directions, diffusion can be made the dominant image contrast mechanism, enabling visualization of variations in diffusion, including their directional dependence.

A variety of studies designed to assess the clinical value of diffusion-weighted imaging have been performed over the last ten years and interest in the technique is increasing.[1] Much work remains to be done in implementing and understanding diffusion-weighted imaging, but the technique appears to have considerable potential for improving the sensitivity of MR imaging to specific diseases of the central nervous system.

Restricted diffusion

Diffusion is most appropriately described in statistical terms. We can define the conditional probability $P(\mathbf{r}_0; \mathbf{r}, t)$ as the probability that a molecule initially at position $\mathbf{r}_0$ arrives at another position r after a time t. In a homogeneous fluid of infinite extent, P is a Gaussian function such that

$$P = (4\pi Dt)^{-3/2} \exp\left[-\frac{(\mathbf{r} - \mathbf{r}_0)^2}{4Dt}\right], \qquad (1)$$

where D is the diffusion coefficient. If distance is measured in millimeters and time in seconds, then D has units of mm^2/s. The diffusion coefficient is a measure of mobility at the molecular level, and varies inversely with viscosity. For pure water at 37°C, $D = 3.4 \times 10^{-3}$ mm^2/s.

Since each molecule follows a random path, the distance travelled in any given time as a result of diffusion varies widely for different molecules. However, it is useful to calculate the average distance l, that molecules travel in a time t, and this is given by the Einstein equation

$$l = \sqrt{6Dt} \qquad (2)$$

if motion in three dimensions is considered, and

$$l = \sqrt{2Dt} \qquad (3)$$

if movement in only one direction is considered.

When diffusion is restricted by barriers such as cell boundaries $P(\mathbf{r}_0; \mathbf{r}, t)$ becomes geometry-dependent and ceases to be a pure Gaussian function of distance. As a consequence, the conventional definition of the diffusion coefficient breaks down, since it is no longer simply a property of the diffusing medium alone. On very short timescales, molecules may diffuse as if they were in a homogeneous fluid, but over progressively longer times more and more of them diffuse far enough to encounter a barrier that hinders their further movement. A practical solution to this difficulty is to replace D by the apparent diffusion coefficient D^*, whose magnitude depends on the time interval over which diffusion is monitored, T_d (the diffusion time). Depending on the symmetry of the barriers to diffusion, D^* may or may not be directionally dependent.

The manner in which D^* varies with T_d depends on the nature of the barriers, including their geometry, permeability and spacing. However, in general, D^* is smaller than the unrestricted value of D, and decreases monotonically from a value close to D for values of T_d near zero to a small limiting value as T_d tends to infinity (Fig. 4.1). This decrease in D^* with T_d is the basic contrast mechanism in restricted diffusion imaging. By an appropriate choice of the pulse timing of diffusion-sensitive imaging sequences, T_d can be selected to reveal highly restricted diffusion in some tissues or in a particular direction within a tissue (small D^*) while still retaining much less restricted diffusion (relatively large D^*) in other tissues or another direction within a tissue. Thus T_d is a key parameter for determining the extent to which diffusion reveals cellular structure.

Diffusion sensitive pulse sequences

Early measurements of diffusion employed a Hahn spin echo collected in the presence of a constant

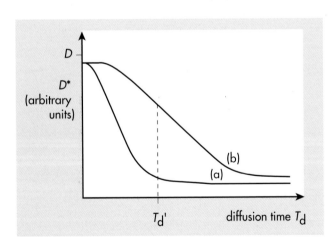

Figure 4.1

Variation of apparent diffusion coefficient D^* with diffusion time T_d. Curve (a) illustrates highly restricted diffusion while (b) shows a moderately restricted pattern. At diffusion time T_d', strong contrast would be seen between (a) and (b), with (a) giving a higher signal intensity than (b).

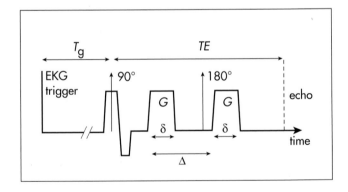

Figure 4.2

Diffusion-weighted spin echo sequence: Following the EKG trigger after a delay T_g, there is a 90° slice-selective pulse followed by either a selective or nonselective 180° pulse. Additional diffusion sensitizing gradients of magnitude G, duration δ and separation Δ are applied along the chosen axis, which is the direction of slice selection in this example. The gradient pulses need not be symmetrically disposed on either side of the 180° pulse.

applied gradient.[2] For a homogeneous liquid, the amplitude of the echo is reduced by a factor R (in addition to the usual T_1 and T_2 effects) given by

$$R = \exp - [\frac{1}{12}\gamma^2 G^2 (TE)^3 D^*], \tag{4}$$

where γ is the gyromagnetic ratio, G is the applied constant field gradient and TE is the echo time. The nominal diffusion time T_d is equal to $TE/3$ with this sequence, forming an undesirable link between contrast due to restricted diffusion and that due to T_2 relaxation.

In 1965 Stejskal and Tanner[3,4] introduced the pulsed gradient spin echo (PGSE) technique, in which sensitivity to diffusion is provided by gradient pulses placed on either side of the 180° refocusing pulse (Fig. 4.2). Neglecting terms due to small slice-selection and space-encoding gradients, the diffusion attenuation factor R with this sequence is then given by

$$R = \exp - [\gamma^2 G^2 \delta^2 (\Delta - \frac{1}{3}\delta)D^*] \tag{5}$$

$$= \exp - (bD^*), \tag{6}$$

where G is the amplitude of the gradient pulses, δ is their duration and Δ is the time between their leading edges. For the PGSE sequence, $T_d = \Delta - \frac{1}{3}\delta$. The composite parameter b (the diffusion sensitivity parameter)[5] determines the overall signal attenuation (in conjunction with D^*), and has units of s/mm². The choice of b value is determined by the required sensitivity to D or D^*. Typically b is chosen to be approximately $1/D^*$.

The PGSE technique has a number of advantages. It decouples diffusion contrast from T_2-dependent contrast, since R no longer depends on TE. In addition, by using very narrow pulses (making δ small in comparison with the average time required to diffuse between barriers), it enables the diffusion time to be determined precisely. This facilitates measurement of barrier spacing and apparent diffusion coefficients.[6,7]

Finally, the use of pulsed gradients separates the diffusion sensitization from the applied radiofrequency (rf) pulses and the data acquisition, so allowing the diffusion weighting to be changed without affecting other sequence properties such as slice thickness and voxel size. In clinical applications this is perhaps the most significant advantage. Since the gradient available on most standard imaging machines (typically about 10–20 mT/m) necessitates the use of broad pulses to achieve the required sensitivity, the PGSE may in practice appear rather similar to the constant-gradient method.

A PGSE sequence can be implemented either as a conventional sequence with one phase mode acquired per TR or with more sophisticated data acquisition such as fast spin echo or echo planar imaging. Artifacts produced by involuntary subject motion are a major problem with diffusion-weighted imaging. Careful positioning and immobilization of the subject and/or the use of rapid sequence or artifact control measures such as cardiac gating, navigator echoes or line scanning methods are essential.

Image contrast

In view of the additional factors that affect image contrast, PGSE sequences need to be labeled, not only by such parameters as TR and TE, but also by the direction of the applied gradients, T_d (which determines the extent to which restrictions are probed) and the overall sensitivity to diffusion, b. In this chapter the following convention is used:

SE/TR/TE/direction:
X, Y or Z sensitizing gradients/T_d/b.

TR and TE are given in milliseconds. The direction of the sensitizing gradient is given as X, Y or Z (Fig. 4.3). The diffusion time T_d is quoted in milliseconds and the diffusion sensitization parameter b in s/mm². In the absence of diffusion sensitizing gradients, the imaging sequences employed had b values of less than 5 s/mm².

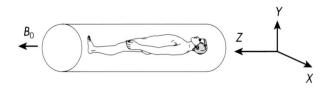

Figure 4.3

Orientation of the patient with respect to the static magnetic field B_0 and the X, Y and Z axes.

In some ways the parameters T_d and b play roles analogous to the window level and width functions used to optimize the display of MR images. T_d can be set to a value at which D^* for a particular tissue is relatively small, resulting in a bright region for that tissue on the images, while D^* for another tissue is relatively large, giving a dark appearance.

Assuming that, in the absence of restriction, cellular water has a diffusion coefficient similar to that of free water, and using a conservative range of values for T_d (from 1 to 100 ms) from equation (3), the range of scale lengths that can be probed by diffusion-weighted sequences is about 2.5–25 μm. This is of considerable importance, since these distances are appropriate for studying effects due to cell structure, and are comparable to the diameter of myelinated axons in the central nervous system.

Standard whole body imaging machines may be unable to achieve the shorter range of T_d values (with useful values of b) without modification to their gradient system. As a consequence, some tissues or directions within tissues may always exhibit highly restricted diffusion when studied with commonly available PGSE sequences. Likewise, T_2-dependent signal decay may make useful imaging of some issues impossible at very long values of T_d.

The parameter b sets the overall level of attenuation, and determines the dynamic range of the images. For example, with $T_d \approx 50$–100 ms, a b value of 1510 s/mm^2 is sufficient to suppress virtually all signals except those from highly restricting structures such as appropriately oriented axons.

was reduced. The same general type of fixation was used on the 1.0 T system.

Cardiac gating on alternate beats (or every fourth beat for rapid pulse rates) with a delay of 200–700 ms from the R wave was employed to time the pulse sequences into mid and late diastole. Images were of 128 × 256 matrix size except where specifically labelled 256 × 256. Two or four excitations were used in each study, with a slice thickness of 4–8 mm.

The basic pulse sequence is illustrated in Fig. 4.2. TE values of 130 or 200 ms were used with the conventional whole body gradient coils. T_d values of 44, 65, 85 and 103 ms were available with the conventional gradient coils. b values of 550 or 600 mm^2/s (TE = 130 and 200 ms) as well as 1100 mm^2/s (TE = 200 ms) and 1510 mm^2/s (TE = 200 ms) were used.

First-order gradient moment nulling[8] was implemented on the Z axis in the coronal, sagittal and transverse planes. The extra gradients lead to a reduction in T_d value to 44 ms from 85 or 103 ms for TE = 200 ms sequences.

A purpose-design small gradient coil set of 300 mm internal diameter was employed for some head studies. This set provided approximately four times the gradient strength of the standard set. With this system, it was possible to obtain b values of 550 mm^2/s with a TE of 80 ms and a T_d of 27 ms. The gradient set was only suitable for imaging heads and limbs in adults, although whole body examinations of infants are possible with this system.

Unsensitized control sequences that were comparable in all respects except for the additional diffusion sensitizing gradients were available to match all PGSE sequences.

Implementation

Two MR systems were used in these studies. One was a Picker prototype and operated at 0.15 T. The other was a standard Picker HPQ system operating at 1.0 T. On the 0.15 T system a whole body gradient coil set of 490 mm internal diameter was used for most studies, and provided a gradient strength of up to 16 mT/m. Quasispherical head receiver coils were used for all studies in this system, with the addition of padded foam to increase patient comfort and a plastic bag containing polystyrene beads, which was evacuated to assist with head fixation. The receiver coils were supported so that rocking motion with respiration

Anatomic considerations

Diffusion-weighted imaging allows the components of the medullary core of the cerebrum to be distinguished. The medullary core can be considered in three parts: association, commissural and projection fibers.

Association fibers connect regions of the cortex within a hemisphere and can be divided into short association fibers (which connect adjacent gyri via subcortical U fiber tracts) and long association fibers. The latter are present in three main bundles: (i) the uncinate fasciculus, (ii) the arcuate fasciculus and (iii) the cingulum. The latter two fasciculi run mainly in the anteroposterior direction, as do smaller tracts such as the superior occipitofrontal tract. Connections between the temporal and parietal lobes tend to run in a caudocephalic direction, while those between the frontal and temporal lobes typically run obliquely within the uncinate fasciculus.

Commissural fibers form the interhemispheric connections of the cortex of both hemispheres. These can be homotopic or heterotopic depending whether or not corresponding or noncorresponding parts of gray matter are connected. These fibers run within coronal planes for at least part of their course.

Projection fibers are those tracts that provide the major input and output channels of the brain, and include pathways such as the corticospinal tracts. These fibers tend to have a caudocephalic course, and are often seen well in the coronal plane as they pass through the internal capsule. The projection fibers for special senses such as vision and olfaction connect the end organ with the appropriate cortex, and may be seen in transverse or oblique transverse planes.

In humans there are about one million fibers in each corticospinal tract, of which 700 000 are myelinated; 90% of the myelinated fibers are between 1 and 4 µm in diameter. Most of the remaining fibers are 5–10 µm in diameter, but the 40 000 fibers from the Betz cells are much larger, being 10–22 µm in diameter. By comparison, fibers of the spinocerebellar tract are 11–20 µm in diameter, and unmyelinated fibers are generally 1–4 µm in diameter. The size of fibers corresponds closely to estimates of the range of dimensions that can be probed with diffusion-weighted imaging as described previously (i.e. 2.5–25 µm).

To highlight a particular tract using diffusion-weighted imaging, it is necessary that sufficient fibers run perpendicular to the gradient being used (Figs 4.4 and 4.5). The density of fibers varies more than tenfold between major tracts[9,10] (Table 4.1), and some may contain an insufficient number of fibers to give high contrast with surrounding tissue.

It is essential that the correct imaging plane be selected (Table 4.2) and that the patient be appropriately positioned and immobilized. If a number of tracts with differing orientations are interdigitated then the selection of b and slice thickness is crucial. Diffusely spread fiber tracts such as the geniculocalcarine projections or the corona radiata may require a thick slice and a large b value for successful imaging.

Diffusion-weighted imaging is sensitive to small deviations from ideal alignment. This is readily seen in the signal intensity of the splenium of the corpus callosum in the transverse plane, which varies dramatically with increasing angulation of the fibers to the direction of the sensitizing gradient. Because

Table 4.1 Density of fibers in major brain pathways[10]

Structure	Number of fibers/mm²
Optic nerve	500 000
Anterior commissure	800 000
Fornix	200 000
Corpus callosum	340 000
Mammilothalamic tract	150 000
Cerebral peduncle	75 000
Spinal cord	75 000

of the complex pathway of many tracts and their oblique orientation to most conventional imaging planes, only part of a tract may be highlighted in any given image.

Myelination

Anistropic change is readily seen in the major tracts of the adult brain. Also of interest is the fact that anisotropic change can be seen in tracts in which myelin is not demonstrable with conventional T_1-weighted sequences (Fig. 4.6). It has been suggested that this may be due to a few layers of myelin that are sufficient to restrict diffusion but insufficient to shorten T_1. However, similar changes have been seen in unmyelinated nerves, so that ordered structure alone may be sufficient to produce anisotropy.[11]

Pathological considerations

The use of PGSE sequences to assess apparent diffusion coefficients D^* in the brain is still at an early stage of development, but some data are now available.

There are only a limited number of reports on the value of D^* of brain in which the direction of the fibers is taken into account. The values of D^* for white matter are variable, but lower values are

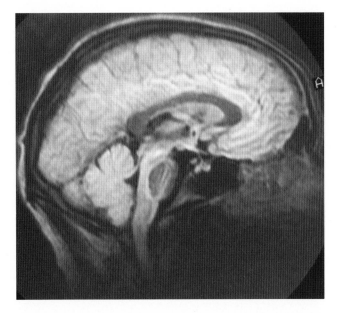

a

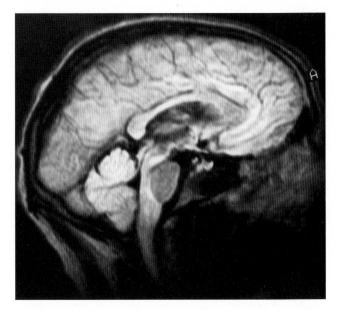

b

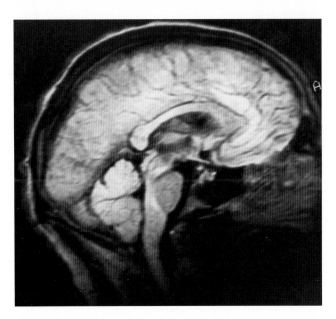

c

Figure 4.4

Normal volunteer (male aged 49 years): SE ≈ 1500/130/X/44/550 (a), SE ≈ 1500/130/Y/44/550 (b) and SE ≈ 1500/130/Z/44/550 (c) images. Image (a) clearly shows a low-signal corpus callosum. Images (b) and (c) show a high signal from corpus callosum. The corticospinal tracts are seen within the pons in (a) but not in (b) or (c).

generally reported for fibers transverse to the sensitizing gradient than for those parallel to the sensitizing gradient. There are also variations in D^* when different values of T_d are used, as well as differences that depend on whether or not cardiac gating is employed.[12] Many reports of pathologic cases in the literature do not make clear the direction of the relevant fiber pathways.

The most studied experimental pathology has been acute infarction, and the fact that D^* decreases in the initial phases and returns to normal later has been established in cat and rat models as well as in humans[13–20] The basis for this is still a matter of speculation. As a result of the decrease in D^*, PGSE sequences produce an increase in signal initially, and this may be apparent before changes

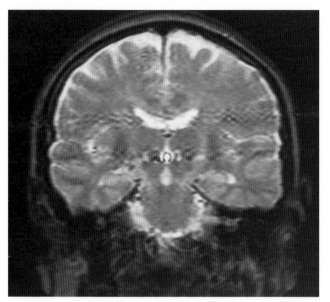

a

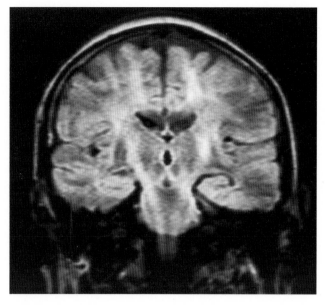

b

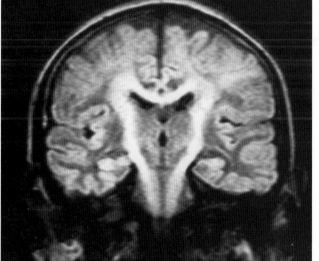

c

Figure 4.5

Normal volunteer (male aged 49 years): SE ≈ 1500/130 (a), SE ≈ 1500/130/X/44/550 (b) and SE ≈ 1500/130/Y/44/550 (c) images. The corpus callosum has a low signal in (b), but is highlighted together with the corticospinal tracts in (c).

appear with conventional T_2-weighted spin echo sequences. This may be due to microvacuolation from swelling of mitochondria, reduction in vascular pulsation, decrease in extracellular fluid as a consequence of cellular swelling, or other mechanisms.

In chronic infarction values of D^* have generally been elevated or within the normal range.

Brain death is a situation in which D^* is decreased.[21] Measurements have been obtained within a few minutes of cessation of cardiac pulsation in cat and rat models. The mechanism for this is not clear at present. Cell shrinkage may occur soon after death, and microvacuolation or astrocytic swelling can be a very acute process, which could retain water in a highly restricted state.

Table 4.2 Orientation and relative sizes of tracts and nerves of the brain

Tract or nerve	Orientation						
	Trans	Coron	Sagit	Obliq trans	Obliq coron	Obliq sagit	Size
Callosum	X	X	X				Large
Splenium of corpus callosum	X	X	X	X			Medium
Genu of the corpus callosum	X		X				Medium
Cingulum	X	X	X				Medium
Fornix	X	X	X	X			Medium
Internal capsule		X		X		X	Medium
External capsule		X		X			Small
Extreme capsule		X		X			Medium
Crus cerebri		X		X			Large
Superior occipitofrontal fasciculus	X	X	X				Small
Superior longitudinal fasciculus	X	X	X				Large
Inferior occipitofrontal fasciculus		X	X	X	X		Large
Perpendicular fasciculus		X					Small
Optic nerve				X		X	Small
Optic tract				X		X	Small
Geniculocalcarine tract	X			X			Medium
Olfactory bulb	X		X				Small
Forceps major				X			Medium
Forceps minor				X			Medium
U fibers	X	X	X	X	X	X	Small
Uncinate fasciculus						X	Medium
Mamillothalamic					X		Medium
Anterior commissure		X	X				Medium
Posterior commissure			X				Small
Pyramidal tracts	X	X	X				Medium
Pyramidal decussation		X					Medium
Lateral lemnisci	X		X				Medium
Medial lemnisci	X		X				Medium
Trapezoid body	X						Small
Superior cerebellar peduncle			X	X			Small
Middle cerebellar peduncle	X						Medium
Pontine transverse	X	X	X				Medium
Pontine longitudinal	X	X	X				Medium

Reports of tumors indicate both an increase and a decrease in D^*.[22,23] The increase in D^* is greatest within cystic components. Arachnoid cysts have higher values of D^*, approaching those of CSF and water. Primary lymphoma is notable for the fact that it is associated with a reduction in D^*. A treated case of multiple sclerosis showed a normal value of D^*, but this was elevated one month after steroid treatment was stopped. In chronic plaques of multiple sclerosis D^* is increased, which is consistent with a less effective myelin barrier to diffusion.[24,25]

Vasogenic edema generally has an increased D^* compared with brain in the initial phase, but may return to normal in time.[26]

In summary, approximate values of D^* in normal subjects appear to be about 0.8×10^{-3} mm^2/s for gray matter, 0.5×10^{-3} mm^2/s for white matter with

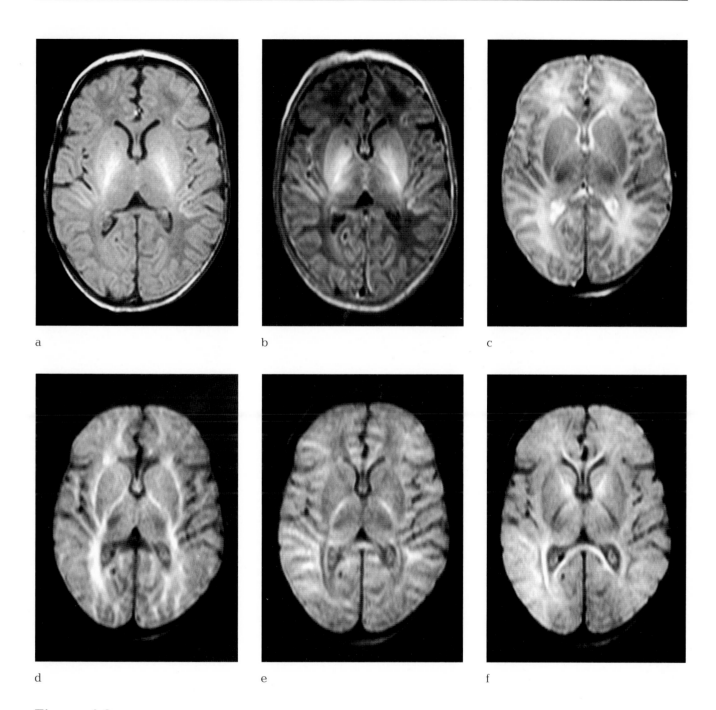

a b c

d e f

Figure 4.6

Normal term infant. SE ≈ 860/20 (a), IR 3800/30/950 (b), SE ≈ 1600/200 (c) SE ≈ 1600/200/X/65/1600 (d), SE ≈ 1600/200/Y/65/1600 (e) and SE ≈ 1600/200/Z/65/600 (f) images. On the T_1-weighted images, myelin is only seen in the posterior limb of the internal capsule (a,b). Marked anisotropy is seen in the posterior limbs of the internal capsule (d,e,f). Anisotropic changes are also seen in the hemispheres (d,e,f), where no evidence of myelination is seen on the conventional (non-diffusion-weighted) images. This may be due to very early myelination or ordered structures in nerves.

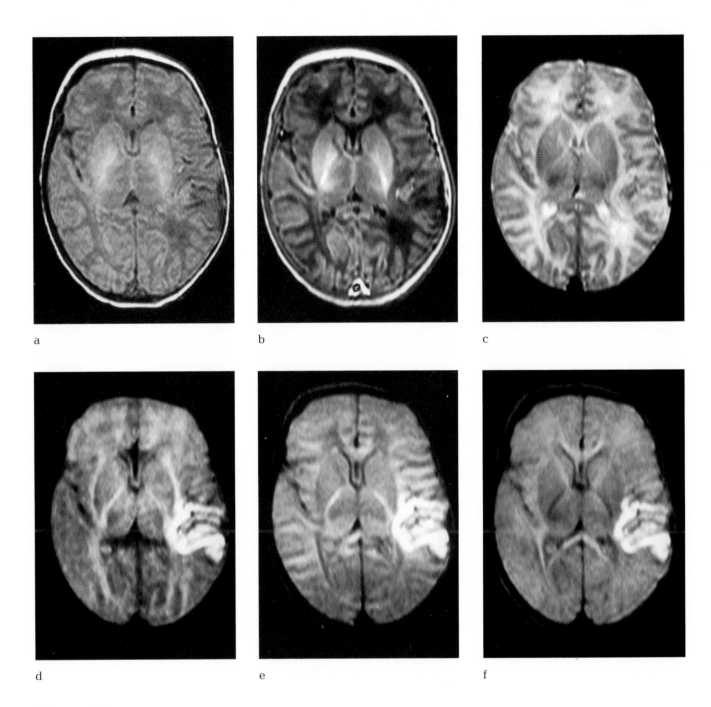

a   b   c

d   e   f

Figure 4.7

Neonatal infarction. Initial scan on day one: SE 820/20 (a), Inversion recovery IR 3800/30/950 (b), SE 1500/200 (c), SE ≈ 1500/200/X/65/600 (d), SE ≈ 1500/200/Y/65/600 (e) and SE ≈ 1500/200/Z/65/600 (f) images. The infarction is poorly seen in (a), (b) and (c) but is readily seen on the diffusion-weighted images (d), (e) and (f).

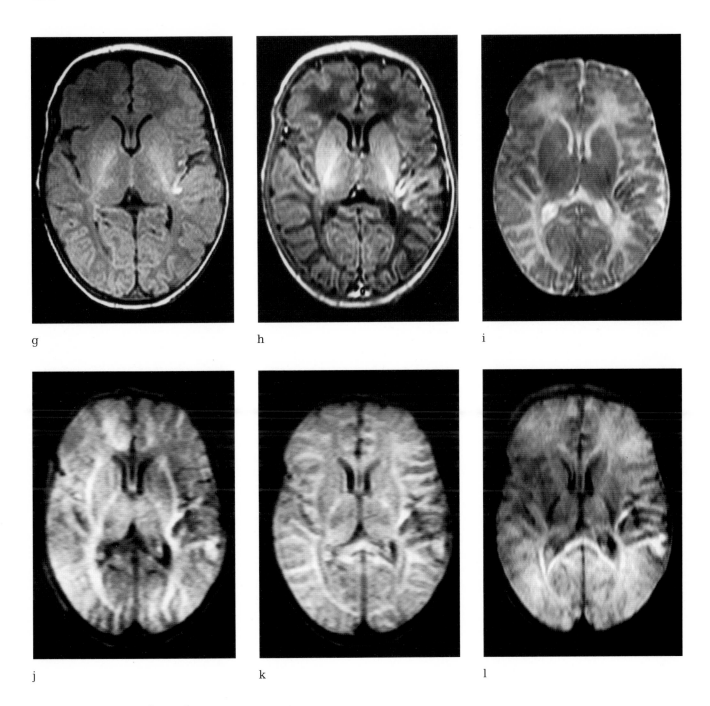

g h i

j k l

Figure 4.7 *continued*

The same patient six days later. SE 820/20 (g),
IR 3000/30/950 (h), SE ≈ 1500/200 (i), SE ≈
1500/200/X/65/600 (j), SE ≈ 1500/200/Y/65/600 (k) and
SE ≈ 1500/200/Z/65/600 (l) images. The infarct has
developed short-T_1 and short-T_2 components at its
margins, and has become more obvious on (h) and (i).
It is now much less obvious on the diffusion-weighted
images (j), (f) and (l).

sensitizing gradients transverse to the fiber direction, 10^{-3} mm^2/s for white matter with sensitizing gradients parallel to the fiber direction. A review of the literature shows that D^* is decreased in acute stroke and brain death, primary lymphoma and some stages of haemorrhage, but is normal or increased in many other conditions. These include chronic infarction, some tumors, cysts, vasogenic edema and most cases of multiple sclerosis. The degree of diffusion anisotropy present in pathologic tissues or lesions has not been assessed in detail in studies performed to date.

Whether the value of D^* for a lesion appears increased or decreased may depend on whether the lesion is compared with gray matter or white matter, as well as on the predominant fiber direction in relation to the sensitizing gradient direction. With diffusion-weighted imaging, it may be possible to radically change the contrast between a lesion and white matter simply by changing the direction of the sensitizing gradient.

Diffusion-weighted pulse sequences are usually heavily T_2-weighted by virtue of their large values of TE. A decrease in D^* in a lesion produces a relative increase in signal, whereas an increase in D^* produces a relative decrease in signal. Thus in acute stroke and brain death a relative increase in signal would be expected with diffusion-weighted imaging, but in chronic infarction, most tumors, edema and multiple sclerosis a relative reduction in signal would generally be expected. The net contrast difference obviously depends on whether gray matter or white matter is the reference tissue and what value of D^* for white matter is relevant, as well as on any anisotropy of diffusion within the lesion itself.

Infarction

Lack of blood or oxygen to the brain may result in focal infarction with damage confined to the territory of a single artery.

Studies of stroke models of middle cerebral artery infarction in cats and of global hypoxic ischemic injury in gerbils have shown that diffusion-weighted MRI can detect change within minutes of the onset of injury—which is well before conventional MRI shows changes. Areas of abnormality shown in this way subsequently become visible on conventional scans. Early changes have also been detected in acute infarction in both adults and infants (see Fig. 4.7). These evolve over a period of several days. Studies correlating these changes with difference in perfusion are in progress.

Animal studies have shown a reduction in the extent of the abnormality detected with diffusion-weighted imaging in stroke models following treatment with cerebroprotective agents. Diffusion-weighted MRI may be of critical importance for early diagnosis if new therapies of this type are used for treatment of hypoxic ischemic injury.

Hypoxic ischemic injury

In hypoxic ischemic injury (HII) damage is more generalized than in focal infarction. The symptomatology of these two conditions can overlap, and both may evolve over several days, making early diagnosis and clinical grading difficult. Focal infarction generally has a good prognosis, whilst the more severe forms of HII have a very poor outcome. Cranial ultrasound and X-ray computed tomography are generally not diagnostic of either condition in the first few days of life, and conventional T_1- and T_2-weighted MR imaging studies have not been performed in the very early neonatal period. The need for early and accurate diagnosis in these conditions has increased, because new forms of therapy may soon be available for HII, and these are likely to require administration within 6–8 h of birth before the onset of irreversible brain damage in order to be effective.

Our findings in babies with HII (see Fig. 4.8) confirm an initial decrease in D^* (relative signal increase) in the lesions followed, by a gradual increase in D^* and changes in T_1 and T_2 over a period of days or weeks in severe cases. This is consistent with animal data, though the timescale of changes is slower. We do not have a definitive explanation for this, but with animal experiments the injury is accurately timed, whereas with our infant data the injury may have occurred slowly or intermittently, and no definite timing of events is possible. This is true for both focal infarction and global injury.

Multiple sclerosis

Studies on multiple sclerosis have been of interest. The contrast developed by lesions depends on the

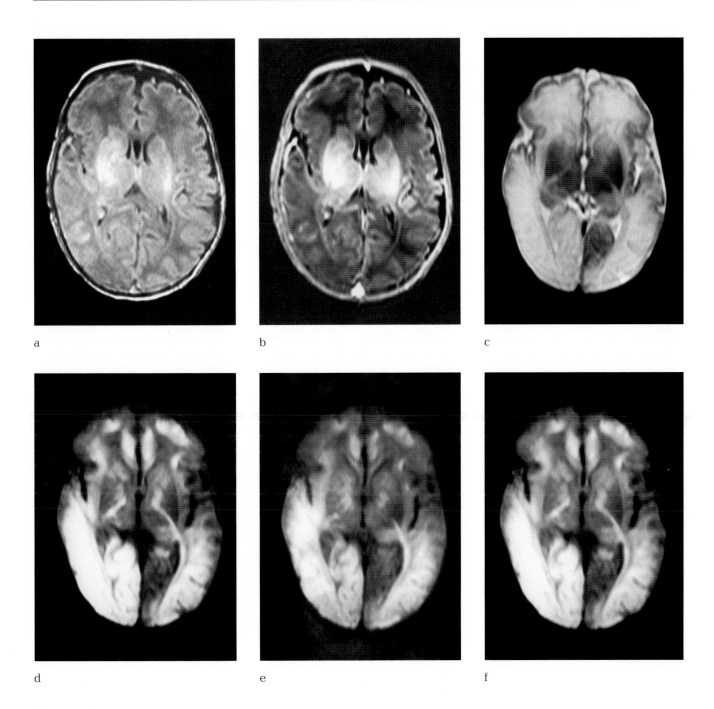

a b c

d e f

Figure 4.8

Hypoxic ischemic injury (HII). Examination on day one: SE 820/20 (a), IR 3800/80/950 (b), SE ≈ 1800/200 (c), SE ≈ 1500/200/X/65/600 (d), SE ≈ 1800/200/Y/65/600 (e) and SE ≈ 1500/200/Z/65/600 (f) images. The area of abnormality is poorly demonstrated in (a). There is evidence of more general involvement in (b) and (c), but the changes are most obvious (high-signal areas) in the diffusion-weighted images (d), (e) and (f).

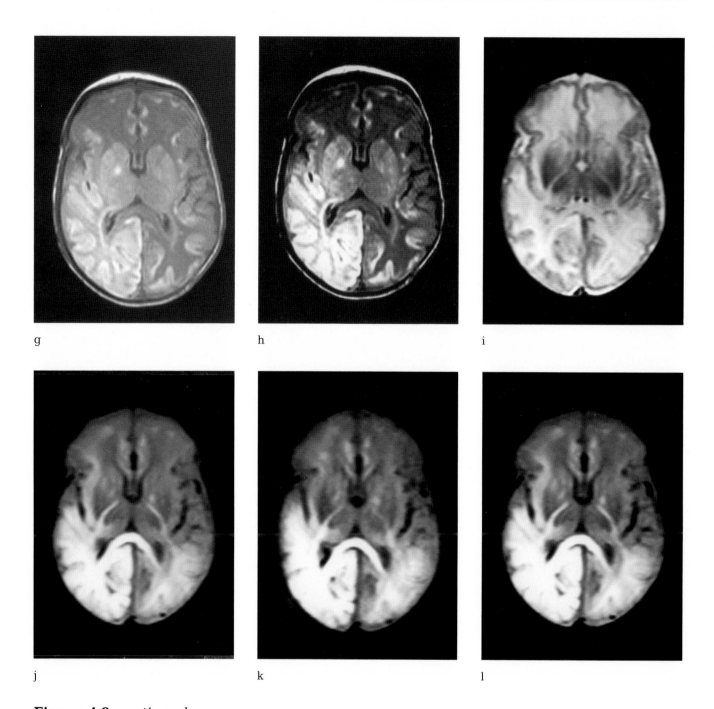

g   h   i

j   k   l

Figure 4.8 *continued*

Examination on day three: SE 820/20 (g),
IR 3800/30/950 (h), SE ≈ 1500/200 (i), SE ≈
1500/200/X/65/600 (j), SE ≈ 1500/200/Y/65/600 (k) and
SE ≈ 1500/200/Z/65/600 (l) images. The areas of
abnormality have developed a short T_1 (g,h). The area
of abnormality on the diffusion-weighted images (j),
(k) and (l) has decreased.

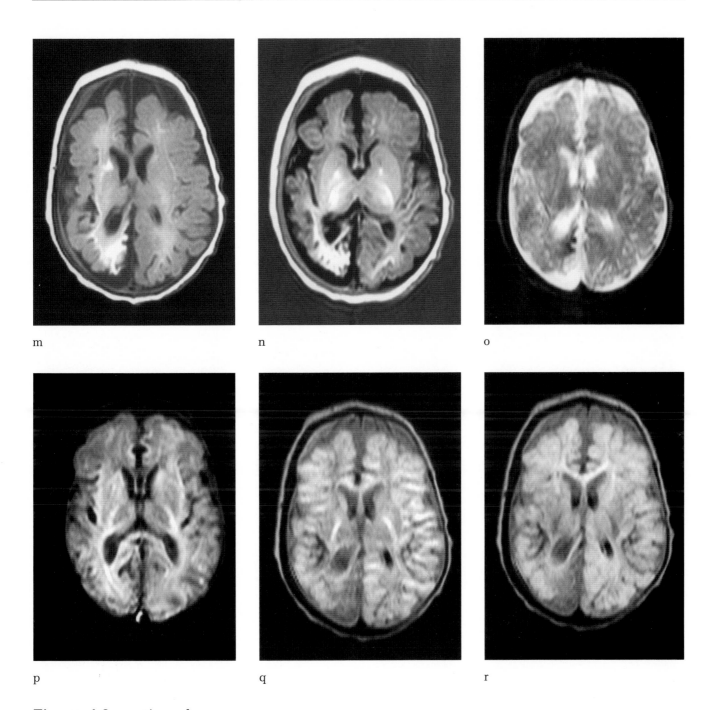

m   n   o

p   q   r

Figure 4.8 *continued*

Examination at two months: SE 820/20 (m),
IR 3800/30/950 (n), SE ≈ 1500/200 (o), SE ≈
1500/200/X/65/600 (p), SE ≈ 1500/200/Y/65/600 (q) and
SE ≈ 1500/200/Z/65/600 (r) images. The brain is
atrophic. The high-signal areas on the diffusion-
weighted images have decreased, and some
anisotropic change is now apparent (p, q, r).

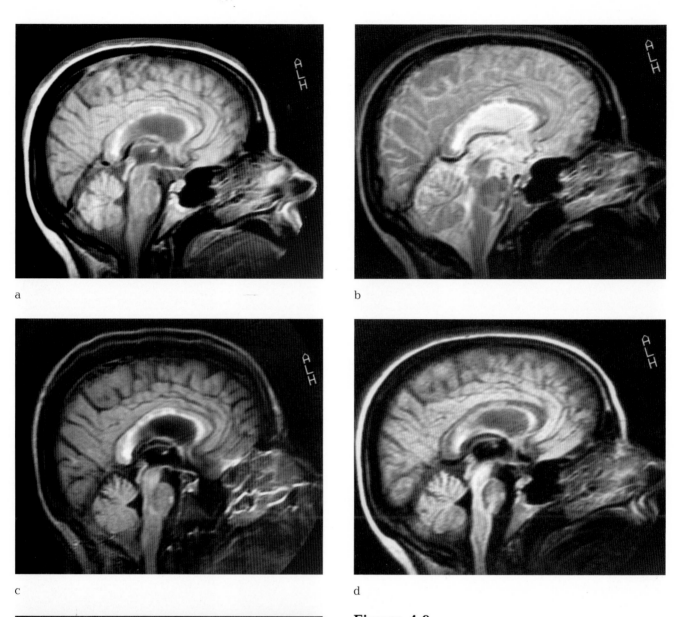

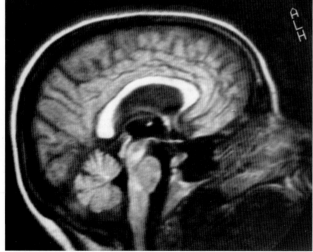

Figure 4.9

Multiple sclerosis. SE 2500/20 (a), SE 2500/80 (b),
FLAIR IR 6000/130/2100 (c), SE ≈ 1500/130/X/44/500
(d) and SE ≈ 1500/130/Y/44/500 (e) images. The
lesions in the corpus callosum are highlighted in (a),
(b) and (c). They are seen against the low signal of the
corpus callosum in (d), but not in (e).

orientation of white matter tracts relative to the gradients (Fig. 4.9). With gradients perpendicular to the predominant fiber direction, the lesions are poorly seen (e.g. the corpus callosum in Fig. 4.9e). With gradients parallel to the fibers, they are readily seen (Fig. 4.9d). In general, the D^* of lesions is increased relative to that of perpendicular white matter fibers.

While differences are relatively easy to demonstrate when there are a large number of parallel fibers, when there is a considerable mix of fiber directions image contrast properties are more difficult to predict.

Tumors

While lymphoma and subacute hemorrhage within tumors may show a reduction in D^*, in general D^* is increased in most tumors relative to gray matter and mixed-direction white matter. As a result, tumors tend to be seen with somewhat lower contrast than with equivalent non-diffusion-weighted pulse sequences. See Fig. 4.10.

Relationship of diffusion-weighted images to the FLAIR pulse sequence

Both diffusion-weighted sequences and FLAIR sequences usually employ a long TE and display a low signal intensity in the CSF. These features produce similarities in image appearance.[27]

Diffusion weighted PGSE sequences require a long TE when using conventional imaging gradient strengths ($\approx$10–20 mT/m) in order to obtain useful values of the diffusion sensitivity parameter b (i.e. about 300–800 s/mm²). Shorter values of TE are possible with insertable gradient sets that have higher gradient strength (of the order of 40 mT/m), and TE values of 120–200 ms are frequently used. These provide high T_2 weighting. With the FLAIR sequence, large TE values are an option that is frequently used to produce heavy T_2 weighting.

The CSF signal suppression can be produced either by free diffusion in the presence of a gradient (with diffusion-weighted PGSE sequences) or by an inversion pulse and subsequent use of the null point (as with FLAIR sequences). When the CSF signal is higher than that of brain, artifacts and partial volume effects between it and the brain may simulate the high signal that many lesions produce with heavy T_2 weighting. Suppressing the signal from CSF by either technique eliminates this problem.

The long values of TE used for diffusion-weighted imaging provide high sensitivity to the many disease processes in which T_2 is increased, and this, coupled with the CSF artifact suppression, may produce improved lesion conspicuity. This can be achieved with increased T_2 weighting and CSF suppression alone, as produced by FLAIR sequences, rather than with the diffusion sensitization of PGSE sequences (Figs 4.9 and 4.10).

The use of long TE with both diffusion weighting and the FLAIR sequences results in highlighting of certain specific white matter tracts that contain long T_2 components. These include the posterior corpus callosum, parietopontine, occipitothalamic and corticospinal tracts as well as the superior and inferior cerebellar peduncles, medial lemnisci and medial longitudinal fasciculi (Fig. 4.11). These are tracts that myelinate early.[28] The frontopontine tracts, anterior commissure, occipitofrontal fasciculi and pontine part of the middle cerebellar peduncles do not show this effect using TE values of 160–240 ms.

Tracts that do not show evidence of long T_2 components using long-TE FLAIR sequences are less easily highlighted with diffusion-sensitized sequences. Studies of excised nerve fibers using Carr–Purcell sequences have demonstrated that the multi-exponential decay exhibited by white matter shows anatomic variations, with tissue from different locations showing distinctly different T_2 distributions.

The high signal seen in some of these tracts with diffusion-weighted images has been attributed to a diffusion effect rather than recognized as a result of the heavy T_2 weighting.

Diffusion weighting can either increase or decrease lesion conspicuity. A reduced apparent diffusion coefficient, as in subacute stages of hemorrhage, leads to a relatively higher signal from the lesion than the surrounding brain and an increase in lesion conspicuity. If diffusion is greater for the lesion than for normal brain (as is the case with many pathologies), conspicuity may be reduced relative to the FLAIR sequence. The detailed changes that occur depend on the direction of the gradient as well as the relative proportions of white matter fibers parallel or perpendicular to it.

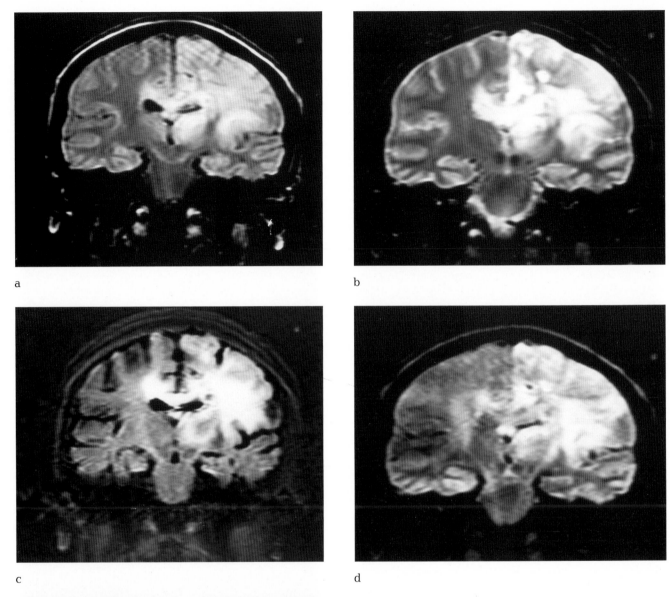

a

b

c

d

e

Figure 4.10

Infiltrating glioma. SE 2500/20 (a), SE 2500/80 (b),
FLAIR 600/160/2100 (c), SE ≈ 1500/130/X/44/500 (d)
and SE ≈ 1500/130/Y/44/500 (e) images. The tumor is
highlighted in all five images. CSF signal is reduced in
(a), (c), (d) and (e). The corticospinal tracts are
highlighted in (e). The FLAIR image shows similarities
to the diffusion-weighted images.

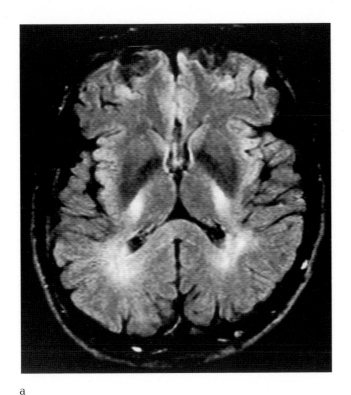

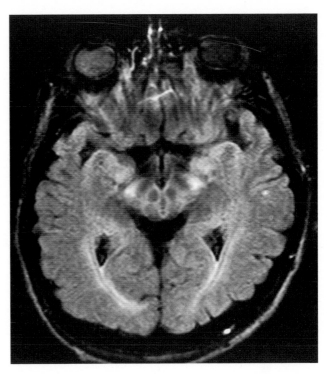

a   b

Figure 4.11

Normal male (49 years). Tranverse FLAIR
(IR 6000/200/2100) images of the brain (a) and (b).
High signal is seen in the parietopontine corticospinal
and occipitothalamic tracts.

Conclusions

Diffusion-weighted imaging provides a fascinating conjunction between the microscopic motion of water, the properties of myelinated nerve fibers, gross anatomy of the brain, and changes in water diffusion in disease.

More studies will be required in order to fully exploit the technical developments and to optimize different values of T_d and b for different tissues and diseases. Increased T_d results in an increased range of the distances that may be probed, and it is possible that relatively large values will be needed to demonstrate anisotropic diffusion in large myelinated fibers. Large values of T_d necessitate high values of TE, which result in a relatively low signal-to-noise ratio.

While large values of b result in greater contrast, they generally require a long TE and produce increased vulnerability to motion artifacts. They may also attenuate signals from tracts with low fiber density reducing the areas in which anisotropic contrast can be seen. Implementation of gradient moment nulling techniques produces better control of motion artifacts, but at the cost of lower b values per unit time.

Small gradient coils offer a wider range of options, since they produce higher gradient strength and enable lower values of TE to be used, with a corresponding increase in signal-to-noise ratio. The fact that the coils are remote from the magnet bore reduces eddy current problems. The major disadvantage is that they limit imaging of adults to the brain and limbs.

More detailed study of anatomic structures will be of considerable interest, and the development of characteristic imaging planes and direction sensitization will help in consistently obtaining images of particular tracts.

Diffusion contrast will need to be optimized in relation to the highly T_2-dependent nature of PGSE sequences. This will also require a more detailed knowledge of how D^* changes in disease. Although excellent experimental work has been done in conditions such as acute infarction, the information available in even the common neurological conditions is quite sparse. The degree to which D^* is anisotropic in lesions needs to be established.

The development of a wider variety of fast forms of imaging[29,30] besides echo planar imaging has extended the range of application of diffusion-weighted imaging, and the increasing availability of these techniques is encouraging.

References

1. Le Bihan D (ed), *Diffusion and perfusion: magnetic resonance imaging*. Raven Press, New York, 1995.

2. Hahn EL, Spin echoes. *Phys Rev* 1950; **80**: 580–94.

3. Stejskal EO, Tanner JE, Spin diffusion measurements: spin echoes in the presence of a time dependent field gradient. *J Chem Phys* 1965; **42**: 288–92.

4. Stejskal EO, Tanner JE, Use of spin echo in pulsed magnetic field gradient to study anisotropic restricted diffusion and flow. *J Chem Phys* 1965; **43**: 3579–603.

5. Le Bihan D, Lallemand D, Grenier P et al, MR imaging of intravoxel incoherent motions. Application to diffusion and perfusion in neurologic disorders. *Radiology* 1986; **161**: 401–7.

6. Thompsen C, Henriksen O, Ring P, In vivo measurement of water self diffusion in the human brain by magnetic resonance imaging. *Acta Radiologica Scand* 1987; **28**: 353–61.

7. Le Bihan D, Breton E, Lallemand D et al, Separation of diffusion and perfusion in intravoxel coherent motion MR imaging. *Radiology* 1988; **168**: 497–505.

8. Pattany PM, Phillips JJ, Chiu LC et al, Motion artefact suppression technique (MAST) for magnetic resonance imaging. *J Comput Assist Tomogr* 1987; **11**: 369–77.

9. Blinkov SM, Glezer II, *The human brain in figures and tables: a quantitative handbook*. Plenum, New York, 1968.

10. Tomasch J, A quantitative analysis of the human anterior commissure. *Acta Anat (Basel)* 1957; **30**: 902–6.

11. Wimberger DM, Roberts TP, Barkovich AJ et al, Identification of 'premyelination' by diffusion weighted MRI. *J Comput Assist Tomogr* 1995; **19**: 28–33.

12. Chien D, Buxton RB, Kwong KK et al, MR diffusion imaging of the human brain. *J Comput Assist Tomogr* 1990; **14**: 514–20.

13. Chien D, Kwong KK, Buonanno FS et al, MR diffusion imaging of cerebral infarction. *Abstracts 7th Ann Mtg Soc Magn Reson Med, San Francisco, 1988*, 889.

14. Kucharzcyk J, Mintorovitch J, Moseley M, In vivo diffusion/perfusion MR imaging of acute cerebral ischemia. In: *Future directions in MRI of diffusion and microcirculation* (ed D Le Bihan) 214–18. Society of Magnetic Resonance in Medicine, Berkeley, 1990.

15. Moonen CTW, de Vleeschouwer MHM, DesPres D et al, Restricted and anisotropic displacement of water in healthy cat brain and in stroke by NMR diffusion imaging. *Abstracts 7th Ann Mtg Soc Magn Reson Med, New York, 1990*, 1124.

16. Knight R, Ordidge RJ, Helpern JA et al, The evolution of ischemic damage in rat brain measured quantitating with diffusion maps. *Abstracts 7th Ann Mtg Soc Magn Reson Med, New York, 1990*, 376.

17. Maeda M, Itoh S, Ide H et al, Acute stroke in cats: comparison of dynamic susceptibility-contrast MR imaging with T_2- and diffusion-weighted MR imaging. *Radiology* 1993; **189**: 227–32.

18. Warach S, Chien D, Li W, Ronthal M, Edelman RR, Fast magnetic resonance diffusion weighted imaging of acute human stroke. *Neurology* 1992; **42**: 1717–23.

19. Kucharczyk J, Vexler ZS, Roberts TP et al, Echo-planar perfusion-sensitive MR imaging of acute cerebral ischaemia. *Radiology* 1993; **188**: 711–17.

20. Cowan FM, Pennock JM, Hanrahan JD et al, Early detection of cerebral infarction and hypoxic ischaemic encephalopathy in neonates using diffusion weighted magnetic resonance imaging. *Neuropediatrics* 1994; **25**: 172–5.

21. Turner R, Le Bihan D, Moonen CTW, Hedges LK, Snapshot diffusion imaging of cat brain death. *Abstracts 7th Ann Mtg Soc Magn Reson Med, New York, 1990*, 316.

22. Hooper J, Rajan S, Rosa L, Le Bihan D, Application of diffusion imaging to monitor tumor growth and response to chemotherapy. *Abstracts 7th Ann Mtg Soc Magn Reson Med, New York, 1990*, 316.

23. Tsuruda JS, Chew WM, Norman D, Moseley ME, Clinical usefulness of 'diffusion weighted' MR imaging of extra-axial brain tumors. *Abstracts 8th Ann Mtg Soc Magn Reson Med, Amsterdam, 1989*, 1003.

24. Mikulis D, Chien D, Kwong K et al, Diffusion magnetic resonance imaging in multiple sclerosis. *Abstracts 7th Ann Mtg Soc Magn Reson Med, San Francisco, 1988*, 762.

25. Larsson HBW, Christiansen P, Thomsen C et al, In vivo measurement of water self diffusion in patients with chronic multiple sclerosis. *Abstracts 7th Ann Mtg Soc Magn Reson Med, New York, 1990*, 150.

26. Sevick RJ, Karuda F, Mintorovitch J et al, Cytoxic brain edema: assessment with diffusion weighted MR imaging. *Radiology* 1992; **185**: 687–90.

27. Oatridge A, Hajnal JV, Cowan FM et al, MRI diffusion weighted imaging of the brain: contributions to image contrast from CSF signal reduction, use of long echo time and diffusion effects. *Clin Radiol* 1993; **47**: 82–90.

28. Cowan FM, Pennock JM, Schwieso J, Holland A, Early myelination and high signal intensity on heavily T2–weighted fluid attenuated inversion recovery (FLAIR) sequences: evidence for primitive myelination. *Abstracts 12th Ann Mtg Soc Magn Reson Med, New York, 1993*, 1457.

29. Butts K, De Crespigny AC, Moseley ME, Diffusion-weighted interleaved echo-planar techniques with navigation for imaging stroke. *Radiology* 1995; **197**: 390.

30. Sinha U, Sinha S, Single-slot diffusion MR imaging with HASTE. *Radiology* 1995; **197**: 391.

5

Magnetization transfer contrast

Joseph V Hajnal and Graeme M Bydder

Introduction

Magnetization transfer (MT) is a useful mechanism for manipulating tissue contrast. This chapter reviews the basic theory behind the technique, shows how both the available longitudinal magnetization and the T_1 of tissues can be changed with MT, and illustrates how these effects can be used with different pulse sequences to produce high levels of tissue contrast.

In essence, protons in tissues can be described as existing in two pools. The first or 'free' pool consists of mobile protons such as those in water. This pool has a narrow spectral line and a relatively long T_2. It provides the bulk of the signal detected with conventional whole body magnetic resonance (MR) systems. The second or 'bound' pool consists of protons bound in proteins, other large macromolecules and membranes. This pool has a very broad spectral line and a very short T_2. It is said to be 'NMR-invisible' in MRI, because its signals are not directly detectable with conventional imaging techniques.

Magnetization can be transferred from one pool to the other by dipole–dipole interaction between spins or transfer of nuclei by direct chemical means. Because the widths of the resonance lines of the two pools are very different, it is possible to substantially saturate the bound pool by applying an off resonance rf pulse while leaving the free pool virtually unaffected. This process can very largely destroy the magnetization in the bound pool, so there is little or no transfer of magnetization from it into the free pool. As a result, the available longitudinal magnetization within the free pool is reduced and its T_1 is decreased.

These changes can be used in the design and application of pulse sequences to produce substantial changes in tissue contrast.

Basic theory

The behavior of systems in which two distinct pools of spins (conventionally labelled A and B) undergo magnetization transfer has been analyzed by Forsen and Hoffman,[1] and the following discussion draws heavily on their work.

In the present context the A pool refers to NMR-visible protons (e.g. those contained in free water and some lipid-containing tissues). Other protons including those in bound water, macromolecules and membranes, are assigned to the B pool. Although the B pool is treated as a single entity, it consists of protons in heterogeneous chemical environments. The two pools have approximately the same central resonant frequency, but are distinguished by the fact that the A pool has a narrow linewidth (with a large value of T_2) while the B pool has a broad linewidth (with a very short T_2) (Fig. 5.1). Pool B is said to be NMR-invisible, since it is not detected with conventional pulse sequences because its T_2 is too short (typically <1 ms).

Key parameters used to describe the two pools are listed in Table 5.1. The longitudinal magnetization in pool A is denoted by M_A, and that in pool B by M_B. These have fully relaxed values M_{A0} and M_{B0}. M_{A0} is the maximum magnetization directly

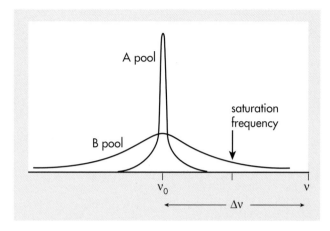

Figure 5.1

Model system showing the spectra of two resonance lines, which are both centered at the same Larmor frequency, ν_0. The A pool has a narrow line, which is associated with a long T_2, and the B pool has a broad line, which is associated with a short T_2. By applying rf irradiation at a frequency offset of $\Delta\nu$ it is possible to substantially saturate the broad resonance of the B pool while hardly affecting the A pool.

available from the tissue using conventional MRI. M_{B0} is not normally detected, and its value is not required for what follows.

The spin–lattice relaxation times of each pool in the absence of exchange are donated by T_{1A} and T_{1B} respectively. The relaxation of the magnetization in pools A and B towards equilibrium occurs both through intrinsic spin–lattice relaxation within each pool (described by the time constants T_{1A} and T_{1B} respectively) and by transfer of magnetization between the pools. This transfer occurs by through-space, dipole–dipole interactions between spins or by physical transfer of nuclei as a result of chemical exchange.

The proportion of the magnetization in pool A transferred to pool B per unit time is specified by the rate constant $K_{A\rightarrow B}$ and vice versa. The reciprocals of these rate constants give the lifetimes τ_A and τ_B of spins in each of the pools before transfer to the other pool. Thus

$$K_{A\rightarrow B} = 1/\tau_A \qquad (1)$$

and

$$K_{B\rightarrow A} = 1/\tau_B. \qquad (2)$$

The A pool loses an amount of magnetization $M_A K_{A\rightarrow B} = M_A/\tau_A$ to the B pool per unit time, but gains magnetization $M_B K_{B\rightarrow A} = M_B/\tau_B$ from the B pool per unit time. At equilibrium, these rates of loss and gain are equal.

Putting this more formally, the rate of change of magnetization in the A pool, dM_A/dt, is given by

$$\frac{dM_A}{dt} = (M_{A0} - M_A)K_A - M_A K_{A\rightarrow B} + M_B K_{B\rightarrow A} \qquad (3)$$

or

$$\frac{dM_A}{dt} = \frac{M_{A0} - M_A}{T_{1A}} - \frac{M_A}{\tau_A} + \frac{M_B}{\tau_B}, \qquad (4)$$

where M_{A0} is the value of the longitudinal magnetization at equilibrium and K_A is the rate constant for intrinsic relaxation. Corresponding equations describe the rate of change of magnetization in the B pool.

In general, if the magnetization in either pool is perturbed (for example by the rf pulses used in conventional MRI), changes occur in both pools and the recovery of each pool to the equilibrium state is bi-exponential. The normally observed spin–lattice relaxation constant for a given tissue, T_{1obs}, is a mono-exponential approximation to this behavior. Although T_{1obs} is a measured property of the visible pool A, it is also affected by the presence of pool B.

A special case occurs when one pool, say B, is held in a state of saturation. This is a state in which there are equal populations of spins in both available energy levels, resulting in no net magnetization, so that $M_B = 0$. True saturation is difficult to achieve, but by applying rf irradiation over a long period, the longitudinal magnetization is continually rotated into the transverse plane, where it continuously dephases. The end result is very little longitudinal magnetization and very little coherent transverse magnetization. Because of the broad spectrum of pool B, it is possible to selectively irradiate it by using an rf pulse offset by $\Delta\nu$ (Fig. 5.1), which has a negligible effect on the A pool. An alternative approach exploits the great disparity in the T_2 values of the two pools, and uses on-resonance rf to perturb and then return the magnetization in pool A, which saturates pool B.[2,3] We assume that as soon as the saturating pulse begins, the magnetization in the B pool is destroyed.

When the magnetization in the B pool, M_B, is reduced to zero, the terms containing M_B on the right-hand sides of equations (3) and (4) disappear, so that transfer from the B pool to the A pool ceases. However, there is still transfer of magnetization from the A pool to the B pool. While the B

Table 5.1 Parameters used to describe the free (A) and bound (B) pools

	Pool A Free, NMR-visible	Pool B Bound, NMR-invisible
Resonance peaks	Narrow, 10–100 Hz	Very broad, 10 000–50 000 Hz
Transverse relaxation time T_2	Tens or hundreds of ms	Very short, <1 ms
Longitudinal magnetization	M_A	M_B
Longitudinal magnetization with full recovery (without saturation)	M_{A0}	M_{B0} (not required)
Longitudinal magnetization with full recovery (with saturation applied)	M_{asat}	0
Longitudinal relaxation time T_1 in the absence of exchange	T_{1A}	T_{1B}
Rate constant for intrinsic relaxation	$K_A = 1/T_{1A}$	$K_B = 1/T_{1B}$
Lifetime of spins in pool	τ_A	τ_B
Rate constant for magnetization transfer	$K_{A \to B} = 1/\tau_A$	$K_{B \to A} = 1/\tau_B$
Magnetization exchanged per unit time	$M_A K_{A \to B} = M_A/\tau_A$	$M_B K_{B \to A} = M_B/\tau_B$
Longitudinal relaxation time T_1 observed by conventional MRI without saturation	T_{1obs}	—
T_1 observed with saturating rf pulse applied	T_{1sat}	—

pool is held at saturation, the recovery of the magnetization in the A pool is characterized by a new time constant, T_{1sat}, given by

$$\frac{1}{T_{1sat}} = \frac{1}{T_{1A}} + \frac{1}{\tau_A} \qquad (5)$$

The value of T_{1sat} is different from T_{1obs}. Combining (4) and (5) and integrating,

$$M_A = (M_{A0} - M_{Asat}) \exp\left(-\frac{t_{sat}}{T_{1sat}}\right) + M_{Asat}, \qquad (6)$$

where t_{sat} is the time for which the B pool has been held at saturation and

$$M_{Asat} = \frac{T_{1sat}}{T_{1A}} M_{A0}. \qquad (7)$$

M_{Asat} is the final equilibrium longitudinal magnetization that the A pool would attain if the B pool

were held in a state of saturation indefinitely. Thus, when the saturating rf is applied, the equilibrium longitudinal magnetization M_{A0} is reduced exponentially to a lower value M_{Asat} with a time constant T_{1sat}. This is illustrated in Fig. 5.2, where the curve shows the decay of M_{A0} during saturation. The above situation describes the position when there has been no recent rf pulse applied to the tissue, so that M_A is fully recovered to the value M_{A0} when saturation of the B pool begins.

If the saturating rf is applied immediately following a 90° pulse, M_A is initially zero and recovers with time constant T_{1sat} towards a final value of M_{Asat} (Fig. 5.3). Curve I shows recovery without the saturating rf and curve II shows recovery with a saturation rf applied.

If the saturating rf is applied immediately following a 180° pulse, the magnetization begins at a value of $-M_{A0}$ and recovers with time constant T_{1sat} towards a lower value M_{Asat} (Fig. 5.4). Curve I

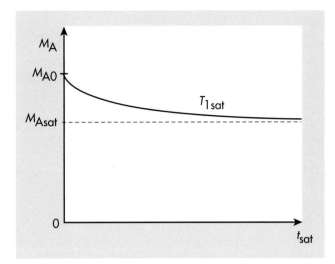

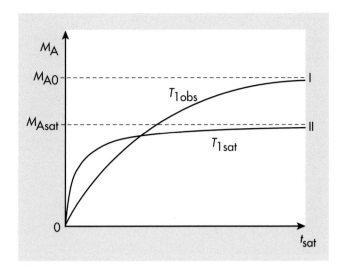

Figure 5.2

Change in longitudinal magnetization M_A with application of an off-resonance saturating rf for a time t_{sat}. M_{A0} decays exponentially with time constant T_{1sat} towards a lower value M_{Asat}.

Figure 5.3

Recovery of the longitudinal magnetization M_A after a 90° pulse: (I) in the absence of a saturating pulse and (II) in the presence of a saturating pulse applied for a time t_{sat}. In case I M_A recovers exponentially towards the value M_{A0} with time constant T_{1obs}. In case II (with the saturating pulse) M_A recovers with a shorter time constant, T_{1sat}, towards a lower value, M_{Asat}.

shows recovery without the saturating rf and curve II shows recovery with the saturating rf applied.

To summarize, the changes induced by saturating the B pool of spins for a time t_{sat} are as follows:

(a) The observed relaxation time of the A pool is changed from T_{1obs} to a new value T_{1sat} as soon as saturation begins.

(b) The MR signal obtainable from the visible pool, which normally has a fully relaxed magnetization M_{A0}, is reduced toward a new value M_{Asat} with time constant T_{1sat}. After a 90° or 180° pulse, the longitudinal magnetization relaxes towards the new value M_{Asat} with time constant T_{1sat}.

Thus saturation of the invisible macromolecule pool reduces the available longitudinal magnetization and reduces the longitudinal relaxation time T_1. In contrast, T_2 is not usually changed under the saturating conditions generally employed to manipulate magnetization transfer.

Choice of B_1 amplitude and frequency offset $\Delta\nu$ to saturate the B pool

Ideally the off-resonance irradiation should fully saturate the B pool and negligibly saturate the A pool. Although this is unlikely to be fully achieved in practice, highly selective saturation conditions can be obtained using an appropriate combination of offset frequency $\Delta\nu$ and rf amplitude B_1. Eng et al[4] have determined optimum combinations for these parameters theoretically using estimates of the spin–lattice and spin–spin relaxation times of the two pools and assuming that both pools have a Lorentzian lineshape. In view of the diverse environments of the spins that contribute to the B pool, it is uncertain what its lineshape is, and so a more empirical approach may be more appropriate.

To determine a suitable combination of $\Delta\nu$ and B_1, measurements of signal strength in regions of

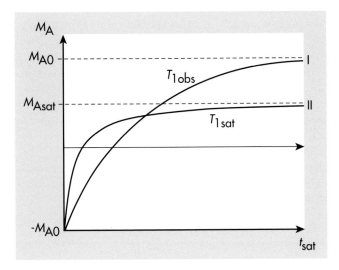

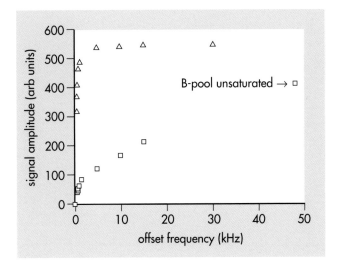

Figure 5.4

Recovery of the longitudinal magnetization M_A after a 180° pulse: (I) in the absence of a saturating pulse and (II) in the presence of a saturating pulse applied for a time t_{sat}. In case I M_A recovers from $-M_{A0}$ exponentially towards the value M_{A0} with time constant T_{1obs}. In case II (with the saturating pulse) M_A recovers exponentially from $-M_{A0}$ with a shorter time constant, T_{1sat}, towards a lower value, M_{1sat}.

Figure 5.5

Signal amplitude (squares) versus offset frequency for muscle in a normal volunteer. The data was collected at 0.15 T using the spin echo sequence shown in Fig. 5.8 with $B_1 = 17\ \mu\text{T}$ and $t_{sat} = 560$ ms (or approximately $3.7T_{1sat}$ in this case). The data point labelled 'B pool unsaturated' was obtained without applying the saturating rf pulse. For comparison data from a water phantom are also displayed (triangles). The water shows only the effects of direct saturation at low offset frequency for this value of B_1, and does not show any effect due to magnetization transfer.

interest within chosen tissues need to be made as $\Delta\nu$ or B_1 is varied. A typical curve for the signal from muscle as a function of offset frequency with B_1 approximately equal to 17 µT is shown in Fig. 5.5. Starting at the large-frequency-offset end of the graph, the initial changes in signal strength, as $\Delta\nu$ is decreased, result predominantly from progressive saturation of the macromolecular (B) pool. This effect gives way to direct saturation of the visible (A) pool as $\Delta\nu$ becomes small, finally resulting in saturation of both pools as $\Delta\nu$ approaches zero. The lack of an intermediate plateau region in which the signal is almost constant indicates that there is no range of frequency offsets for which saturation of the B pool is effectively complete and therefore unchanging, while the A pool is still negligibly saturated. Altering the magnitude of B_1 displaces the central portion of the curve, but does not result in increased selectivity of the saturation. However, it is possible to find operating conditions in which a low value of B_1 is combined with a small offset

frequency to achieve the desired degree of saturation with minimal rf dose to the subject.[5]

The lack of a regime in which M_{Asat} is insensitive to choice of $\Delta\nu$ and B_1 means that the measured tissue relaxation parameters (T_{1sat}, T_{1A} and τ_A) will be dependent to some degree on the operating conditions. The degree of direct rf saturation of the visible A pool can be estimated assuming a Lorentzian lineshape using the following relation:

$$R \approx \frac{1}{1 + (\gamma B_1/\Delta\nu)^2\ T_1/T_2} \tag{8}$$

where R is the fractional reduction of magnetization produced by partial saturation of the A pool, γ is the gyromagnetic ratio, and T_1 and T_2 take their observed values under the prevailing conditions. Thus the appropriate value of T_1 is T_{1sat}. For typical operating conditions of $B_1 = 17$ µT, $\Delta\nu = 5$ kHz and $T_{1sat}/T_2 \approx 1.8$ (which is an appropriate value for muscle), $R = 0.96$, i.e. only 4% of the

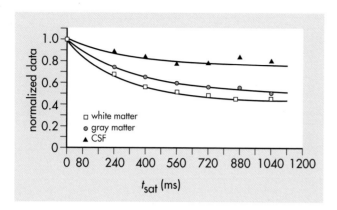

Figure 5.6

Normalized signal strength data M_{Asat}/M_{A0} measured in regions of interest in the brain of a normal volunteer as a function of the duration of the off-resonance irradiation t_{sat} using the SE sequence with $B_1 = 17\,\mu T$ and $\Delta\nu = 5$ kHz. As t_{sat} is increased from zero, the available magnetization decreases exponentially towards a lower value, M_{Asat}, as predicted by equation (6). The solid lines are three-parameter nonlinear least squares fits to the data using this equation. The data were acquired at 0.15 T.

magnetization in the A pool is lost as a direct result of the off-resonance rf.

Measurements of M_{Asat}/M_{A0}, T_{1sat}, T_{1A} and τ_A in normal volunteers

Figure 5.6 shows the measured signal of gray matter, white matter and CSF, relative to that obtained with no saturating rf (M_{Asat}/M_{A0}), as a function of t_{sat}. In each case the data were from a single adult subject using multiple regions of interest. The solid lines show a three parameter nonlinear least-squares fit to the data using equation (9).

Average values obtained from measurement at 0.15 T for the parameters T_{1A}, T_{1sat} and τ_A for gray and white matter from normal volunteers are shown in Table 5.2. Gray and white matter each

showed a reduction in available magnetization, to between 40 and 50% of their usual fully relaxed values once equilibrium was established. Likewise, their spin–lattice relaxation times were correspondingly reduced by 110 and 80 ms respectively. For comparison, typical values of T_{1obs} obtained by standard sequences without saturating the macromolecular pool are included in Table 5.2.

The values of T_{1A}, the spin–lattice relaxation time in the absence of exchange, are much smaller than would be obtained from pure water. This indicates that there may be significant relaxation mechanisms in addition to, and independent of, the magnetization transfer process.

Data from CSF were variable, and the parameters of the fitted curve are not statistically significant. It is probable that the data were contaminated by partial-volume effects from the brain and other tissues in the measured voxels.

A detailed theoretical and experimental treatment of MT in ex vivo samples from animals has been provided by Morrison and Henkleman.[6]

Magnetization transfer pulse sequences

As shown in the previous section, the incorporation of prolonged selective rf saturation pulses results in a significant reduction in the available magnetization and the observed T_1 of gray and white matter. Since the spin–lattice relaxation time changes to T_{1sat} immediately upon saturation of the B pool, but M_A only approaches M_{Asat} (and recovers again) exponentially, it is possible to vary the effects of these two parameters semi-independently by applying the saturating rf pulse at different stages of a pulse sequence. The application of saturating rf for gradient echo[7-9] and SE pulse sequences is shown in Figs 5.7 and 5.8 respectively.

Figure 5.9 illustrates various ways in which saturating rf pulses can be added to IR sequences.[10] Sequence (a) has no additional rf. In sequence (b) saturating rf is only applied during the TI period of an IR sequence, and in (c) there is an additional period of saturating rf prior to the start of the sequence to allow the magnetization time to decay towards M_{Asat} before it is inverted. Sequence (d) has a period of saturating rf prior to the inversion pulse, but none in the TI period.

Table 5.2 Relaxation times and T_{1sat}/T_{1A} calculated from pooled data from normal adult volunteers

	T_{1obs} (ms)	T_{1sat} (ms)	T_{1A} (ms)	τ_A (ms)	T_{1sat}/T_{1A}
White matter[a]	350	270±10	670±30	470±50	0.40±0.02
Gray matter[a]	450	340±40	710±10	650±14	0.48±0.06

[a] Three examinations.

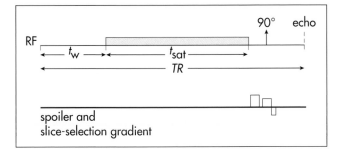

Figure 5.7

Gradient echo sequence with variable duration off-resonance rf (shaded). t_w is the waiting time, t_{sat} is the duration of the saturating pulse and TR is the repetition time.

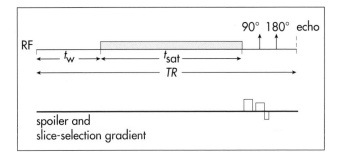

Figure 5.8

SE sequence with variable duration off-resonance rf (shaded region). t_w is the waiting time, t_{sat} is the duration of the saturating pulse and TR is the repetition time. Spoiler and slice selection gradients are applied.

Effects of MT on normal and abnormal tissue, the MT ratio (MTR)

For a specific pulse sequence and MT regime, it is possible to define the MT ratio (MTR)[11,12] such that

$$\text{MTR} = \frac{M_0 - M_s}{M_0} \qquad (9)$$

where M_0 is the magnetization without the offset irradiation and M_s is that obtained with the same sequence with the extra irradiation applied. The actual value of the MTR depends on the operating field strength and the pulse sequence, as well as the frequency, amplitude and duration of the

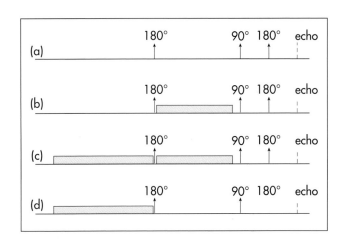

Figure 5.9

IR sequences with different distributions of saturating rf (shaded regions): (a) standard IR sequence; (b) off-resonance rf in the TI period only; (c) off-resonance rf before inversion pulse and in the TI period; (d) off-resonance rf before the inversion pulse only.

Table 5.3 Values of MTR at 0.1 T[13]

White matter	0.43
Gray matter	0.42
CSF	0.07
Pituitary adenoma	0.37
Meningioma	0.34
Craniopharyngioma	0.11
Astrocytoma grade I–II	0.14
grade III–IV	0.28
Edema in white matter	0.24

saturating irradiation. It reflects both the decrease in longitudinal magnetization and the decrease in T_1.

Tissues or fluids that show little or no MT effect (such as CSF) have a value of M_s equal to M_0, so their MTR is low. Tissues with a large MT effect (e.g. white matter) have a high MTR. It is also possible to produce MTR images based on this concept. On these images high signal (light gray) represents a high MTR (e.g. white matter), while low signal represents little or no MT effect (e.g. CSF). MTRs obtained under specific conditions at 0.1 T for tumors have been published by Lundblom[11] (Table 5.3).

Table 5.4 Values of MTR at 1.5 T[14,28]

White matter	0.42
Gray matter	0.39
Multiple sclerosis	0.25
Normal-appearing white matter	0.40
Optic nerve: normal side	0.48
affected side	0.20
Cerebral hemorrhage: acute	0.27
subacute/chronic	0.07
HIV infection:	
normal-appearing white matter	0.40
normal-appearing gray matter	0.36
Metastases (and edema)	0.27
Adjacent normal-appearing white	
matter	0.31–0.37

The MTR for white matter is slightly greater than that for gray matter. The MTRs for all tumors were less than normal brain. Those for pituitary adenomas and meningiomas were higher than those for astrocytomas. Edema in white matter occupied an intermediate position.

Another body of results have come from Grossman et al[12] in Philadelphia operating at 1.5 T (Table 5.4). In multiple sclerosis, hemorrhage and other conditions the MTR was reduced. Normal-appearing white matter had a reduced MTR in multiple sclerosis and metastatic disease, but was not reduced in asymptomatic AIDS.

The MTR from pathological tissues is reduced compared with that of white and gray matter. With this knowledge, it is possible to illustrate the contrast behavior of different pulse sequences, as shown in the next section.

Contrast properties of difference pulse sequences

For the purposes of this section, it is assumed that all disease processes will produce a reduction in MT relative to white and gray matter. Pathologic lesions have then been divided into two groups: those with a short T_1 and those with a long T_1 relative to white and/or gray matter. Contrast curves showing longitudinal magnetization M_A followed at the time of the 90° pulse by M_{xy} have been drawn for spin echo and IR (short-TI) sequences.

A T_1-weighted spin echo sequence is shown in Fig. 5.10 with pathological tissue (P) having a longer T_1 and T_2 than gray or white matter.

Application of MT produces a net loss of contrast (Fig. 5.10b).

For the case in which the lesion has a shorter T_1 than gray or white matter (e.g. subacute hematoma and early calcification) application of the MT pulse produces an increase in contrast (Fig. 5.11).

The case of a T_2-weighted sequence with a pathological lesion with a long T_1 and T_2 is shown in Fig. 5.12. Application of MT produces a net increase in contrast.

Finally, the case of a STIR sequence is illustrated for a lesion with a longer T_1 and T_2 than brain (Fig. 5.13). MT produces a net increase in lesion contrast.

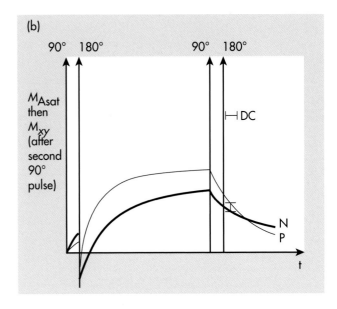

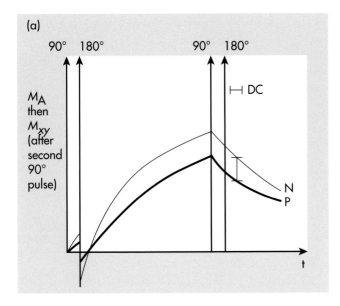

Figure 5.10

Contrast behavior for a T_1-weighted SE sequence without (a) and with MT (b). M_A then M_{xy} are plotted against time for normal (N) and pathological (P) tissue. The pathological tissue is assumed to have longer T_1 and T_2 than the normal tissue and to display less MT effect (i.e. its reduction in T_1 and available longitudinal magnetization are assumed to be less than for the normal tissue). The 90° and 180° pulses are shown together with the data collection (DC). The saturation pulse is applied between the first 180° pulse and the second 90° pulse (b). Contrast between N and P is indicated by the vertical distance between the two curves at the time of data collection. Comparison of (a) and (b) shows that MT produces a reduction in lesion contrast.

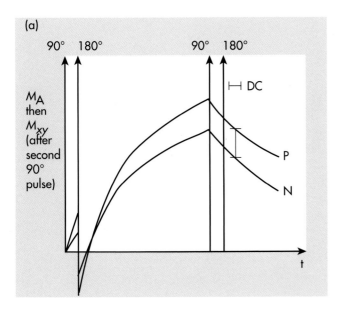

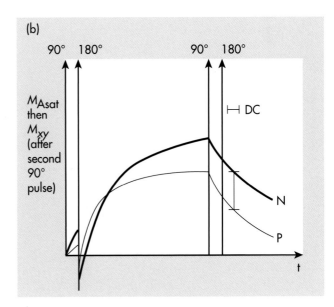

Figure 5.11

Contrast behavior for a T_1-weighted SE sequence without (a) and with MT (b). M_A then M_{xy} are plotted against time for normal (N) and pathological (P) tissue. The pathological tissue is assumed to have shorter T_1 and T_2 than normal tissue and to display less MT effect. Application of the MT pulse in (b) increases the contrast (vertical distance between P and N at the time of data collection, DC) in (b).

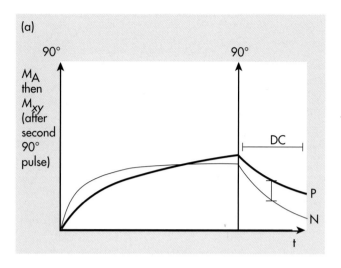

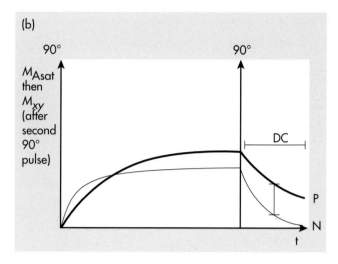

Figure 5.12

Contrast behavior for a T_2-weighted SE sequence. M_A then M_{xy} are plotted against time for normal (N) and pathological (P) tissue. The pathological tissue is assumed to have longer T_1 and T_2 than the normal tissue and to display less MT effect. The saturation pulse is applied for time t_{sat} in (b). Contrast between N and P is indicated by the vertical height between the curves at the time of data collection (DC). Comparison of (a) and (b) shows that MT produces an increase in lesion contrast.

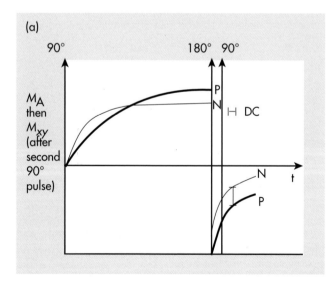

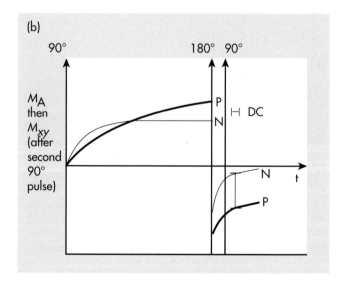

Figure 5.13

Contrast behavior for a STIR sequence. M_A then M_{xy} are plotted against time for normal (N) and pathological (P) tissue. The pathological tissue is assumed to have longer T_1 and T_2 than normal tissue and to display less MT effect. Contrast between N and P as shown by the vertical line at data collection (DC) is increased in (b).

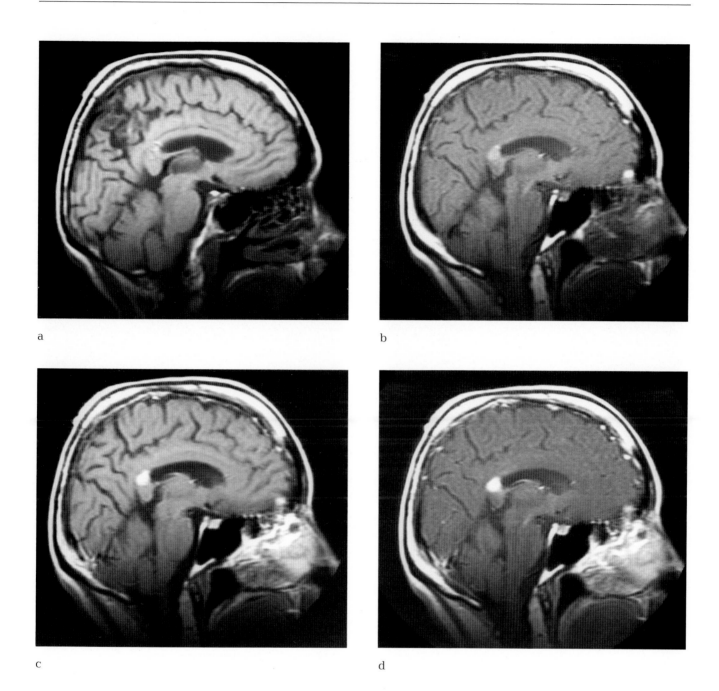

a

b

c

d

Figure 5.14

Ependymoma: T_1-weighted SE (SE720/20) without (a) and with application of saturating rf (b); repeated SE720/20 (c) and SE720/20 with saturating rf (d) following i.v. gadolinium-DTPA. Application of saturating rf in (b) increases the conspicuity of the lesion in the posterior corpus callosum. The lesion is enhanced in (c), but is seen with greatest conspicuity in (d).

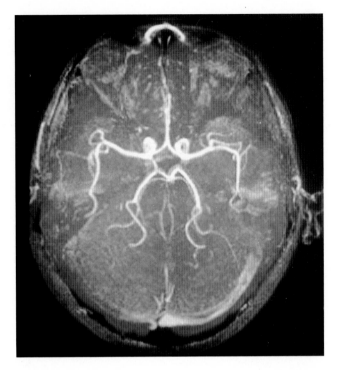

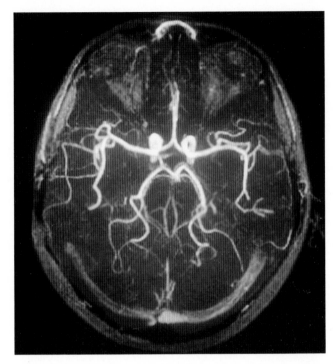

a

b

Figure 5.15

Time-of-flight angiogram: standard sequence (a) and
sequence with addition of saturating rf (b). The
conspicuity of the small vessels is increased in (b).

Contrast agents

MT has been used to improve the conspicuity
produced by contrast enhancement with intravenous gadolinium chelates since the early
1990s.[13-16] MT operates synergistically. With a T_1-
weighted spin echo sequence, it decreases the T_1
of the lesion, and so increases its signal intensity.
It also decreases the signal from the surrounding
brain. Both effects may increase the conspicuity of
the lesions (Fig. 5.14).

In general, gadolinium-DTPA (Gd-DTPA)
would be expected to affect the free pool rather
than the bound pool, but the degree to which this
occurs also depends on other factors, such as
whether or not it crosses the blood–brain barrier.
If T_{1A} is reduced by Gd-DTPA then the absolute
effect of MT is likely to be reduced. On the other
hand, if the signal intensity of a tumor is

increased by Gd-DTPA and the signal intensity of
normal brain is reduced by MT, lesion conspicuity may be increased.

Clinical applications

MT has been used in angiography to decrease the
background signal from gray and white matter,
and thus increase the conspicuity with which small
vessels are seen (Fig. 5.15).[17-19] The result is based
on the fact that blood displays a smaller MT effect
than brain. This technique is now in general use.

Another general application of MT is to increase
the conspicuity with which short-T_1 lesions are
seen with T_1-weighted sequences.[20] These lesions
usually have a signal equal to or greater than that

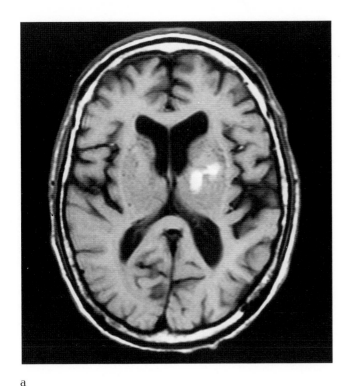

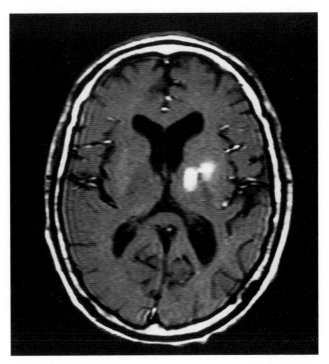

a

b

Figure 5.16

Basal ganglia calcification (short T_1): SE720/20
sequence without (a) and with saturating rf (b). The
conspicuity of the lesion is increased in (b).

of surrounding brain. MT reduces the brain signal
and increases the contrast with which the lesions
are seen. The cases illustrated here are of calcification in the basal ganglia (Fig. 5.16) and chronic
hepatic encephalopathy (Fig. 5.17).

Other abnormalities that have been demonstrated in this way include subacute hematoma,
fatty lesions and hamartomas.

Cerebral infarction is a disease where the lesion
has an increase in T_1 and T_2, and conspicuity can
be increased.[21,22] This may be important in acute
infarction, where lesions are not seen well with
conventional T_2-weighted sequences. MT has also
been of value in Wallerian degeneration when
other sequences failed to show the changes. In
the illustration of neonatal cerebral infarction the
T_2-weighted sequences are relatively insensitive,
but the lesion is more clearly shown posteriorly
than with the MT T_1-weighted spin echo (Fig.
5.18).

Increased conspicuity can also be produced with
hemorrhage.[23]

Multiple sclerosis (MS) was one of the earliest
applications of MT. The technique was initially
used to increase the conspicuity of lesions (Fig.
5.19), but more recently it has been used to differentiate between different forms of the disease.[24-26]
Individual lesions may show differences between
edematous (higher-MTR) and demyelinating
(lower-MTR) components. Abnormalities in normal-
appearing white matter have been demonstrated.

Benign tumors usually show a larger MT effect
than malignant tumors, and low-grade tumors
show a larger MT than high-grade tumors.[11,27]
Contrast can be increased, but the details depend
on whether the tumor has a longer or shorter T_1
than the surrounding brain. Meningeal enhancement may be seen more clearly (Fig. 5.20).

Malignant tumors may be seen with greater
conspicuity[27] (Figs. 5.21 and 5.22).

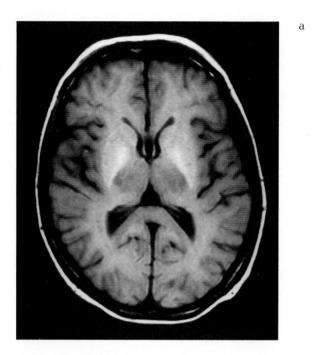

a

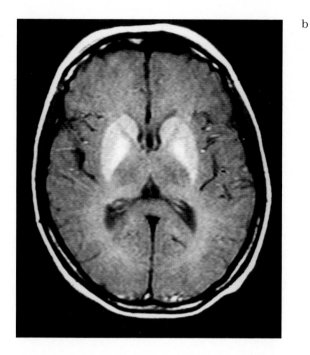

b

Figure 5.17

Chronic hepatic encephalopathy SE720/20 sequence without (a) and with saturating rf (b). The globus pallidus has a high signal in (a). The whole of the lentiform nuclei and the heads of the caudate nuclei have a high signal in (b).

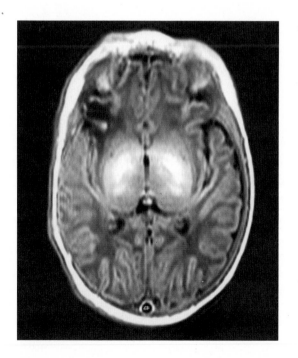

a

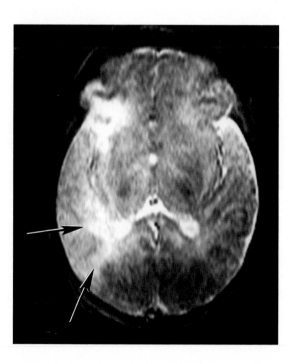

b

Figure 5.18

Neonatal cerebral infarction: IR3000/30/950 (a) and MT SE2000/20 (b) scans. The posterior area of infarction is better seen in (b) (arrows).

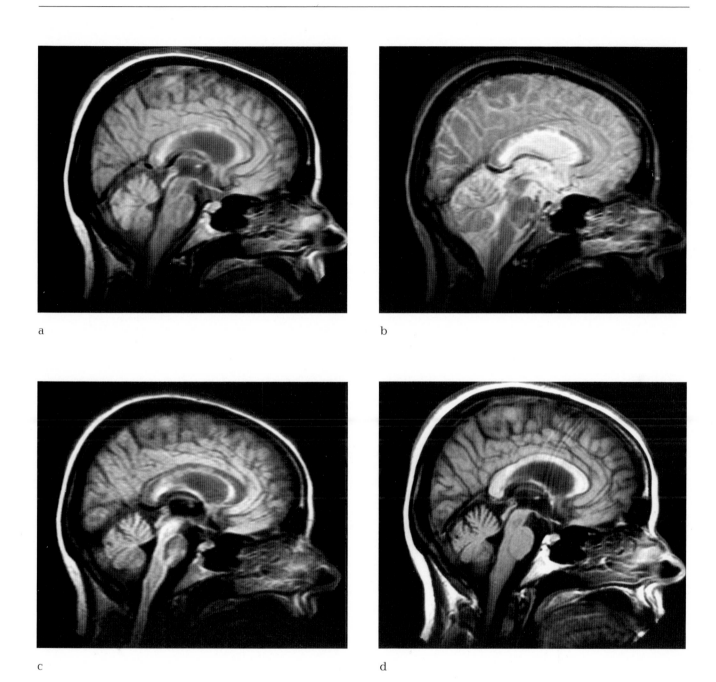

a

b

c

d

Figure 5.19

Multiple sclerosis: SE2500/20 (a), SE2500/80 (b), FLAIR6000/130/2100 (c), SE76020 (d), MT-SE760/20 (e), SE760/20 without contrast enhancement (f) and MT-SE760/20 with contrast enhancement (g). The application of saturating rf from (d) to (e) improves the conspicuity of the lesion in the corpus callosum. MT with contrast enhancement improves the conspicuity of the lesion in the pons (arrow), which is best seen in (g).

continued

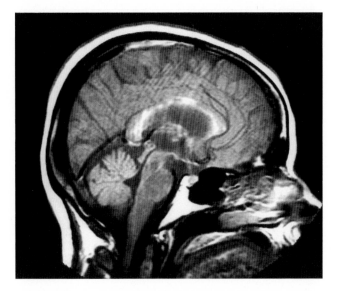

e

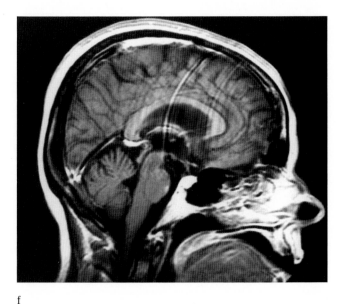

f

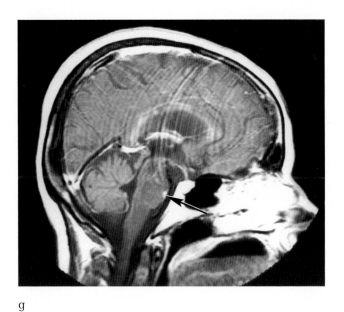

g

Figure 5.19 *continued*

Simple cysts typically show little or no MT effect. If they are isointense on a T_2-weighted sequence, they can readily be shown (Fig. 5.23).

Spinal cord

Finelli et al[28] have also shown that it is possible to increase the conspicuity of a variety of lesions in the spinal cord.

Safety

From the earliest days of this technique, there have been concerns about the rf power deposition or other adverse effects arising from the prolonged rf exposure. It is possible to keep the specific absorption rate within approved guidelines by using rf pulses that are only slightly off-resonance and so require much lower amplitude (and power). This means that the A pool may be partially saturated. By using approaches of this type, MT has been successfully applied between 0.1 and 1.5 T. However the number of slices may need to be

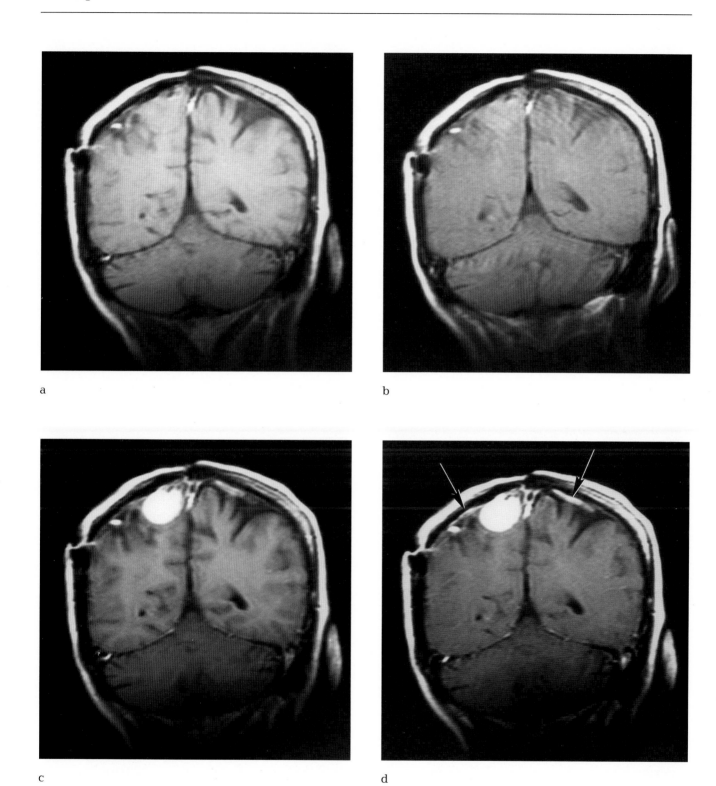

a

b

c

d

Figure 5.20

Recurrent meningioma: SE720/20 (a), MT-SE72/20 (b),
SE720/20 after enhancement (c) and MT-SE720/20
after enhancement (d). The meningeal enhancement is
best seen in (d) (arrows).

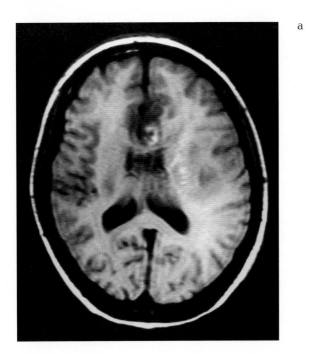
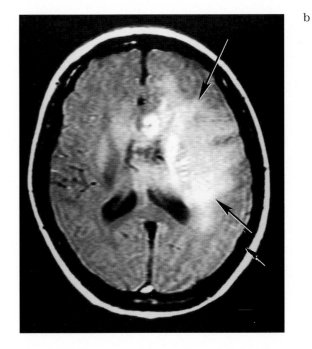

Figure 5.21

Astrocytoma: SE720/20 (a) and MT-SE720/20 (b). The
lesion is seen more clearly in (b) (arrows).

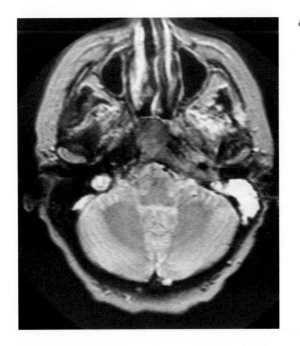
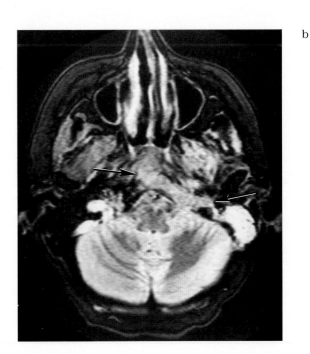

Figure 5.22

Metastases in the skull base: SE2500/80 (a) and MT-
STIR 2500/30/130 (b). The tumor (arrows) has a relatively
higher signal in (b). Fluid is seen in the left mastoid sinus.

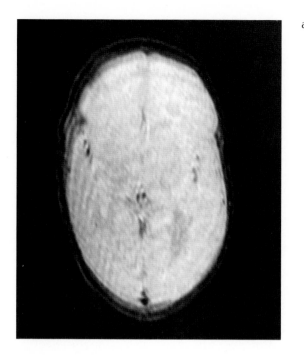 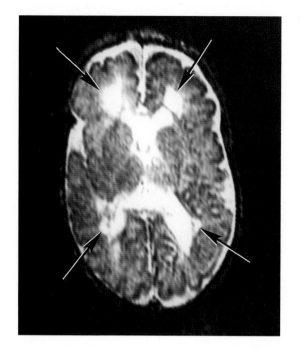

Figure 5.23

Periventricular cysts: SE2500/80 (a) and MT-SE250080 (b) images. The signal for the brain is reduced in (b), rendering the cysts more obvious (arrows).

limited, and attention to safety is necessary in implementing and operating MT sequences.

Summary

The two-pool model provides a valuable explanation of the changes in tissue contrast produced by off-resonance saturating pulses. These are explicable in terms of a reduction in both the available magnetization and T_1. The experimental data provides a specific guide to sequence design.

With sequences such as T_1-weighted SE, MT can produce an increase or decrease in lesion contrast, depending on the T_1 of the lesion. The contrast of 'proton density' or mildly T_2-weighted spin echo sequences may be increased for long-T_1 and long-T_2 lesions.

The IR pulse sequence is sensitive both to changes in the available longitudinal magnetization and to changes in T_1. The effects of reduction in available magnetization and decrease in T_1 may be synergistic in reducing tissue signal intensity with the STIR[17,18] pulse sequence. Applying MT to a STIR sequence may allow the same or higher tissue contrast to be achieved with a shorter echo time (and hence less vulnerability to motion artifacts), while still allowing the fat signal to be suppressed.

In most pathologies the MT process is less effective, so that the reduction in T_1 and available magnetization is less than that in normal tissue. The effect of MT is to increase the conspicuity developed by gadolinium chelates with T_1-weighted sequences.

Applications to date have included angiography, short-T_1 lesions, vascular disease, multiple sclerosis and tumors of the brain, as well as spinal cord disease. Quantitative approaches using the MTR may help in characterizing lesions.

Acknowledgements

We wish to thank the Medical Research Council and the Department of Health for their continued support.

References

1. Forsen S, Hoffman RA, Study of moderately rapid chemical exchange reactions by means of nuclear magnetic double resonance. *J Chem Phys* 1963; **39**: 2892–901.

2. Pike GB, Hu B, Glover GH, Enzmann DR, Magnetic resonance angiography. *Magn Reson Med* 1992; **25**: 372–9.

3. Hua J, Hurst GC, Analysis of on-and-off resonance magnetization transfer techniques. *J Magn Reson Imaging* 1995; **5**: 113–20.

4. Eng J, Ceckler TL, Balaban RS, Quantitative ^{1}H magnetization transfer imaging in vivo. *Magn Reson Med* 1991; **17**: 304–14.

5. Balaban RS, Ceckler TL, Power and frequency dependence of magnetization contrast (MTC) generation. *Abstracts 10th Ann Mtg Soc Magn Reson Med, San Francisco, 1991*, 1213.

6. Morrison C, Henkleman RM, A model of MT in tissue. *Magn Reson Med* 1995; **33**: 475–82.

7. Wolff SD, Eng J, Balaban RS, Magnetization transfer contrast: method to improve contrast in gradient-recalled echo images. *Radiology* 1991; **179**: 133–7.

8. Ordidge RJ, Knight RA, Helpern JA, Welch KMA, Magnetization transfer contrast in FLASH MR imaging. *J Magn Reson Imaging* 1991; **1**: 147.

9. Jones RA, Southern TE, A magnetization transfer preparation scheme for snapshot FLASH imaging. *Magn Reson Med* 1991; **19**: 483–8.

10. Hajnal JV, Baudouin CJ, Oatridge A et al, Design and implementation of magnetization transfer pulse sequences for clinical use. *J Comput Assist Tomogr* 1992; **16**: 7–18.

11. Lundborn N, Determination of magnetization transfer contrast in tissue MR imaging study of brain tumors. *AJR* 1992; **159**: 1279–85.

12. Grosman RI, Gomori JM, Ramer KN et al, Magnetization transfer: theory and clinical application in neuroradiology. *Radiographics* 1994; **14**: 279–90.

13. Tanttu JI, Sepponen RE, Lipton MJ et al, Synergetic enhancement of MRI and Gd-DTPA and magnetization transfer. *J Comput Assist Tomogr* 1992; **16**: 19–24.

14. Elster AD, King JC, Mathews VP, Hamilton CA, Cranial tissues: appearance of gadolinium-enhanced and non-enhanced MR imaging with magnetization transfer contrast. *Radiology* 1994; **190**: 541–6.

15. Finelli DA, Hurst GC, Gullapali RP, Bellon EM, Improved contrast of enhancing brain lesions on post gadolinium and weighted spin echo images with use of magnetization transfer. *Radiology* 1994; **190**: 553–9.

16. Mathews VP, Elster AD, Fing JC et al, Combined effects of magnetization transfer and gadolinium in cranial MR imaging and MR angiography. *AJR* 1995; **164**: 169–72.

17. Petrie GB, Hu BS, Glover GH et al, Magnetization transfer time of flight magnetic resonance angiography. *Magn Res Med* 1992; **25**: 372–9.

18. Atkinson D, Brant-Zawadski MN, Gillan GD et al, Improved MR angiography: magnetization transfer suppression with variable flip angle excitation and increased resolution. *Radiology* 1994; **190**: 890–4.

19. Dousset V, Franioni J-M, Degnese P et al, Use of magnetization transfer contrast to improve cerebral 3D MR angiography. *Neuroradiology* 1994; **36**: 188–95.

20. deSouza NM, Hajnal JV, Baudouin CJ, Potential for increasing conspicuity of short T_1 lesions in the brain using magnetization transfer imaging. *Neuroradiology* 1995; **37**: 278–83.

21. Mehta RC, Pike GB, Haros SP, Enzmann DR, Central nervous system tumor, infection and infarction: detection with gadolinium-enhanced magnetization transfer MR imaging. *Radiology* 1995; **195**: 41–6.

22. Mathews VP, King JC, Elster AD, Hamilton CA, Cerebral infarction: effects of dose and magnetization transfer saturation on gadolinium-enhanced MR imaging. *Radiology* 1994; **190**: 547–52.

23. Mittle RL Jr, Gomori JM, Schnall MD et al, Magnetization transfer effects in MR imaging of in vivo intracranial hemorrhage. *AJNR* 1993; **14**: 881–91.

24. Tanttu JI, Sepponen RE, Foust RJ, Kinnunen E, MR of multiple sclerosis plaques at 0.1 T: correlation between magnetization transfer contrast, $T_1\rho$ dispersion, T_1 values and intensity as T_2 weighted images. *Abstracts 9th Ann Mtg Soc Magn Reson Med, New York, 1990*, 356.

25. Loevner LA, Grossman RI, Cohen JA et al, Microscopic disease in normal-appearing white matter on conventional MR images in patients with multiple sclerosis: assessment with magnetization-transfer measurements. *Radiology* 1995; **196**: 511–15.

26. Heihle JF, Lenkinski RE, Grossman RJ et al, Correlation of spectroscopy and magnetization transfer imaging in the evaluation and demyelinating lesions and normal appearing white matter in multiple sclerosis. *Magn Reson Imaging* 1994; **32**: 285–93.

27. Boorstein JM, Wong KT, Grossman RI et al, Metastatic lesion of the brain: imaging with magnetization transfer. *Radiology* 1994: **191**: 799–803.

28. Finelli DA, Hurst GC, Karaman BA et al, Use of magnetization transfer for improved contrast in gradient echo MR images of the cervical spine. *Radiology* 1994; **193**: 165–71.

6

Contrast properties of the inversion recovery sequence

Ian R Young, Graeme M Bydder and Joseph V Hajnal

Introduction

The inversion recovery (IR) pulse sequence has been used to provide heavily T_1-weighted images since the earliest days of clinical MR. It was used in the first studies that showed an advantage of MR over X-ray computed tomography (CT).[1] The sequence produced high contrast between normal and pathological tissues that had a prolonged T_1, and was the single most effective imaging technique available from 1980 to early 1982.

The introduction of the heavily T_2-weighted spin echo (SE) sequence into clinical practice in 1982[2-4] provided a very useful approach for disease detection based on differences in T_2. This has since become the mainstay of clinical diagnosis in the brain and spinal cord. T_1-weighted SE sequences also provided a method for obtaining T_1-weighted images that were lower in contrast than IR sequences, but were quicker. As a result, there was less need for the IR sequence.

MR studies from 1980 to early 1982 only involved a single slice, and were performed at low fields (0.04–0.15 T). After this time, there was a general tendency to increase operating field strength, which increases tissue T_1 and prolongs the time required for the IR sequence for equivalent image contrast. Multislice techniques were also implemented during this time, and these required slice-selected 180° pulses. While slice-selected 90° pulses were easy to implement, it took some time to achieve this with 180° pulses. Also, the IR sequence, with its relatively long interval between the initial 180° pulse and the subsequent 90° pulse, was more difficult to interleave into a multislice format than conventional SE sequences.

For these reasons, the conventional IR pulse sequence was displaced as the principal pulse sequence used for diagnostic purposes, but it continued to have many applications when high T_1-weighted contrast was desired, such as in detecting contrast enhancement[5] or in demonstrating myelination in infants.[6,7]

A particular variant of the IR sequence in which the timing of the initial inversion pulse was set to null the signal from fat (which has a very short T_1) and TE was chosen to provide very high lesion contrast proved to be very useful in head, neck and spine applications.[8,9] This short-inversion-time IR (STIR) sequence combined fat suppression with high lesion contrast, and did not require the careful shimming needed with frequency-selective fat suppression techniques. The sequence was particularly well suited to mid- and low-field applications where chemical shift techniques for fat suppression are difficult or impossible to implement.

The capacity of the IR sequence to null fluids has also been exploited in the form of the fluid attenuated IR (FLAIR) sequence, where CSF is suppressed and mild or heavy T_2 weighting (long TE) is used to detect lesions in the brain and spinal cord.[10,11]

Both fluid suppression and fat (or white matter) suppression can be combined in the form of the double inversion recovery (DIR) sequence, which can be used, for example, to isolate the cerebral cortex.[8,12]

With the development of faster imaging techniques for clinical use, such as the RARE sequence,[13] the rapid gradient echo sequence,[14,15] combinations of these,[16] and echo planar imaging,[17] there has been renewed interest in the use of the IR sequence. With these sequences, the time penalty associated with the IR sequence is no longer felt so acutely. Also, many of the faster sequences have unfavorable contrast properties that can be modified to make them more useful by application of an appropriately timed inversion pulse prior to the data collection. The clinical uses of these sequences parallel those previously developed with slower versions of the IR sequence, but they have the substantial advantage that they can be performed much more rapidly. Details of both the fast spin echo sequence and echo planar imaging are given in other chapters in this book.

The flow effects of the IR inversion recovery sequence have never received the same attention as those of the SE sequence, but are now achieving more recognition. Inversion pulses have been used to label inflowing blood outside of the slice of interest as a measure of tissue perfusion.[18]

In the following section the basic form of the IR sequence is described, followed by outlines of the STIR, FLAIR, DIR and other forms of the IR sequence.

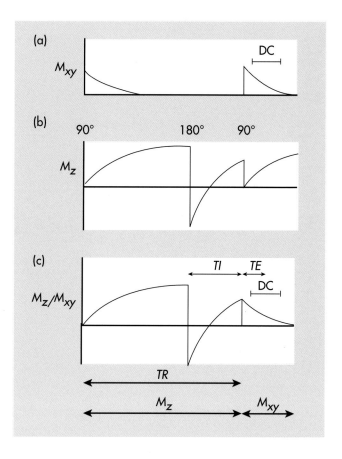

Figure 6.1

Changes in M_{xy} (a) and M_z (b) with time in the IR sequence (medium-TI) using gradient echo data collection (DC). (c) shows M_z initially, then M_{xy} in the last segment. The 90° pulse of the preceding cycle is shown at A and that of the cycle under study at B. The cycle repetition time is TR.

The basic form of the inversion recovery sequence

The dependence of signal intensity seen with the IR sequence on proton density, T_1 and T_2 can be described in mathematical terms using the Bloch equations, but for simplicity a qualitative description of the IR sequence is used in this chapter. (The specific relationships are given in the Appendix.) The proton magnetization induced in the patient by the static magnetic field can be represented by a vector $\mathbf{M}$. The component of the magnetization in the transverse plane at any given time is then represented by M_{xy}, and that in the longitudinal direction at the same time by M_z. The effect of a 90° pulse is to rotate M_z into the transverse plane to become M_{xy}.

Following the 90° pulse, M_z increases exponentially from zero with time constant T_1 (Fig. 6.1b) and M_{xy} decays exponentially with time constant T_2 (Fig. 6.1a). A 180° pulse inverts M_z to become $-M_z$ and it then recovers with a time constant T_1 but initially at *twice* the rate for the earlier longitudinal recovery after the 90° pulse. At the next

90° pulse, M_z is rotated to become M_{xy}. M_{xy} then decays exponentially with time constant T_2. Using a gradient echo (or SE) data collection, the signal is collected at a mean time TE after the 90° pulse, and the cycle is repeated.

A composite diagram following first M_z then M_{xy} after the second 90° pulse can be used to represent the 'potential signal intensity' at various stages of the sequence (Fig. 6.1c). The size of the received signal and ultimately the signal intensity or voxel value in the image is proportional to M_{xy} at the time of data collection (DC). M_{xy} is also proportional to tissue proton density.

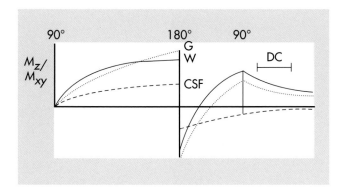

Figure 6.2

Changes in M_z/M_{xy} with time in the IR sequence (medium-TI) for white matter (W), gray matter (G) and CSF, using gradient echo data collection (DC). The signal intensity on the image is proportional to the height of M_{xy} at the middle of DC. White matter is highest, followed by gray matter, then CSF.

Times labeled TI and TE are shown in Fig. 6.1(c). TI is the inversion time between the inverting 180° pulse and the following 90° pulse, and TE is the time from the last 90° pulse to the following echo. TR is the duration of each cycle of the sequence.

Using Fig. 6.1(c) as a model of the IR sequence, we can next compare the signal intensities of white matter (which has a relatively short T_1), gray matter (which has a longer T_1) and CSF (which has a very long T_1) as in Fig. 6.2. The observed signal intensity is proportional to the height of M_{xy} at the time of DC, and it can be seen that the shorter T_1 of white matter results in a higher signal intensity than for gray matter. The very long T_1 of CSF results in a low signal intensity, which may be negative as in Fig. 6.2. The last segment of the decay converges towards zero for both gray and white matter with their positive signal intensities, as well as for CSF with its negative signal intensity. Display of the resultant image after phase-corrected processing (see later) gives white signal intensity for white matter, light gray for gray matter and black for CSF. The signal for gray matter is slightly greater than that for white matter at the time of the 180° pulse because of its greater proton density.

The general rule is that a repetition time TR of at least $3T_1$ should be allowed for recovery of the longitudinal magnetization between the 90° and the last pulse cycle and the following 180° pulse of the next cycle to allow a high level of recovery of M_z, though, in practice, it may be possible to use times less than this. Reducing TR produces a reduction in signal intensity for tissues with a long T_1, though there is little effect on tissues with a short T_1 where TR is still greater than $3T_1$. Reducing TR is therefore used to reduce the relative signal intensity of tissues or fluids such as CSF that have a very long T_1.

There are two types of image reconstruction available: *phase-corrected*, where positive values of signal intensity are shown positive and negative values appear negative, and *magnitude*, where the magnitude of the signal is used irrespective of its sign. CSF appears dark with phase-corrected processing, but may show a 'rebound' with a lighter central area with magnitude processing. The signal intensities follow directly from considering Fig. 6.2.

The 90° pulse in the IR sequence is always slice-selected, though for single scans the 180° pulse(s) need not be. However, when the IR sequence is used to obtain an interleaved set of slices, the 180° pulse(s) must be slice-selected. When the 180° pulse is slice-selected, it is possible for flowing blood to experience only part of the IR sequence, depending on where it is at the time of the inversion pulses. For example, blood flowing into a slice may only experience a 90° pulse and behave as though it is being imaged with a partial saturation sequence, producing a high signal intensity rather than the usual low signal intensity.

In initial studies the data collection (DC) was achieved with a single phase-encoding step after each 90° pulse. It is also possible to collect data with multiple phase-encoding steps and thus decrease the scan time. Thus, the rapid gradient echo sequences can be used to acquire data for a whole image in one or two seconds as a comprehensive data collection. The term magnetization preparation' has been applied to the use of the IR (and other pulse sequences) in this context. The magnetization-prepared rapid acquisition gradient echo (MP-RAGE) sequence has proved particularly useful in producing highly T_1-weighted volume images of the brain.[19] The rapid acquisition with relaxation enhancement (RARE) sequence employs multiple phase-encoding steps with repeated 180° SE pulses. The echo planar imaging technique typically acquires all the data for one image in a single shot, with data being acquired for 40–200 ms.

The contrast properties described previously apply to these sequences, though in slightly more complex form. The increase in the duration of DC

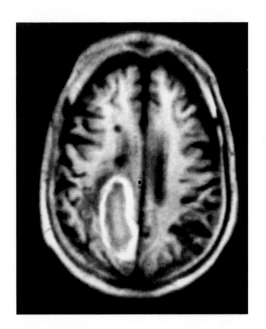
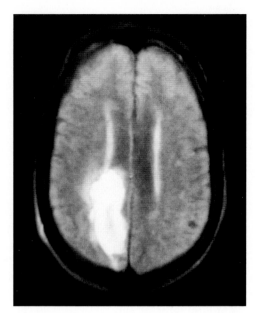

a   b

Figure 6.3

Subacute hematoma
(0.15 T) medium-*TI* IR
sequence: transverse
IR1500/44/500
(IR*TR/TE/TI*) (a) and
SE1500/80 (b) scans.
There is high
gray–white matter
contrast. The rim of the
hematoma has a short
T_1 and a high signal
rim in (a).

means that *TI* and *TE* are not so precisely defined. These fast forms of the IR sequence are now receiving greater emphasis, and are very likely to be the way in which this sequence will be used in the future.

It is useful to consider three main variants of the IR sequence according to their values of *TI*:

(i)   the medium-*TI* inversion recovery sequence (e.g. *TI* of 200–800 ms);
(ii) the short-*TI* (STIR) sequence (e.g. *TI* of 80–150 ms);
(iii) the long-*TI* (FLAIR) sequence (e.g. *TI* of 1500–2500 ms).

These will be dealt with in the next three sections. Since tissue T_1 values increase with field strength, the appropriate values of *TI* for use in each group also increase with field strength (although least for the long-*TI* (FLAIR) sequence).

The medium-*TI* IR sequence

The working rule to obtain an image with good contrast between two tissues of different T_1 values is to choose a value of *TI* intermediate between the

T_1 values of the two tissues of interest (neglecting the effects of proton density and T_2). Thus at 0.15 T satisfactory contrast between white matter (T_1 = 350 ms) and gray matter (T_1 = 450 ms) is achieved with a *TI* of about 400 ms. Note that the signal intensity is not maximal at this point, so the image appears noisier than that obtained with, for example, *TI* = 500 ms, where the signal is higher (although the gray/white matter contrast is less). In theory, maximum contrast is obtained when *TI* is about 0.69 times the average of the T_1 values for the two tissues, but the signal levels in this case are close to zero, so maximizing the appearance of the noise of the image. Note that the *TI* for optimum contrast between gray matter and a tumor or an infarct (which have an increased T_1) is greater than that for gray and white matter. These features are illustrated in Fig. 6.3, which shows a subacute hematoma. White matter is white, gray matter is gray, and there is a high level of contrast between them. The hematoma has a high signal intensity.

There are two additional modifying factors. The increased mobile proton density of gray matter relative to white matter results in slightly less tissue contrast. More important is the fact that the T_2-dependent period following the 90° pulse and prior to data collection may produce a *reduction* in net tissue contrast. This is particularly so for lesions that follow the common pattern and have an increase in both T_1 and T_2. Thus the T_2-dependent decay, in the last component of the sequence,

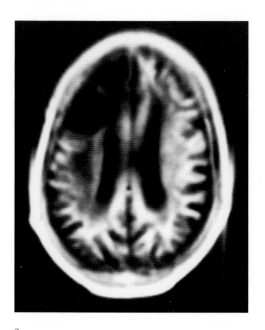

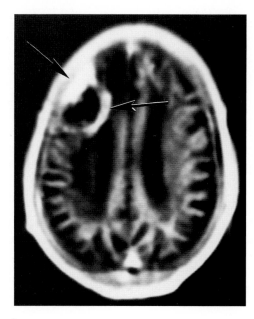

a   b

Figure 6.4

Metastases to the brain
(0.15 T)—the first
patient in whom MR
contrast enhancement
was demonstrated in
the brain (1983):
Transverse medium-*TI*
(IR1400/5/400 scans
before (a) and after i.v.
gadolinium-DTPA
(dimegluminė
gadopentetate) (b).
Ring enhancement
(arrows) is seen around
the low-signal-intensity
tumor (b).

reduces the T_1 contrast developed earlier in the sequence.

The method of image reconstruction and the type of data collection effect the choice of *TE*. *TE* can generally be shorter with projection reconstruction than with 2D Fourier transformation (2DFT), since a single vector encoding gradient is used, without the need for a previous phase-encoding gradient as with 2DFT. A gradient echo data collection can be completed earlier than a SE data collection with the same bandwidth, although the former is more vulnerable to B_0 field inhomogeneities. With the brain ($T_2 \approx 100$ ms) the T_2 dependence of the IR sequence is not such a problem as it is in the body, where values of T_2 are typically half of those in the brain (45–60 ms), making the same IR sequence much more T_2-dependent than when it is used in the brain. The use of low values of *TE* to control this problem then becomes important.

The medium-*TI* IR sequence shows high gray–white contrast in the brain as well as strong sensitivity to pathology. Many lesions have a long T_1 and a low signal intensity with this sequence. The sequence is also very sensitive to contrast enhancement (Fig. 6.4).

The sequence has been of considerable interest in the form of 3D MP-RAGE. This provides high-contrast thin-section 3D images of the brain with sensitivity to pathology comparable to conventional 2D T_2-weighted spin echo sequences, but with the addition of 3D capability and sensitivity

to contrast enhancement with i.v. gadolinium-DTPA (dimeglumine gadopentetate). T_2-weighted 3D volumes have been difficult to achieve, and they are not sensitive to contrast enhancement, so that the 3D MP-RAGE sequence has been proposed as the basic approach for imaging the brain.

The sequence is used in pediatric brain imaging for detecting myelination and subtle pathology in neonates. The brain contains increased water at this age, and lesion contrast obtained from IR sequences for ischaemia and infarction is helpful in this situation.

At lower field there is an advantage in the use of T_1-weighted approaches. The T_1 of tissues is shorter than at high fields, so that *TR* can be shortest and the T_1-weighted contrast may be higher.

The short-*TI* inversion recovery (STIR) sequence

Values of *TI* under discussion here are about 80–150 ms. In the limit where *TI* equals zero (or, from a practical point of view, about 1 ms) the 90° and 180° pulses add to give a 270° pulse, which is

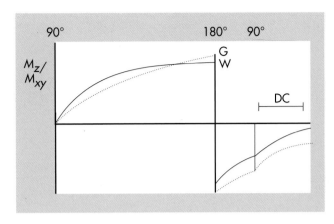

Figure 6.5

Changes in M_z/M_{xy} with time for the STIR sequence. The size of the signal from gray matter (G) is greater than that from white matter (W). When magnitude processing is used, it has a higher signal.

equivalent to a –90° pulse. This is equivalent to a 90° pulse, and the sequence becomes 90° data collection, or the gradient echo sequence. Thus the gradient echo sequence can be regarded as a limiting case of the IR sequence with $TI = 0$. The same reasoning applies when a SE data collection is used, and the IR sequence (with $TI = 0$) becomes equivalent to a standard SE sequence. Using magnitude reconstruction with TI in the range of 80 to about 150 ms, an IR image of the brain appears like an SE one, although with greater gray–white matter contrast. The magnetization curves can be represented as shown in Fig. 6.5.

Note that, following the final 90° pulse, the T_1 contrast and the T_2 contrast are *additive*; i.e. increasing the T_1 of a tissue increases the tissue's relative signal intensity, and so does increasing its T_2. (This is not the case in Fig. 6.2, which illustrates medium values of TI.) The short-TI IR (STIR) sequence is sensitive to changes in T_1 and T_2, and can be used as a screening sequence in the brain in a similar way to the SE sequences with long TE and long TR such as SE2500/80 (Fig. 6.6). To reduce the signal intensity of CSF to less than that of white matter, TR can be shortened to

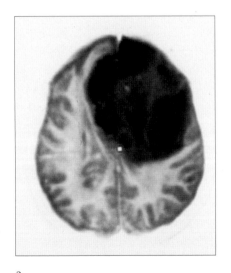

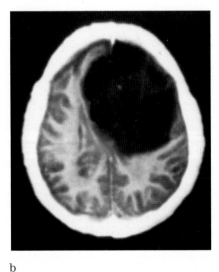

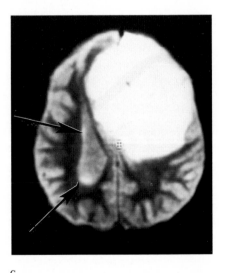

a   b   c

Figure 6.6

Glioma (0.15 T): STIR (IR1500/44/100) sequence, real reconstruction (a), real construction displayed without the surrounding noise (b), and magnitude reconstruction (c). The tumor has a long T_1 and is in low signal in (a) and (b) but is highlighted in (c). Additional lesions are seen in (c) (arrows).

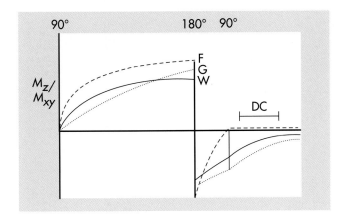

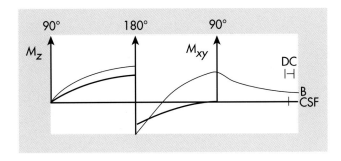

Figure 6.7

Changes in M_z/M_{xy} with time for fat (F), white matter (W) and gray matter (G), using a fat-suppressed STIR sequence. The signal from gray matter is greater than that from white matter. Fat gives no signal.

Figure 6.8

M_z followed by M_{xy} for brain (B) and CSF during the FLAIR sequence. Following the first 90° pulse, the brain recovers more quickly than the CSF. After the 180° pulse, brain largely recovers, but CSF with its long T_1 only reaches zero magnetization when the second 90° pulse is applied. The brain signal then decays with time constant T_2, while the CSF signal remains zero.

1000 ms with a sequence such as IR1000/44/100 (at 0.15 T).

Since many pathological lesions produce an increase in both T_1 and T_2, the addition of these two types of contrast with the STIR sequence produces a high net tissue contrast. This type of sequence also enables some T_1-dependent decay to be substituted for the T_2-dependent decay in the equivalent SE sequence. This is of particular value where the T_1 and T_2 decays of the tissues differ, and explains why the gray–white matter contrast of this sequence is greater than that of the equivalent SE sequence.

It is also possible to choose particular values of TI so that the signal intensity of a particular tissue is zero at the time of the 90° pulse. (This occurs at a value of TI that depends on T_1 and TR, but is typically between $0.5T_1$ and $0.65T_1$, with a maximum of $0.69T_1$ for $TR > 3T_1$). At 0.15 T, values of about 100 ms are suitable to eliminate the fat signal (Fig. 6.7), while 255 ms is adequate for white matter. In this situation the tissue signal is said to be 'suppressed'. Suppression or partial suppression of the fat signal is of particular value in imaging of the orbit, head and neck as well as the spine.[20–23]

The STIR sequence provides robust fat suppression at any field strength, though it has the disadvantage that it is insensitive to contrast enhancement unless TR is shortened.[24] Because of difficulties in performing chemical-shift-sensitive

fat suppression, it is the fat-suppression technique of choice at medium and low field strengths.

Long-*TI* or fluid attenuated inversion recovery (FLAIR) sequence

If TI is increased to 2000–2500 ms and TR is suitably extended then the signal from CSF can be reduced to zero while the magnetization from brain very largely recovers (Fig. 6.8). With the signal from CSF very greatly reduced, it is then possible to use echo times of 100–200 ms and develop high contrast without problems from CSF artifacts (Fig. 6.9). The resultant fluid attenuated IR (FLAIR) sequence has been used in the brain in multiple sclerosis, epilepsy (Fig. 6.10) and many other conditions.[10,25–27]

It is particularly useful in regions of the brain where partial volume effects from CSF cause difficulty. Its reduced gray–white contrast (as a result of incomplete recovery of the brain magnetization) provides a bland background against which lesions are readily seen (Figs 6.11 and 6.15). The sequence is also of value in demonstrating low-contrast lesions,[28,29] as well as subarachnoid hemorrhage[30].

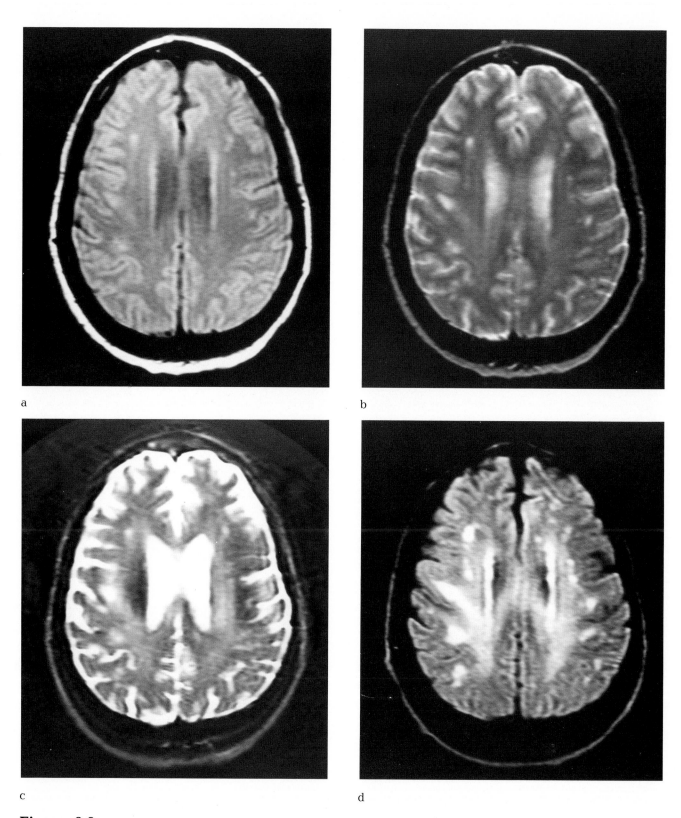

a

b

c

d

Figure 6.9

Viral infection of the brain (1.0 T): SE2500/20 (a), SE2500/80 (b), SE2500/160 (c) and IR 6000/160/2100 (FLAIR) (d) sequences. Deep white matter and periventricular lesions are seen in (a) and (b). Increasing *TE* to 160 ms (c) increases artifacts from the CSF and produces little net benefit. The FLAIR sequence at the same *TE* (160 ms) suppresses the CSF signal and highlights the lesions, which appear more extensive than in (a) or (b).

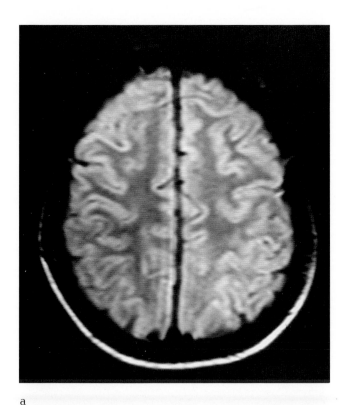

a

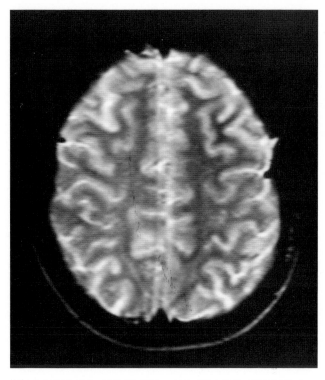

b

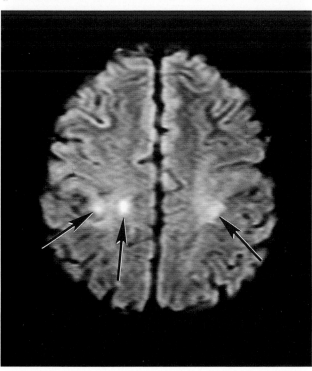

c

Figure 6.10

Multiple sclerosis (1.0 T): SE2500/20 (a), SE2500/80 (b) and IR6000/160/2100 (c) scans. The lesions (arrows) are only seen on (c).

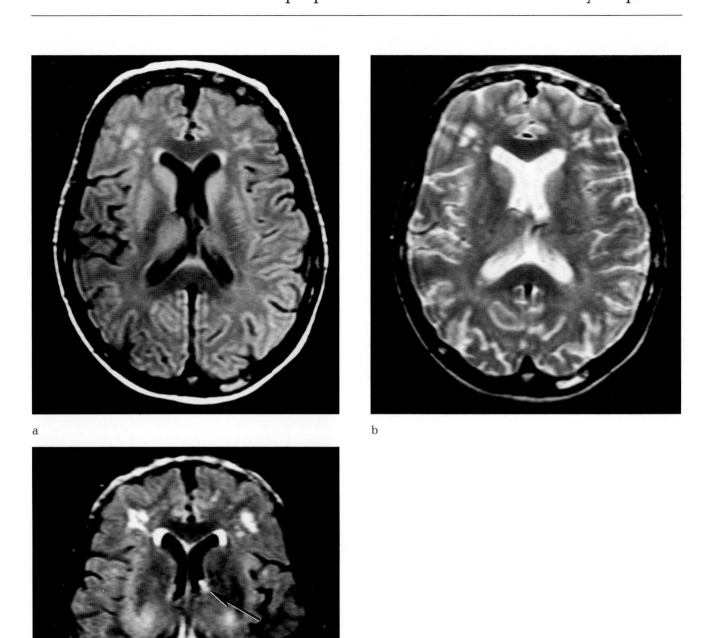

a

b

c

Figure 6.11

Cerebral metastases (1.0 T): SE2500/20 (a), SE2500/80 (b) and IR6000/160/2100 (c) scans. Additional lesions (arrows) are only seen on (C).

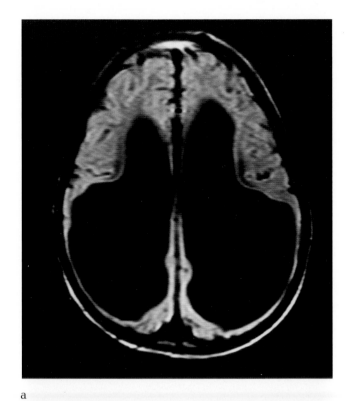

a

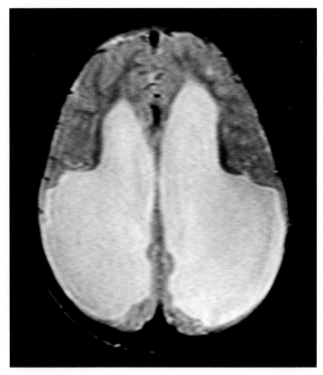

b

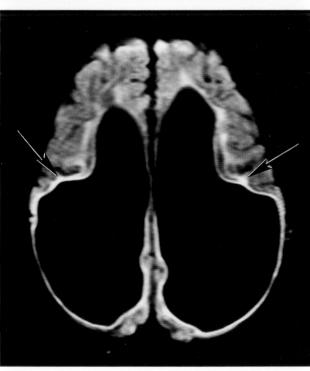

c

Figure 6.12

Hydrocephalus in a 2½ year-old child (1.0 T): SE2500/20 (a), SE2500/80 (b) and IR6000/160/2100 (c) scans. The highlighting around the enlarged ventricles (arrows) is best seen on (c).

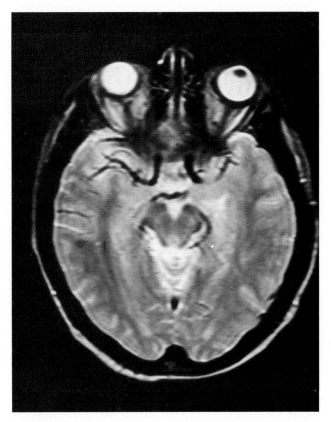

a

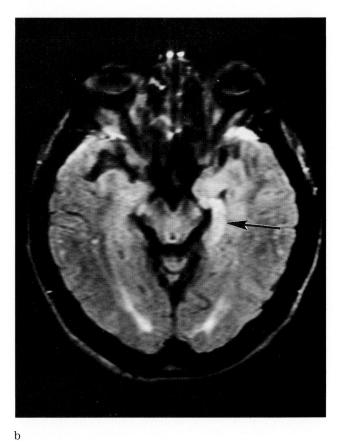

b

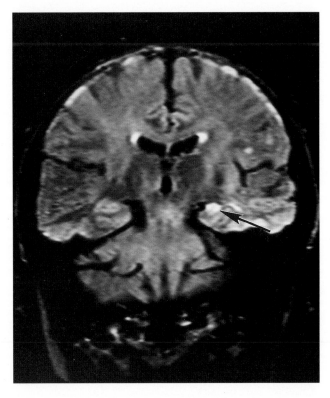

c

Figure 6.13

Epilepsy: mesial temporal sclerosis (1.0 T): transverse
SE2500/80 (a) and IR6000/160/2100 (b) and coronal IR
6000/160/2100 (c) scans. Some dilatation of the
temporal horn is seen in (a). The left hippocampus is
highlighted in (b) and (c) (arrows).

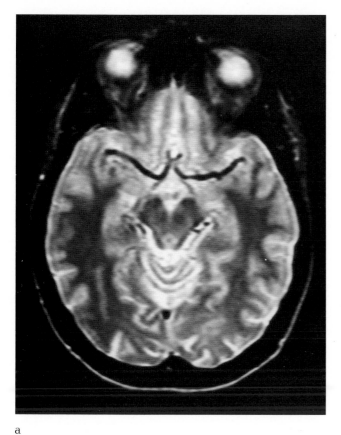

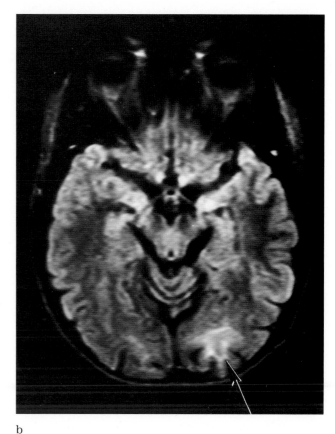

a

b

Figure 6.14

Epilepsy: focal lesion in occipital lobe: SE2500/80 (a) and IR6000/160/2100 (b) scans. The focal lesion (arrow) is only seen on (b).

One of the disadvantages of the sequence is the fact that unwanted CSF may flow into the slice of interest during the *TI* period when a slice-selected initial inversion pulse is used. This effect can be reduced by increasing the width of the initial inversion pulse or using a non-slice-selected pulse. In the spine, this latter technique is the preferred approach to imaging of the spinal cord. Increased sensitivity to MS lesions has been described using this technique.[31] In addition, the sequence is very sensitive to intramedullary tumors, cysts and syrinxes (provided they have a very long T_1) (Figs 6.16–6.18).

The double IR (DIR) sequence

The double IR sequence combines the features of the FLAIR and STIR sequences. It can be used to simultaneously suppress short-T_1 tissue (e.g. fat, white matter and gray matter) as well as long-T_1 tissue or fluid (e.g. CSF), and its applications follow from this. (Fig. 6.19).

It can be used to isolate the cerebral cortex by nulling white matter and CSF (Fig. 6.20).

The DIR sequence suffers from a low signal-to-noise ratio, and is likely to have specialized applications only.

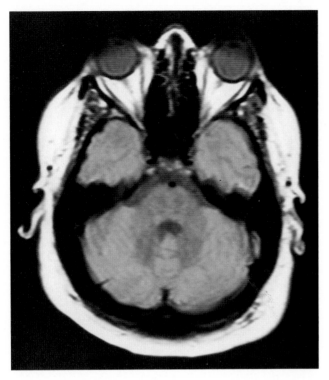

a

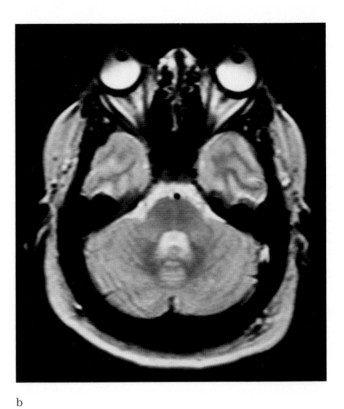

b

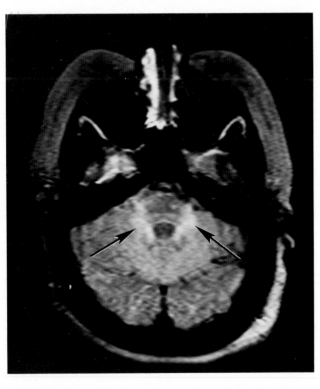

c

Figure 6.15

Sarcoidosis with bilateral VIIth nerve palsy: SE2500/20 (a), SE2500/80 (b) and IR6000/160200 (c) scans. The abnormalities (arrows) are only seen on (c).

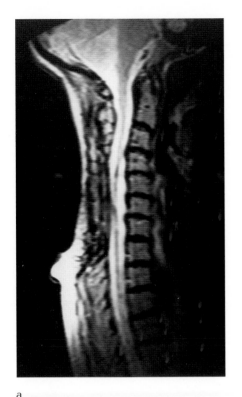
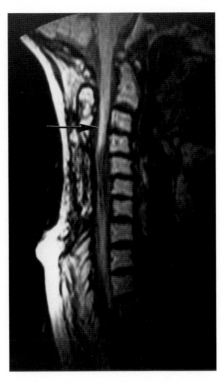

a   b

Figure 6.16

Postoperative ependymoma
(1.0 T): SE2500/80 (a) and
IR6000/30/2100 (b) scans. The
cavity at the site of surgery has
low signal. An area of gliosis or
residual or recurrent tumor is
highlighted (arrow).

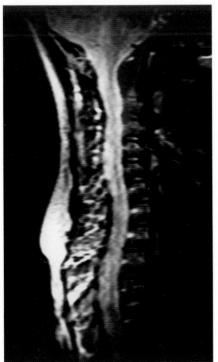
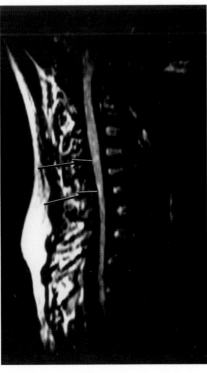

a   b

Figure 6.17

Multiple sclerosis (1.0 T):
SE2500/80 (a) and
IR6000/90/2100 (b) scans. No
lesions are seen in (a), but
highlighted areas can be seen in
(b) (arrows).

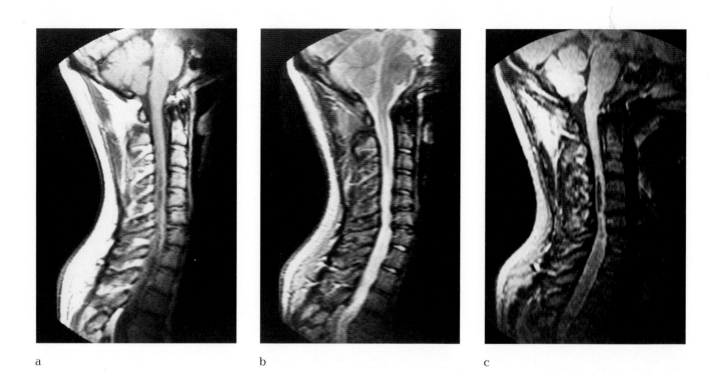

a   b   c

Figure 6.18

Syringomelia (1.0 T): SE540/20 (a), SE2500/80 (b) and
IR6000/90/2100 (c) scans. The cavity is best outlined in
(c).

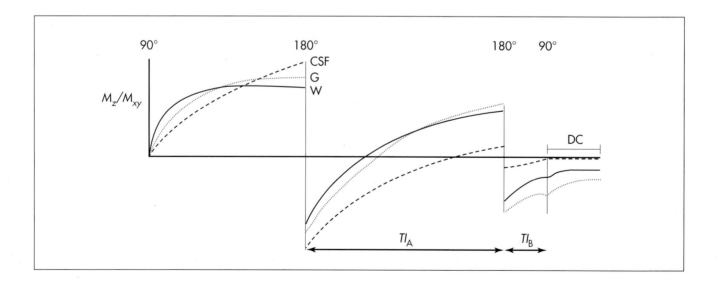

Figure 6.19

The double IR (DIR) sequence: M_z followed by M_{xy}.
This sequence combines the FLAIR and STIR
sequences. Note that after the first 180° pulse, the CSF
is allowed to recover beyond the null point before
being inverted a second time and nulled at the time of
the second 90° pulse. Gray (G) and white (W) matter
are shown. The first inversion time is TI_A and the
second inversion time is TI_B.

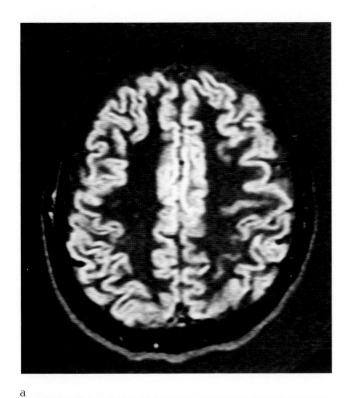

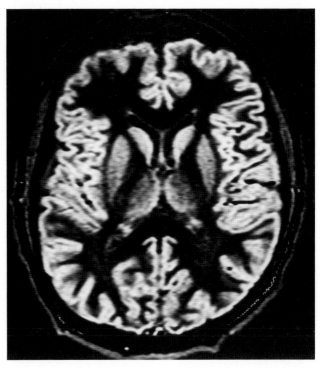

a

b

Figure 6.20

Normal transverse head scan (1.0 T):
DIR3000/20/2300/245 scans at two levels (a) and (b).
The gray matter has been isolated, and gives a high
signal. The complex folding of the cortex is readily
seen.

Other variants of the IR sequence

A variant of the STIR sequence of interest is the
SPIR (spectral presaturation IR) sequence, which
employs a frequency-selective inversion pulse to
invert the magnetization of protons in fat but not
that of protons in water.[32] TI is then selected to null
the fat signal, and any pulse sequence can be used
subsequently to image the remaining water selectivity. This sequence provides fat suppression, and
can be used in a T_1-weighted form to provide
sensitivity to contrast enhancement. It has the
disadvantages that it requires a high field and
good shimming for successful chemical-shift-
sensitive fat suppression. Applications to date have
mainly been in the spine.

Magnetization transfer (MT) can also be used
with the IR sequence. Since MT shortens the T_1 of
some lesions, it can be used in the STIR form to
reduce the T_1 of muscle to that of fat so that both
are nulled and blood vessels can be seen (i.e. MT-
STIR angiography). It can also be used to
markedly reduce the signal from gray and white
matter in the brain in order to increase lesion
contrast (Fig. 6.21).

One approach to the assessment of tissue perfusion is to image the brain and then apply an inversion pulse out of slice for a second image and
finally subtract the two.[18] The inverted spins
change the brain signals as a function of the rate
of blood flow, the distance the blood travels, the
T_1 of blood, the fraction of blood in the tissue, and
other factors. The technique has been applied to
the brain,[33-35] but there is an essential requirement

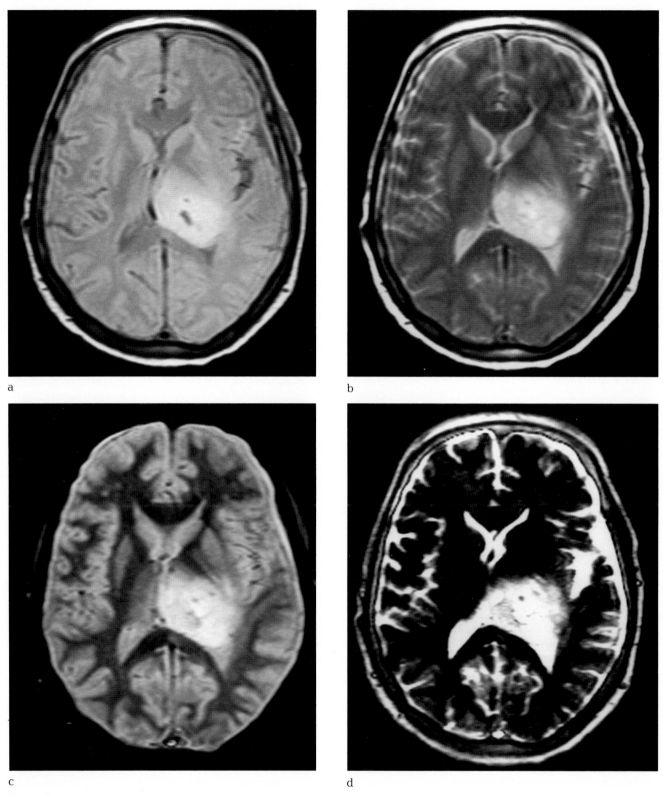

a

b

c

d

Figure 6.21

Thalamic glioma (1.0 T): transverse SE2500/16 (a), MT-SE2500/16 (b), STIR2500/16/130 (c) and MT-STIR2500/16/130 (d) scans. MT alone drops the signal from gray and white matter more than from tumor, increasing the lesion contrast from (a) to (b).

The STIR sequence (c) shows the tumor with higher contrast. The MT-STIR sequence virtually reduces the gray and white matter signal to zero, leaving only the tumor and CSF (d).

to ensure that the detected signals are not due to CSF flow. When the inversion is performed over the carotid and vertebral arteries beneath the skull base, this can readily be achieved. If it involves a comparison of slice-selected and non-slice-selected pulses in the brain, considerable care may be necessary to control or eliminate effects due to CSF flow.

Conclusions

Different aspects of each of the common forms of the IR sequences have been described, and a unified approach to understanding the contrast developed by each of them has been outlined. The IR sequence is versatile, and can provide high tissue contrast by several different mechanisms, the most important of which are heavy T_1 and/or T_2 weighting and nulling of unwanted signals from fat and/or fluid.

Appendix

The following are some useful relationships for the inversion recovery sequence (using the notation given in the figures—specifically Fig. 6.1c).

For the standard inversion recovery sequence:

$$M_{xy} = M_{zmax} \left[1 - 2 \exp\left(-\frac{TI}{T_1}\right) + \exp\left(-\frac{TR}{T_1}\right) \right]$$
$$\times \exp\left(-\frac{TE}{T_2}\right),$$

where M_{zmax} is the fully recovered z magnetization. TE is the time to the echo, regardless of whether it is fixed by a gradient-recalled or spin echo.

At cancellation of a tissue ($M_{xy} = 0$),

$$1 + \exp\left(-\frac{TR}{T_1}\right) = 2 \exp\left(-\frac{TI}{T_1}\right).$$

In the case where $TR \gg T_1$,

$$TI = T_1 \ln (0.5) = 0.69 T_1.$$

This relationship applies equally to STIR and FLAIR sequences.

The relationship for the DIR sequence (see Fig. 6.19) is

$$M_{xy} = M_{zmax} \left\{ 1 - 2 \exp\left(-\frac{TI_B}{T_1}\right) \left[1 - \exp\left(-\frac{TI_A}{T_1}\right) \right] \right.$$
$$\left. + \exp\left(-\frac{TR}{T_1}\right) \right\} \exp\left(-\frac{TE}{T_2}\right).$$

TI_A is the interval between the first and second 180° pulses, and TI_B is the interval between the second 180° pulse and the 90° pulse.

References

1. Young IR, Hall AS, Pallis CA et al, Nuclear magnetic resonance imaging of the brain in multiple sclerosis. *Lancet* 1981; **ii**: 1063–6.

2. Crooks LE, Arakawa M, Hoenninger J et al, Nuclear magnetic resonance whole-body imager operating at 3.5 Kgauss. *Radiology* 1982; **143**: 169–74.

3. Bailes DR, Young IR, Thomas DJ et al, NMR imaging of the brain using spin-echo sequences. *Clin Radiol* 1982; **33**: 395–414.

4. Bydder GM, Steiner RE, Young IR et al, Clinical NMR imaging of the brain: 140 cases. *AJR* 1982; **139**: 215–36.

5. Graif M, Bydder GM, Steiner RE et al, Contrast enhanced MRI of malignant brain tumors. *AJNR* 1985; **6**: 855–62.

6. Levene MI, Whitelaw A, Dubowitz et al, Nuclear magnetic resonance imaging of the brain in children. *Br Med J* 1982; **285**: 774–6.

7. Johnson MA, Pennock JM, Bydder GM, Clinical NMR imaging of the brain in children: normal and neurologic disease. *AJNR* 1983; **4**: 1013–26; *AJR* 1983; **141**: 1005–18.

8. Bydder GM, Young IR, MRI: clinical use of the inversion-recovery sequence. *J Comput Assist Tomogr* 1985; **9**: 659–75.

9. Shields AF, Porter BA, Churchley S et al, The detection of bone marrow involvement by lymphoma using magnetic resonance imaging. *J Clin Oncol* 1987; **5**: 225–30.

10. De Coene B, Hajnal JV, Gatehouse P et al, MR of the brain using fluid attenuated inversion recovery (FLAIR) pulse sequences. *AJNR* 1992; **13**: 1555–64.

11. White SJ, Hajnal JV, Young IR, Bydder GM, Use of fluid attenuated inversion recovery sequences for imaging the spinal cord. *Magn Reson Med* 1992; **28**: 153–62.

12. Redpath TW, Smith FW, Imaging gray brain matter with a double inversion pulse sequence to suppress CSF and white matter signals. *MAGMA* 1994; **2**:451–5.

13. Hennig J, Naureth A, Friedburgh H, RARE imaging: a fast imaging method for clinical MR. *Magn Reson Med* 1986; **3**: 823–33.

14. Haase A, Matthaei D, Bantkowski R et al, Inversion recovery snapshot FLASH MR imaging. *J Comput Assist Tomogr* 1989; **13**: 1036–40.

15. Mugler JP, Brookeman JR, Three dimensional magnetization-prepared rapid gradient-echo imaging (3D MP RAGE). *Magn Reson Med* 1992; **15**: 152–7.

16. Feinberg DA, Oshio I, GRASE (gradient and spin echo) MR imaging: a new fast clinical imaging technique. *Radiology* 1991; **181**: 597.

17. Mansfield P, Morris PG, *NMR imaging in biomedicine*. Academic Press, New York, 1982.

18. Detre JA, Leigh JS, Williams DS, Koretsky AP, Perfusion imaging. *Magn Reson Med* 1992; **23**: 37–45.

19. Brant-Zawadski M, Gillan GD, Mitz WR, MP RAGE: a three-dimensional, T_1-weighted gradient-echo sequence — initial experience in the brain. *Radiology* 1992; **182**: 769–80.

20. Shields AF, Porter BA, Churchley S et al, The detection of bone marrow involvement by lymphoma using magnetic resonance imaging. *J Clin Oncol* 1987; **5**: 225–30.

21. Smith RC, Reinhold C, Lange RC et al, Fast spin echo STIR imaging. *Radiology* 1992; **184**: 665–9.

22. Stoller DW, Porter BA, Steinkirchner TM, Marrow imaging. In: *MRI in orthopaedics and sports medicine* (ed. DW Stoller). JB Lippincott, Philadelphia, 1993.

23. Panish D, Fulbright R, Sze G et al, Inversion recovery fast spin-echo MR imaging: efficacy in the evaluation of head and neck lesions. *Radiology* 1993; **187**: 421–8.

24. Fleckenstein JL, Archer BT, Barker BA et al, Fast short-tau inversion recovery MR imaging. *Radiology* 1991; **179**: 499–504.

25. Rydberg JN, Hammond CA, Grimm RC et al, Initial clinical experience with a fast fluid-attenuated inversion recovery pulse sequence. *Radiology* 1994; **193**: 173–80.

26. Rydberg JN, Reiderer SJ, Rydberg SH, Jack CR, Contrast optimization of fluid-attenuated inversion recovery (FLAIR) imaging. *Magn Reson Med* 1995; **34**: 868–77.

27. Hashemi RH, Bradley WG, Chen D-Y et al, Suspected MS: MR imaging with a thin section fast FLAIR pulse sequence—initial experience in the brain. *Radiology* 1995; **196**: 505–10.

28. Bergin PS, Fish DR, Shorron SD et al, MRI in partial epilepsy: additional abnormalities demonstrated with the fluid attenuated inversion recovery (FLAIR) pulse sequence. *J Neurol Neurosurg Psych* 1995; **58**: 439–43.

29. Riederer SJ, Jack CR, Grimm RC, New technical developments in magnetic resonance imaging of epilepsy. *Magn Reson Imaging* 1995; **13**: 1095–8.

30. Nogichi K, Ogawa T, Inugani A, Acute subarachnoid haemorrhage: MR imaging with fluid attenuated inversion recovery pulse sequences. *Radiology* 1995; **196**: 773–7.

31. Thomas DJ, Pennock JM, Hajnal JV et al, MRI: use of fluid attenuated inversion recovery (FLAIR) pulse sequences for imaging the spinal cord on MS. *Lancet* 1993; **341**: 593–4.

32. Zee CS, Segall HD, Terk MR et al, SPIR MRI in spinal disease. *J Comput Assist Tomogr* 1992; **16**: 356–60.

33. Edelman RR, Siewert B, Darby DG et al, Quantitative mapping of cerebral blood flow and functional localisation with echoplanar MR imaging and signal targetting with alternating radio frequency. *Radiology* 1994; **192**: 513–20.

34. Kim SG, Quantification of relative cerebral blood flow change by flow sensitive attenuating inversion recovery (FAIR) technique: application to functional mapping. *Magn Reson Med* 1995; **34**: 293–301.

35. Kwong KK, Chesler DA, Weiskoff RM et al, MR perfusion studies with T_1-weighted echo planar imaging. *Magn Reson Med* 1995; **34**: 878–87.

7

Use of MR contrast agents in the brain

William G Bradley, William TC Yuh, Graeme M Bydder

Introduction

The use of gadolinium-based contrast agents in magnetic resonance imaging (MRI) is directly analogous to the use of iodine-based contrast agents in X-ray computed tomography (CT). As a rule, anything that enhances with iodine on CT of the brain enhances on MR with gadolinium. This is particularly true for the original gadolinium chelate Gd-DTPA or gadopentetate dimeglumine (Magnevist: Berlex Laboratories, Wayne, NJ, and Schering AG, Berlin, Germany).[1] This is because ionic iodinated agents (e.g. diatrizoate meglumine (Renografin: Bracco, Princeton, NJ)) have a charge and size similar to those of gadopentetate dimeglumine. Thus lesions producing similar degrees of blood–brain barrier breakdown allow passage of either gadolinium or iodinated contrast medium from the intravascular to the extracellular space with subsequent increased signal intensity or enhancement. Obviously, such lesions must also be perfused (i.e. blood supply to the lesion must be intact) as a prerequisite for enhancement with either agent.[1]

While almost all lesions that enhance visibly with iodinated agents will also enhance with gadopentetate dimeglumine, the converse is not true. As is true for a comparison of unenhanced MR imaging with unenhanced CT in general, posterior fossa enhancement is better appreciated with MR imaging than with CT because of beam-hardening artifacts in the latter.[2]

Similar artifacts may degrade peripheral lesions subjacent to the calvarium. The few situations in which gadolinium enhancement on MR images is less apparent than contrast enhancement on CT scans arise when the enhancement occurs against an already high-signal-intensity background. Thus enhancement of the orbit may be less apparent on non-fat-suppressed T_1-weighted images than on CT scans, since the orbital fat has high signal intensity on T_1-weighted images and low attenuation on CT scans. As another example, evaluation of a subacute hematoma (containing short-T_1, high-signal-intensity methemoglobin) for nodular enhancement (suggestive of a tumor) might be better accomplished with CT than with MR imaging, because the background will have low attenuation on CT scans and high signal intensity on MR images. However, evaluation of an acute hematoma (containing long-T_1, short-T_2, low-signal-intensity deoxyhemoglobin) would be better accomplished with MR imaging than with CT, because the background would have low signal intensity on MR images and high attenuation on CT scans.

There are other essential differences between the contrast agents for CT and MR imaging. Estimates for reactions to the high-osmolar, ionic iodinated contrast agents place the mortality at 1 in 40 000 (25 in 1 million)[3] to 9 in 1 million.[4] Thus far, over 8 million doses of gadolinium have been administered worldwide, with only a single, definite associated death.[5] Death in this case resulted from an immediate, severe asthma attack in a patient known to have asthma. Twelve other severe asthmatic reactions have been documented in persons known to have asthma, two of them resulting in brain injury. However, when these figures are compared with similar numbers of patients receiving iodinated agents, approximately 72 patients in 8 million would have died (using the 9 in 1 million figure) with the latter. Thus ionic (high-osmolar) gadopentetate dimeglumine is clearly safer than ionic (high-osmolar) iodinated agents for contrast-material-enhanced studies of the brain.

Just as the degree of enhancement on CT scans is a function of the dose of iodine delivered, so the degree of enhancement with gadolinium is dose-dependent.[6,7] The two newer nonionic gadolinium chelates are approved for use at two to three times the dose approved for gadopentetate dimeglumine (i.e. standard dose 0.1 mmol/kg; triple dose 0.3 mmol/kg). These nonionic agents are respectively gadodiamide injection (Gd-DTPA-BMA: diethyl-enetriaminepentaacetic acid bis(methylamide)) (Omniscan: Nycomed, Oslo, Norway) and gadoteri-dol (Gd-HP-DO3A: 1,4,7-tris(carboxymethyl)-10-(2'-hydroxypropyl)-1,4,7,10-tetraazacyclododecane) (ProHance: Bracco, Princeton, NJ). The nonionic nondissociating gadolinium chelates have approxi-mately one-third the osmolality of ionic gadopen-tetate dimeglumine, which dissociates into three particles (Gd-DTPA^{2-} and two meglumine cations) in water. Since the morbidity of contrast agents in general is at least partially due to the osmotic load, three times the gadolinium dose of the nonionic chelates (0.3 mmol/kg) can be administered at the same osmotic load (and presumed margin of safety) of single-dose, ionic gadopentetate dimeglumine. With regard to safety, it should also be noted that the usual 20 ml maximum dose of gadopentetate dimeglumine (0.1 mmol/kg) is still one-tenth the osmotic load of 200 ml of Renografin 76 (which has the same osmolality as gadopentetate dimeglu-mine), a common upper limit on contrast agent load for runoff arteriograms. This may partially explain the substantially better morbidity and mortality statistics for any of the three gadolinium chelates relative to the iodinated agents.

With regard to the relative safety of the gadolin-ium chelates themselves, there have not, to our knowledge, been any peer-reviewed comparison studies. The three gadolinium chelates appear to be comparably safe when administered at comparable osmotic loads. The efficacy (i.e. degree of enhance-ment) and the likelihood of a lesion being detected are, however, markedly different depending on the dose of gadolinium given. For that, we need to examine the theoretical basis of lesion detection.

Theory of lesion detection

For a lesion to have the potential of being detected, signal intensity is required that is substantially different from that of the surrounding background. In the experience of one of the authors (WTCY), the lesion-to-background signal intensity ratio (L/B) of a lesion detected with contrast-enhanced MR imaging at a dose of 0.1 mmol/kg ranges from 1.3 to 2.0.[6] Therefore a minimal difference of approximately 30% between signal intensities of lesion and background is required for the lesion to be detected. In normal brain parenchyma, gadolinium does not cross an intact blood–brain barrier to cause an increase in intensity.[8-11] An increased dose of contrast agent, however, will increase the intensity of a lesion that has caused breakdown of the blood–brain barrier. This breakdown will produce increased contrast between the lesion and surrounding normal brain tissue. These relationships have been demon-strated quantitatively[6] (Fig. 7.1).

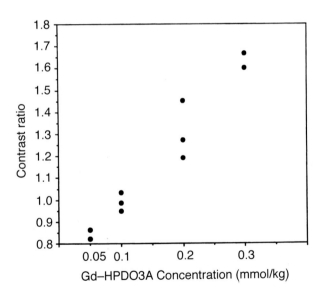

Figure 7.1

Quantitative analysis. Linear relationship between lesion contrast ratio (L/B) and gadoteridol dose ranging from 0.05 to 0.3 mmol/kg is demonstrated ($r = 0.975$). There is no evidence of plateau or decreased contrast at 0.3 mmol/kg. (Reprinted with permission from Yuh et al.[6])

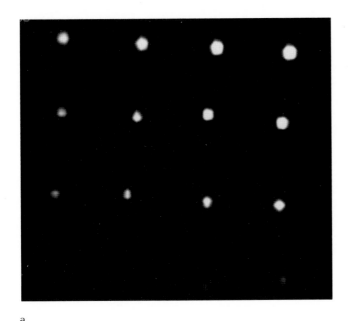

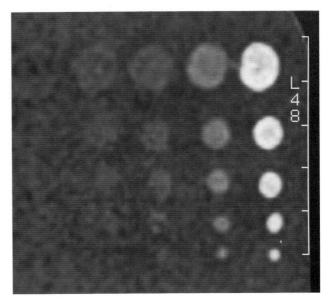

a   b

Figure 7.2

Contrast phantoms. (a) Gd-DTPA phantom experiment shows progressive increment in glass tube diameter from the bottom row to the top row. In each row, the tubes have the same diameter. Similarly, there is a progressive increment in Gd-DTPA concentration from the left column to the right column. Note the increased lesion signal intensity and detectability as the concentration of Gd-DTPA increases. The size of the tube appears smaller at lower concentrations (left) than at higher concentrations (right). (b) Agar gel phantom experiment shows progressive increment in lesion size (bottom (small) to top (large)) and signal intensity (left (low) to right (high)) arranged as in the Gd-DTPA phantom in (a), with the background closely approximating the T_1 and T_2 of normal brain parenchyma. Lesion detectability (bottom right) and delineation (right column) are increased as the lesion contrast increases. Apparent lesion size is gradually reduced (especially of small lesions) as contrast decreases (bottom right). (Reprinted with permission from Yuh et al.[6])

Increased concentration of gadolinium may not increase the contrast of non-central nervous system (CNS) lesions as much as that of CNS lesions. It has been shown that the signal intensity and tissue concentration of gadolinium in normal non-CNS parenchyma are linearly proportional to the dose injected.[12] This relationship is presumably due to the lack of a blood–brain barrier in normal non-CNS tissues. Small gadolinium chelate complexes readily permeate the extracellular space in both normal and pathologic non-CNS tissue, and will therefore enhance both; thus lesion contrast may not increase markedly with increased concentration of gadolinium.[6]

On the basis of the data in Fig. 7.1, a lesion that is minimally detectable at a dose of contrast agent of 0.1 mmol/kg (L/B = 1.3) would have a predicted L/B ratio of 2.3 when imaged after a dose of 0.3 mmol/kg. Thus, for lesions that are minimally

detectable at 0.1 mmol/kg, a high-dose study would yield a lesion signal intensity 130% above the surrounding background signal intensity. An increase in intensity proportional to doses of gadolinium up to 0.3 mmol/kg has also been observed by others.[7,8,13,14] Studies of lesion signal intensity characteristics after a high dose have found a similar proportionality between dose of gadolinium and lesion enhancement.

In addition to contrast, lesion detectability depends on the size of the lesion, as demonstrated in phantom studies.[6] Poorly enhancing, large lesions with low contrast may still be detected. This has been shown by using an agar phantom that was constructed to closely approximate the T_1 and T_2 values of normal brain parenchyma and to have an L/B ratio of up to 2.0, similar to the findings in 0.3 mmol/kg studies (Fig. 7.2). The results of the phantom study demonstrated that

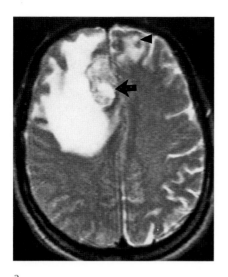
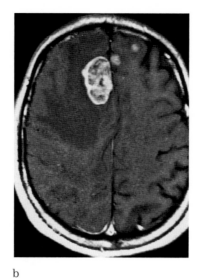
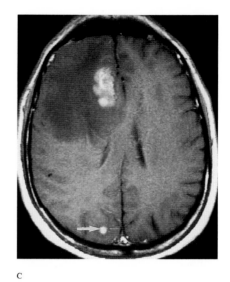

a   b   c

Figure 7.3

Metastatic disease to the brain in a patient with adenocarcinoma of the lung. (a) T_2-weighted image (spin echo (SE) $TR = 2500$ ms/$TE = 90$ ms) shows large parafalcine metastasis (arrow) and smaller left cortical metastasis (arrowhead). (b) T_1-weighted image (SE 500/20 with Gd-DTPA) at the same level as (a), shows three enhancing lesions typical of metastatic disease. (c) At a slightly lower level, an additional 5 mm metastasis to the right parietal lobe is noted (arrow) (SE 500/20 with Gd-DTPA). (Images courtesy of Anton N Hasso, MD, Orange CA.)

large lesions did not require substantial enhancement to be detectable. Small lesions, however, frequently were not associated with marked edema, and required considerable enhancement to be detected. The results of the agar gel phantom study demonstrated that a greater degree of enhancement was necessary for the detection of small lesions and that larger lesions were conspicuous, even with relatively minimal enhancement.

The size of a lesion on an MR image is represented by the total number of pixels that have a higher signal intensity than that of the surrounding background. Because of partial-volume effects, pixels at the periphery of a lesion tend to have lower signal intensity than those in the central portion, and therefore may not have sufficient L/B contrast to be detected. This results in an apparent decrease in lesion size. Since small lesions have a higher percentage of peripheral pixels, partial-volume effects tend to be more critical, and may affect the detectability more than for larger lesions. Increased enhancement in small lesions may be essential to reduce the apparent

decrease in lesion size, and therefore to increase detectability. The results of the agar and glass tube phantom studies (Fig. 7.2) demonstrate several principles:

(a) small lesions require greater enhancement to be detectable owing to partial-volume averaging of peripheral pixels;
(b) lesions that are smaller than a pixel may still be detected if high enough contrast can be obtained;
(c) the apparent size of larger lesions will increase as lesion enhancement increases.

Normal enhancement patterns in the brain

Unlike in other tissues in the body, the tight junctions between the capillary endothelial cells in

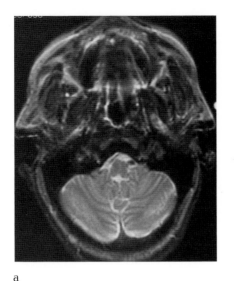
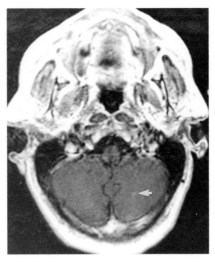
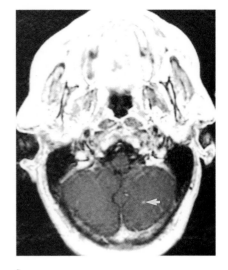

a   b   c

Figure 7.4

Improved confidence in lesion detection with gadoteridol. (a) Axial T_2-weighted image (SE 2350/90) shows no marked abnormality. (b) Axial T_1-weighted initial-dose study (SE 350/15) shows faint pulsation artifact and a small focal area (arrow) with faint enhancement thought to be a possible lesion. (c) High-dose study shows further enhancement and border delineation of this small lesion (arrow) (approximately 1.9 mm). (Reprinted with permission from Haustein et al.[18])

the brain prevent contrast agents from passing through the blood–brain barrier from the intravascular to the extracellular space. Not all parts of the brain, however, have an intact blood–brain barrier, and certainly structures other than brain are visualized on an MR image of the head. Some of these structures may demonstrate enhancement with gadolinium.

Structures in the brain per se without an intact blood–brain barrier include the pituitary gland and stalk (or infundibulum) and the choroid plexus.[1] In addition, enhancement can be seen in the nasal mucosa and in the mucosal lining of the paranasal sinuses. Subtle dural enhancement may be seen normally, particularly on high-field-strength imaging systems.[15] This variation in enhancement with field strength appears to reflect the degree of T_1 weighting achievable, high-field-strength systems typically having shorter TE than those of midfield, low-bandwidth systems. Dural enhancement is less often appreciated on middle-field-strength systems,[16] reflecting the longer TE usually associated with low-bandwidth techniques.

Intraparenchymal tumors

Metastases

Contrasts agents are frequently necessary for lesion detectability and delineation and for optimal treatment of cancer patients with possible brain metastases.[6,17] However, MR images of patients with large metastases may not require contrast enhancement, since the lesions may be detectable on unenhanced MR images because of mass effect and vasogenic edema (Fig. 7.3). Similarly, contrast-enhanced MR imaging may not be required in patients with evidence of multiple (more than two) metastatic lesions demonstrated on unenhanced MR images, because the additional lesions detected with contrast-enhanced MR imaging will probably not affect patient treatment. The purpose of using contrast agents in the evaluation of possible brain metastases is therefore to detect small, early lesions in patients who otherwise appear disease-free or have only a single metastasis demonstrated with other imaging techniques.[17]

In general, tumors such as metastases have an exponential rate of growth. Early metastases may remain small for many years, and may be difficult to detect with routine imaging techniques, including MR imaging studies with a standard dose of 0.1 mmol/kg gadolinium. Recent studies report that CNS lesions imaged with higher doses of gadolinium (0.2 and 0.3 mmol/kg) exhibit greater enhancement.[6,7,17,18] On the basis of the preliminary results in 27 patients with clinical suspicion of brain metastasis, high-dose (0.3 mmol/kg) gadolinium-enhanced MR imaging may have advantages over 0.1 mmol/kg examinations in detecting early and/or small metastases.[17] This is obviously important in the treatment of patients with cerebral metastases.

In a prospective study with nonionic gadoteridol,[17] each patient received an initial injection of 0.1 mmol/kg. An additional dose of 0.2 mmol/kg was administered 30 min later. Images were obtained before, immediately after, and 10 and 20 min after the initial dose. Images were then acquired immediately after the additional dose of gadoteridol. After the additional dose of gadoteridol, there was a marked qualitative improvement in lesion conspicuity and detection (Fig. 7.4). The conspicuity of 80 of 81 lesions was increased in the high-dose studies, and 46 new lesions were detected in 19 of 27 patients.[17]

Quantitative image analysis (Fig. 7.5) demonstrated a significant increase in normalized mean lesion contrast between the routine-dose and high-dose studies (35 lesions identified in 13 patients: $P<0.0001$). The additional information gained from high-dose examinations contributed to a potential modification of treatment in 10 of 27 (37%) patients. This improved lesion contrast on the high-dose images also allowed better definition of lesion borders and visualization of tumor extension beyond the periphery defined with the standard-dose image (Fig. 7.6).

There may be several advantages to the use of gadolinium at high doses (greater than 0.1 mmol/kg) to evaluate CNS metastases:[17]

(a) Inappropriate local therapy for primary neoplasms with unsuspected brain metastases may be reduced.
(b) Isolated brain metastases may be identified and removed surgically and/or given boost radiation therapy.
(c) Patients with a solitary metastasis detected with 0.1 mmol/kg gadolinium and additional metastases detected with higher doses may avoid unnecessary surgical excision and boost radiation therapy.

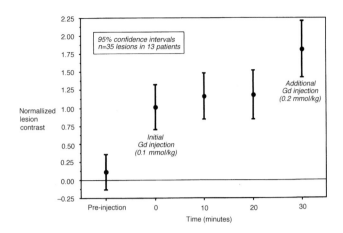

Figure 7.5

Quantitative analysis. Mean normalized lesion contrast and 95% confidence intervals are plotted for a total of 35 lesions identified in 13 patients. The normalized lesion contrast increased significantly ($P < 0.0001$) between precontrast studies and initial-dose studies, and also between initial-dose studies and high-dose studies. Both the 10- and 20-min-delayed examinations demonstrated a slight but significant increase in mean normalized lesion contrast compared with the immediate initial-dose studies ($P < 0.005$). (Reprinted with permission from Yuh et al.[17])

(d) In patients with multiple metastases, the lesions most amenable to uncomplicated diagnostic biopsy may be identified.
(e) Increased lesion delineation may identify an area for diagnostic biopsy that has less surgical morbidity.
(f) The appropriate surgery, radiation therapy and/or chemotherapy may be instituted earlier.

Early work showed that higher doses of gadolinium caused a substantial decrease in signal intensity in the urinary system because of T_2 shortening resulting from the high gadolinium concentration in the urine.[14,19] However, the early contrast-enhanced CNS neoplasm data demonstrate a directly proportional relationship between the lesion contrast ratio and gadoteridol dose up to a dose of 0.3 mmol/kg without evidence of decrease in signal intensity resulting from T_2 shortening (Fig. 7.1).

Gliomas

Gliomas include astrocytomas, ependymomas and subependymomas, the latter arising from the

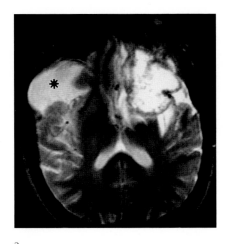
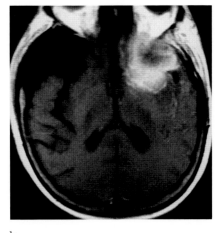
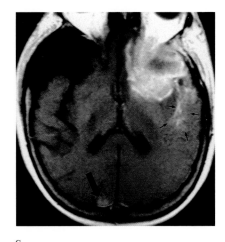

a　　　　　　　　　　　　b　　　　　　　　　　　　c

Figure 7.6

Increased lesion conspicuity and detection. (a) Axial T_2-weighted image (SE 2000/100) shows an area with abnormal signal intensity in the left frontal lobe and a subarachnoid cyst (*) near the temporal lobe. (b) Axial T_1-weighted initial-dose study (SE 583/20) shows an enhancing left frontal lobe mass and the nonenhancing subarachnoid cyst. (c) High-dose study shows slightly greater enhancement, improved border definition and more extensive involvement of the left frontal lobe mass (small arrows) than either the initial-dose or T_2-weighted study. An additional lesion (large arrow) was also detected in the right occipital lobe. (Reprinted with permission from Yuh et al.[17])

ventricular walls. Lower-grade (I and II) gliomas tend not to enhance, while enhancement is almost universally present in anaplastic astrocytomas (grade III) and glioblastomas multiforme (grade IV). Lesions not enhancing on CT scans may not enhance on MR images either (Fig. 7.7).

Gliomas detected in symptomatic patients tend to be large. They are frequently associated with considerable mass effect and vasogenic edema, and are therefore detected readily on unenhanced T_1- and T_2-weighted images. Contrast agents may not be necessary for lesion detection but rather for lesion delineation and specificity (Fig. 7.6). Gadolinium is useful in demonstrating dural spread as well as spread through the cerebrospinal fluid (CSF) spaces, particularly for the higher-grade gliomas. Dural spread of tumor tends to be nodular and localized to the site of origin of the tumor (Fig. 7.8). This should be differentiated from benign meningeal fibrosis, which tends to be generalized and of uniform thickness (Fig. 7.9). (Benign meningeal fibrosis is most often seen after ventricular shunting, and is thought to represent a chemical meningitis resulting from bleeding into the subarachnoid space around the catheter.)

With both delayed imaging techniques and higher doses of contrast medium, improvement in the delineation of gliomas can be achieved. In one study evaluating gliomas with various doses of contrast medium ranging from 0.05 to 0.3 mmol/kg, maximal enhancement of gliomas was seen most frequently on the high-dose, 30-min-delayed images.[20] This is related to a slight but statistically significant temporal increment in lesion contrast on delayed images, similar to that of the metastases shown in Fig. 7.5.

The application of higher doses of gadolinium in the evaluation of gliomas may be useful not only for tumor delineation but also for the demonstration of tumor involvement beyond the zone of apparent abnormality on T_2-weighted images. On standard-dose contrast medium studies, the area of tumor enhancement is usually within the area of abnormal signal intensity demonstrated on T_2-weighted images. However, recent studies with stereotaxic biopsies have confirmed that some gliomas infiltrate and extend beyond the zone of apparent abnormality on T_2-weighted images (Fig. 7.6). This extended zone of enhancement likely represents tumor infiltration, and appears to be

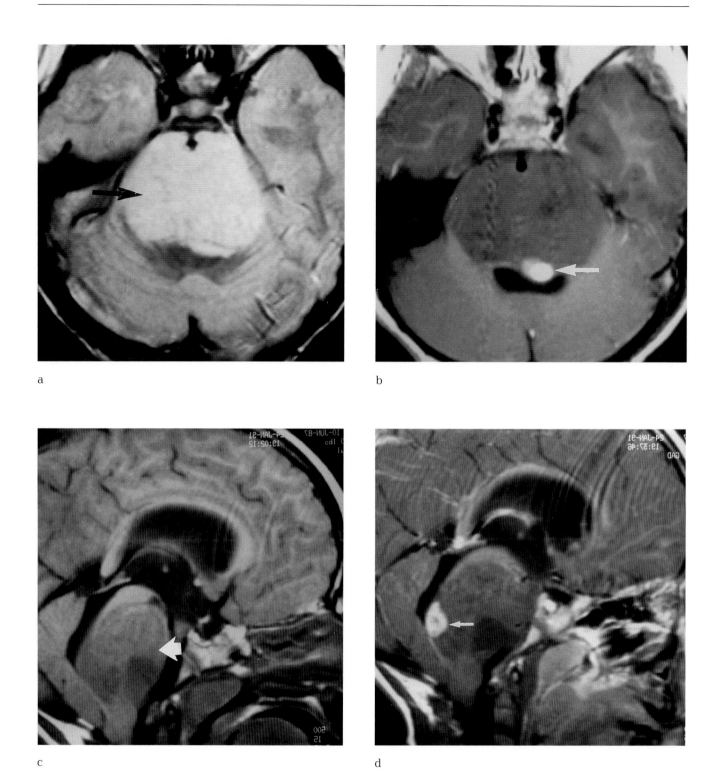

a

b

c

d

Figure 7.7

Low-grade brain stem glioma. (a) T_2-weighted image
(SE 3000/22) shows high signal intensity in a diffusely
enlarged pons (arrow). (b) T_1-weighted contrast-
enhanced image (SE 500/15 with Gd-DTPA) at the same
level as (a) shows only one small focus of nodular
enhancement (arrow); the remainder of the glioma did
not enhance. (c) Unenhanced T_1-weighted sagittal image
(SE 500/15) shows large heterogeneous brain stem tumor
(arrow). (d) Contrast-enhanced T_1-weighted sagittal
image (SE 500/15 with Gd-DTPA) through the same
level as (c) shows only one small focus of enhancement
(arrow); the remainder of the tumor did not enhance.
(Reprinted with permission from Bradley et al[5].)

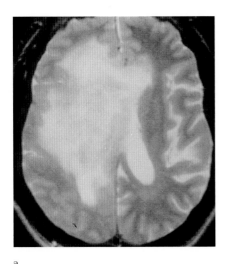
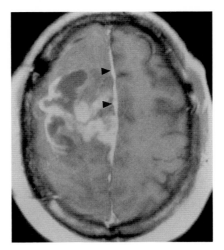
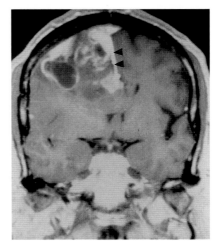

a   b   c

Figure 7.8

Dural spread of glioblastoma multiforme. (a) T_2-weighted image (SE 3000/90) shows large right frontoparietal lesion with surrounding edema. (b) Contrast-enhanced image (SE 500/15) shows heterogeneous enhancement with nodular deposits along the falx (arrowheads). (c) T_1-weighted coronal image (SE 500/15 with Gd-DTPA) shows falcine thickening (arrowheads) and displacement by heterogeneously enhancing mass. (Reprinted with permission from Bradley et al[5].)

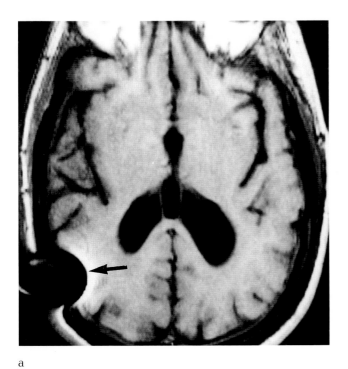
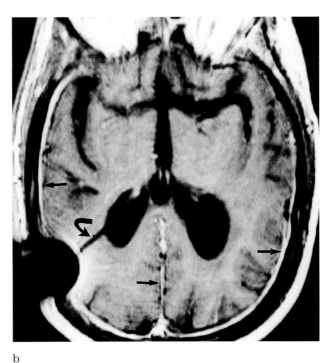

a   b

Figure 7.9

Benign meningeal fibrosis. (a) Precontrast T_1-weighted image (SE 500/15) shows metallic artifacts from shunt reservoir (arrow) and subtle thickening of the dura. (b) After administration of Gd-DTPA (SE 500/15), there is diffuse uniform enhancement of the dura (straight arrows) resulting from chronic shunt therapy. This is presumed to represent chemical meningitis caused by subarachnoid hemorrhage from the shunt (curved arrow). Note the lack of extension into the cortical sulci, which differentiates this dural thickening from a potentially much more serious leptomeningeal process. (Reprinted with permission from Bradley et al[5].)

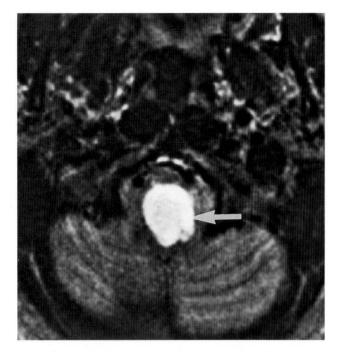

a

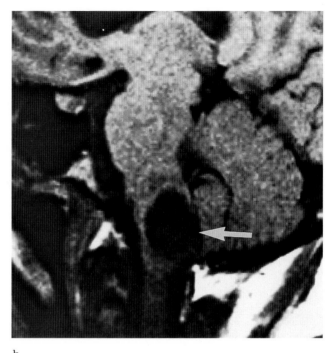

b

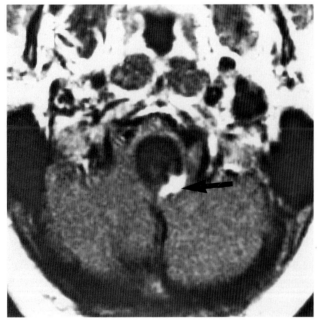

c

Figure 7.10

Hemangioblastoma. (a) T_2-weighted image (SE 2500/90) shows a high-signal-intensity, predominantly cystic lesion in the medulla (arrow). (b) T_1-weighted sagittal image (SE 500/20) shows low-signal-intensity cystic lesion in the medulla (arrow). (c) Gadolinium-enhanced axial image (SE 500/20 with Gd-DTPA) through the same level as (a) shows nodular enhancement (arrow) along the left posterolateral margin of the lesion. (Images courtesy of Anton N Hasso, MD, Orange CA.)

proportional to the gadolinium dose. These preliminary results, based on a small number of patients, suggest that high-dose studies may be useful for patient treatment, such as in biopsy, surgery and radiation planning.[17] This unusual pattern of enhancement demonstrated on the high-dose study without associated increased signal intensity on T_2-weighted images cannot be explained by a breakdown of the blood–brain barrier. A possible explanation is an increase in

blood pooling in these tumors; however, further study is required.

Other intraparenchymal tumors

Hemangioblastomas are typically cystic cerebellar lesions with nodular enhancement (Figs 7.10 and 7.11). Many are associated with similar lesions in

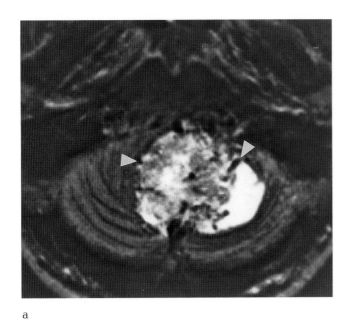

a

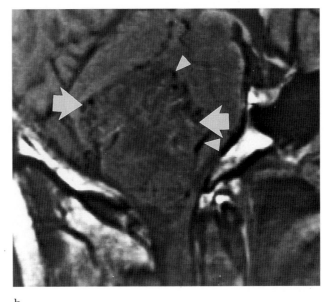

b

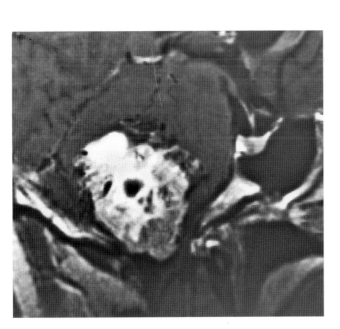

c

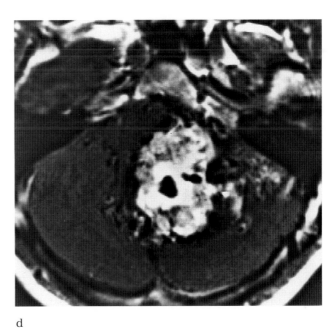

d

Figure 7.11

Hemangioblastoma. (a) T_2-weighted axial image (SE 2500/90) shows high-intensity (cystic) cerebellopontine tumor with multiple flow voids due to enlarged vessels (arrowheads). (b) T_1-weighted sagittal section (SE 500/20) shows large mass (arrows) with peripheral flow voids (arrowheads). (c) Gadolinium-enhanced T_1- weighted image (SE 500/20) demonstrates large enhancing mass with peripheral flow voids. (d) Axial section (SE 500/20 with Gd-DTPA) through the same level as (a) shows enhancing mass with peripheral and central signal voids. (Images courtesy of Anton N Hasso, MD, Orange CA.)

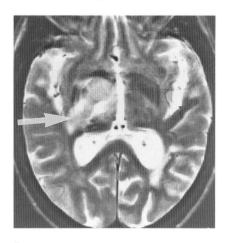
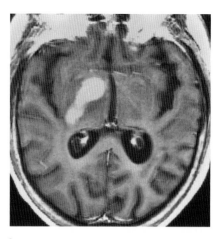
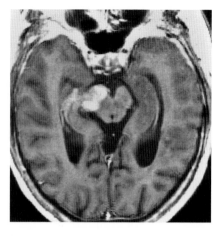

a   b   c

Figure 7.12

Primary thalamic and mesencephalic cerebral lymphoma in a 64-year-old woman. The patient had a history of 'stroke' four months before this study. (a) On unenhanced axial image (SE 2500/90), a mixed, predominantly hyperintense lesion is seen in the right internal capsule and thalamus (arrow). There is slight mass effect on the adjacent ganglionic structures. (b,c) Images (SE 500/20) obtained after administration of contrast material. There is a somewhat lobulated, intensely enhancing lesion involving the right internal capsule, thalamus, subthalamus and upper portion of the midbrain. The focal enhancement in the center of the lesion appears somewhat less (short T_2) in (a). There is slight distortion of the adjacent neural structures. (Images courtesy of Anton N Hasso, MD, Orange CA. Reprinted with permission from Hasso et al.[22])

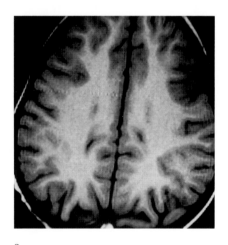
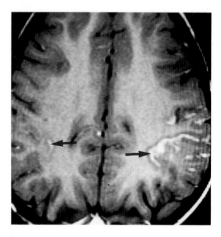
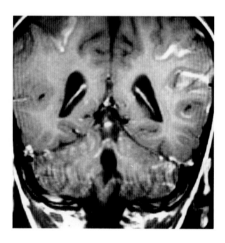

a   b   c

Figure 7.13

Leptomeningeal carcinomatosis from subarachnoid spread of medulloblastoma in a 2-year-old girl. (a) T_1-weighted axial section (SE 600/15) through the centrum semiovale shows no signal abnormality. (b) Gadolinium-enhanced image (SE 500/15) through the same level as (a) demonstrates bilateral enhancement of leptomeninges extending into the sulci characteristic of the leptomeningeal carcinomatosis (arrows). (c) T_1-weighted coronal image (SE 500/15 with Gd-DTPA) demonstrates bilateral leptomeningeal enhancement extending into the cortical sulci. (Reprinted with permission from Bradley et al[5].)

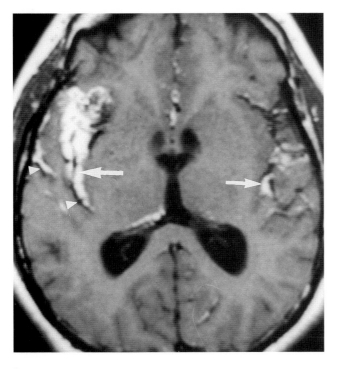
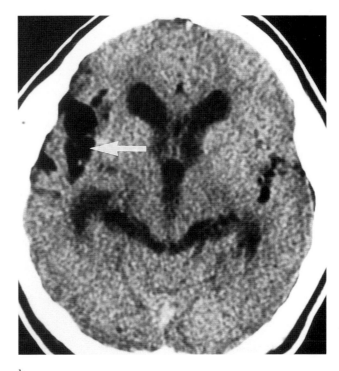

a

b

Figure 7.14

Ruptured dermoid. (a) T_1-weighted unenhanced axial section (SE 500/20) demonstrates high signal intensity extending into the cortical sulci and sylvian cisterns (arrows), simulating leptomeningeal enhancement.

Note the adjacent black lines (arrowheads) of chemical shift artifact. (b) CT scan also demonstrates fatty attenuation in the sulci and sylvian cisterns (arrow). (Reprinted with permission from Bradley et al[5].)

the spinal cord. Approximately one-half of all hemangioblastomas occur in patients with von Hippel–Lindau disease, and one-third of all patients with von Hippel–Lindau disease have hemangioblastomas.[21]

Primary intracranial lymphoma tends to enhance with gadolinium (Fig. 7.12). Such lesions tend to be central and to have a short T_2, with surrounding long-T_2 vasogenic edema. Primary intracranial lymphoma is more prevalent in patients with acquired immunodeficiency syndrome (AIDS).

Meningeal tumors

Metastatic disease to the leptomeninges (leptomeningeal carcinomatosis or carcinomatous meningitis) may not cause abnormal signal intensity on T_1- or T_2-weighted images, and may be seen only on gadolinium-enhanced, T_1-weighted images (Fig. 7.13). When the pial deposits are small (i.e. under 5 mm), there is little invasion of brain parenchyma and therefore no reactive vasogenic edema to prolong T_2. The use of gadolinium is critical in the evaluation of such patients. As is the case with parenchymal deposits, it is highly likely that triple-dose gadolinium will improve the sensitivity of detection of leptomeningeal carcinomatosis compared with single-dose gadolinium. Leptomeningeal deposits may arise from intracranial tumors (astrocytomas, ependymomas, pineoblastomas, medulloblastomas) or extracranial metastases (most commonly carcinoma of the lung and breast, and lymphoma). Leptomeningeal carcinomatosis, which extends into the cortical sulci (Fig. 7.13), must be distinguished from benign meningeal fibrosis, which is confined to the dura, or pachymeninges, and does not extend into the sulci (Fig. 7.9). Leptomeningeal enhancement with gadolinium may be simulated by rupture of fatty dermoid tumors into the subarachnoid space (Fig. 7.14). The latter may be suggested by the lack

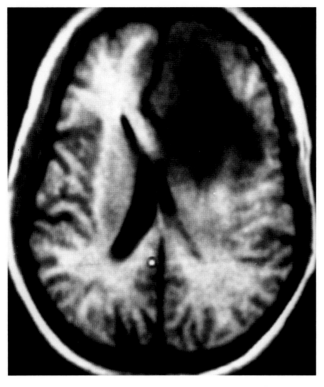

a

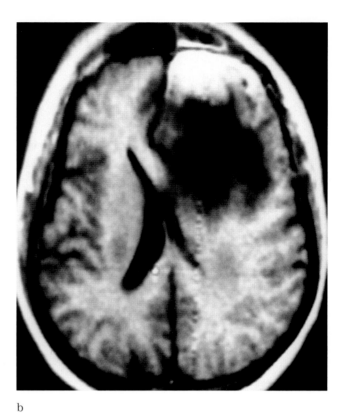

b

Figure 7.15

Meningioma. Images before (a) and after (b) Gd-DTPA administration. Enhancement of the tumor, adjacent dura and mucosa in the frontal sinus is seen in (b) (inversion recovery (IR) $TR = 1500$ ms/$TI = 500$ ms/$TE = 44$ ms). (Reprinted with permission from Bydder.[23])

of normal sinonasal enhancement and the associated chemical shift artifact.

Meningiomas tend to be isointense to brain on both T_1- and T_2-weighted images. This reflects their dense cellularity and relatively low water content (compared with that of gliomas) and similar water content (compared with that of brain). Gadolinium chelates cause intense enhancement (Fig. 7.15) of all but the most densely calcified meningiomas. This property is particularly useful in the preoperative evaluation of meningiomas to define the full degree of any en plaque extension. It should also be noted, however, that there can be adjacent dural enhancement due merely to local inflammation of the dura and not en plaque extension. Thus 'dural tails' may represent either local inflammation or tumor extension.[24] In the parasellar region, meningiomas may be distinguished from macroadenomas of the pituitary by their tendency to encase and narrow the internal carotid artery. When meningiomas invade an adjacent dural sinus, gadolinium-enhanced MR angiography may be necessary to distinguish slow flow, which demonstrates the vessel, from complete occlusion, which does not.[25]

Pituitary adenomas

The normal pituitary gland does not have a blood–brain barrier, and therefore enhances promptly and intensely after administration of contrast medium. The signal intensity of a pituitary adenoma is generally lower than that of the surrounding normal pituitary parenchyma (i.e. the lesion is apparent by 'negative' contrast). Thus the conspicuity of pituitary adenomas increases as L/B decreases. Generally, a low L/B (less than 0.8) is necessary for this type of tumor to be detected.[20] When gadolinium is administered, both the adenoma and surrounding normal pituitary parenchyma enhance. Both high-dose and delayed-imaging techniques cause considerable enhancement of both pituitary adenomas and background pituitary tissue; thus lesion contrast actually decreases as L/B approaches unity. As a result, lesion detectability and conspicuity decrease with increasing dose of contrast medium or with delayed imaging. A fractional-dose (0.05 mmol/kg) technique followed by immediate imaging has been shown to cause a rapid increase in normal pituitary tissue signal intensity and a minor increase in adenoma signal intensity.[26] Thus pituitary adenomas may be best studied with imaging protocols opposite to those applied to intraparenchymal lesions; fractional doses of gadolinium may be more appropriate in the evaluation of such tumors.[20]

When the prolactin level is available prior to MR imaging, the use of gadolinium may be further modified. When the prolactin level is definitely abnormal (>100 ng/ml), MR imaging is often used to confirm the endocrinologists's suspicion of disease. Regardless of MR imaging findings, these microadenomas are treated with bromocriptine. Thus there is no need to use gadolinium in the setting of an abnormal unenhanced study. For equivocal prolactin levels (25–100 ng/ml), MR imaging is useful, because the finding of a focal, nonenhancing, laterally positioned lesion may confirm the physician's impression of prolactinoma and result in treatment. Exceptionally elevated prolactin levels (over 1000 ng/ml) indicate invasion of the cavernous sinus, a diagnosis that can be difficult to make with MR imaging.

Cerebellopontine angle and internal auditory canal lesions

Both cerebellopontine angle (CPA) and internal auditory canal (IAC) lesions (e.g. acoustic neurinomas (Figs 7.16 and 7.17)) are surrounded by a low-signal-intensity background, such as mastoid air cells or CSF (which has an average of 8.4 times less signal intensity than normal brain parenchyma).[20] CPA and IAC lesions therefore have an inherently higher L/B because of this low-signal-intensity background. This allows tumors the same size as the 7th–8th nerve bundle to be seen (Fig. 7.17). In a retrospective review of IAC lesions studied with 0.1 mmol/kg gadolinium, an average L/B of 28 was measured.[20] This degree of lesion contrast far exceeds levels considered minimally detectable for an introparenchymal lesion (L/B >1.2). In prospective studies with fractional doses of gadolinium,[20] an L/B as high as 11.4 could be achieved by using one-eighth of a standard dose (0.0125 mmol/kg) of gadolinium (Fig. 7.18). No substantial increase in tumor contrast was noted visually when the dose was increased from 0.05 to 0.1 mmol/kg, although, quantitatively, L/B was found to increase by an average of 16%.[20] Because IAC lesions may be very small and therefore may require a higher L/B (higher than 1.3) to be detected, we believe that half-dose studies (0.05 mmol/kg), which yield an average L/B ration of 15.4, are sufficient for the evaluation of IAC lesions.

The signal intensity and enhancement pattern of acoustic schwannomas reflect the predominant cell type within the tumor mass. Schwannomas composed of Antoni type A cells typically show scattered areas of low signal intensity of T_2-weighted images because of the large amount of lipid in these cells. Schwannomas composed predominantly of Antoni type B cells may also show decreased signal intensity on T_2-weighted images because of the presence of mucin (Fig. 7.16). However, Antoni type B cell tumors may undergo regressive changes consisting of hyalinization, fatty degeneration and vacuolization that result in an elevated water content, which would tend to prolong the T_2 and increase signal intensity on T_2-weighted images. Such areas of degeneration do not enhance with gadopentetate dimeglumine.

Although small tumors of the IAC can be sensitively demonstrated with a fractional dose of gadolinium chelates, the findings are not specific. Inflammatory cranial neuritis can cause similar degrees of constant enhancement (Fig. 7.19).[27] Unfortunately, there is no reliable method for distinguishing inflammatory from neoplastic causes of enhancement, including location or size, particularly when lesions are small. Thus, in the setting of facial nerve palsy (Bell palsy) or sensorineural hearing loss, cranial neuritis cannot be distinguished from Schwannoma.

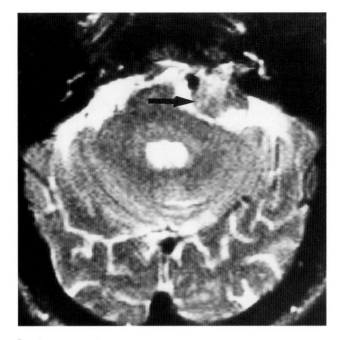

a

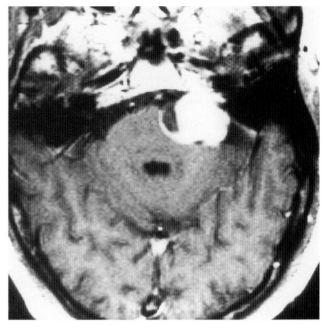

b

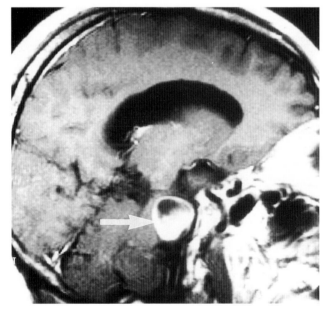

c

Figure 7.16

Acoustic schwannoma in a 68-year-old man. (a) T_2-weighted axial section (SE 2700/90) shows left CPA mass (arrow). (b) T_1-weighted gadolinium-enhanced axial section (SE 600/15) through the same level as (a) shows irregular enhancement of schwannoma. The area of nonenhancement was found to be cystic at pathology and to be rich in Antoni B cells with mucoid degeneration. (c) Left parasagittal section (SE 600/15 with Gd-DTPA) shows mixed solid and cystic acoustic schwannoma (arrow). (Images courtesy of Anton N Hasso, MD, Orange CA.)

Tumor follow-up

After surgery, radiation therapy, or chemotherapy, MR imaging with gadolinium is indicated to follow-up tumor size (Fig. 7.20). It should be realized, however, that recurrent tumor is not all that enhances. Leptomeningeal scarring is quite common after surgery, and local enhancement may persist for years. Unless sequential studies confirm size increase in the region of enhancement, it may be impossible to distinguish recurrent tumor from scar. Radiation necrosis is an entity that can also simulate recurrent tumor, demonstrating enhancement, cyst formation and mass effect. At this time, only positron emission tomography and thallium SPECT can reliably distinguish these.

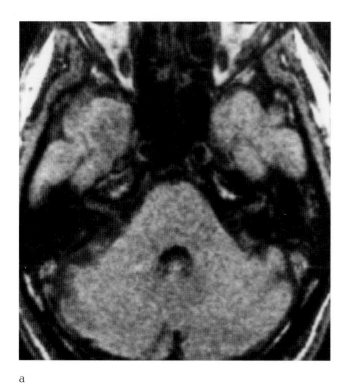

a

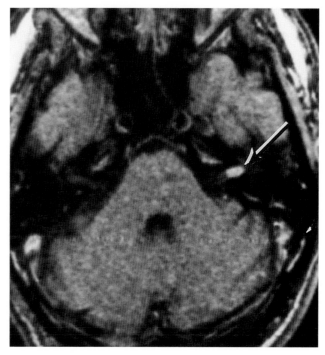

b

Figure 7.17

Acoustic neuroma. Images (gradient echo 300/22, 90° flip angle) before (a) and after (b) Gd-DTPA administration. Enhancement of a left intracanalicular tumor no larger than the 7th–8th nerve bundle is seen on the right in (b) (arrow). (Reprinted with permission from Bradley et al[5].)

Inflammation

Inflammatory conditions sufficient to produce blood–brain barrier breakdown will generally enhance with gadolinium. The acute stage of multiple sclerosis generally shows enhancement (Fig. 7.21), a finding that can be used to follow the activity of the disease. This is particularly important in following the treatment for MS using interferon β-1b (Betaseron, Berlex Laboratories, Wayne, NJ).[28] In one early study,[29] there was good correlation between the site of enhancement and the patient's symptoms. Despite these observations, gadolinium is not generally used to initially detect multiple sclerosis. Our experience with single-dose gadolinium has failed to reveal lesions that were not obvious on images obtained with a long TR, double echo technique (i.e. proton density and T_2-weighted images).

Occasionally, multiple sclerosis can present acutely with a tumefactive form simulating a neoplasm (Fig. 7.21). This may prove particularly confusing when additional white matter lesions are not apparent. Thus, acute tumefactive multiple sclerosis should be considered whenever a 'tumor' is identified in either the brain or spinal cord in a young adult. If surgery is not indicated immediately, repeat examination in 6 weeks (and if necessary again at 12 weeks) may be useful for distinguishing acute tumefactive multiple sclerosis from neoplasm, the former tending to decrease in size over a 6–12 week follow-up. If available, thin-slice fast FLAIR imaging in the sagittal plane has been shown to be more sensitive than traditional long-TR, double spin echo techniques.[30] In one study,[30] thin fast FLAIR images detected lesions consistent with MS in 43% of patients who would have been called normal on routine 5 mm spin echo images.

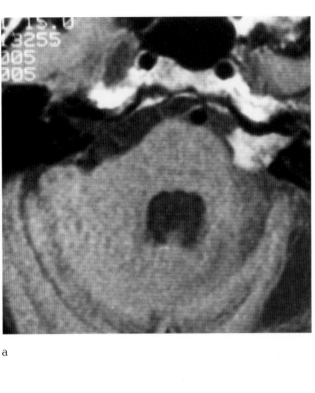

a

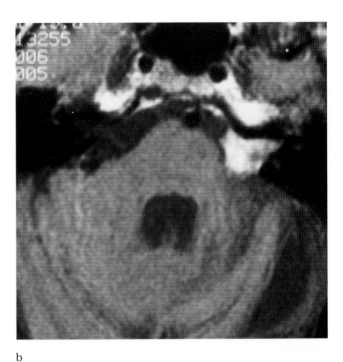

b

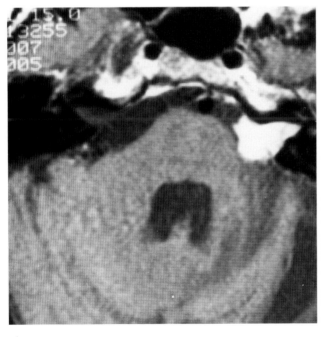

c

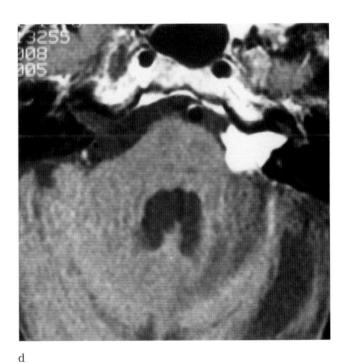

d

Figure 7.18

Fractional-dose studies of acoustic neurinoma. (a) Image was acquired after initial administration of a one-eighth standard dose (0.0125 mmol/kg) of gadolinium. Sequential MR images were then acquired with additional injections of one-eighth, one-quarter and one-half doses at 5 min intervals to achieve cumulative (b) one-quarter (0.025 mmol/kg), (c) one-half (0.05 mmol/kg) and (d) full (0.1 mmol/kg) doses. Substantial lesion contrast (L/B) was obtained even with the one-eighth dose. No additional qualitative improvement of lesion contrast was noted between the half-dose and full-dose studies despite a 100% increase in the dose. (Reprinted with permission from Yuh et al.[20])

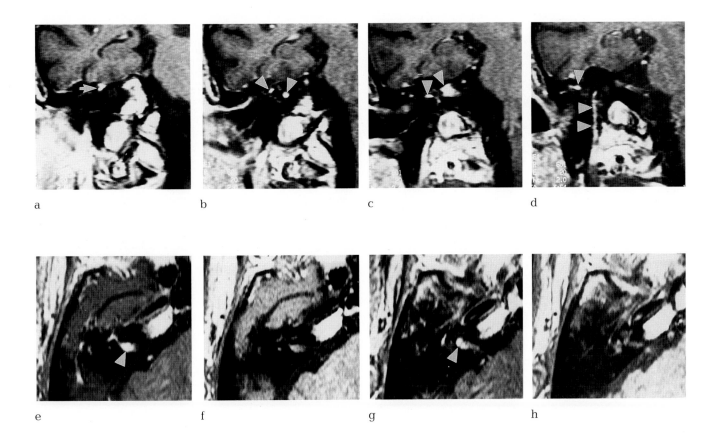

Figure 7.19

Facial neuritis and geniculate ganglionitis in an elderly man with right facial palsy. (a–d) Coronal T_1-weighted images (SE 600/20) of the right temporal bone after intravenous administration of Gd-DTPA.
(a) Anteriormost section shows enhancement within the region of the geniculate ganglion (arrow). (b–d) Serial images from anterior to posterior document enhancement within the proximal intracanalicular portion and distal intratympanic and mastoid portions of the right facial nerve (arrowheads). Axial unenhanced (e) and enhanced (f) sections through the intracanalicular portion of the facial nerve show abnormal enhancement (arrowhead in (f)) due to facial neuritis. Unenhanced (g) and enhanced (h) axial sections through the geniculate ganglion also show abnormal enhancement (arrowhead in (h)). (Images courtesy of Anton N Hasso, MD, Orange CA. Reprinted with permission from Hasso et al.[29])

Acute disseminated encephalomyelitis (ADEM) is a postviral autoimmune leukoencephalopathy generally occurring three weeks after an exanthemous viral infection or a vaccination. This condition in clinically difficult to distinguish from an acute viral meningoencephalitis, and therefore MR imaging findings are critical in the treatment of such patients. While viral encephalitis (e.g. herpes) tends to involve an entire lobe, acute disseminated encephalomyelitis is generally confined to the white matter, where it may enhance with gadolinium. Since this is an autoimmune, potentially steroid-responsive inflammatory condition, it is important to suggest the diagnosis so that proper therapy can be instituted.

Infection

Not all infections enhance with gadolinium. Indolent parenchymal infections such as progressive multifocal leukoencephalopathy (PML) in AIDS (acquired

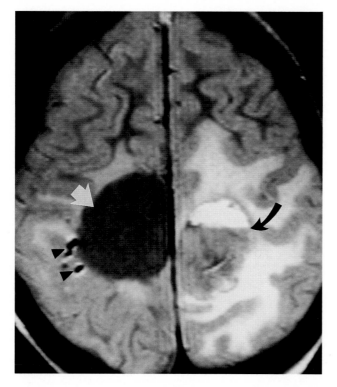

a

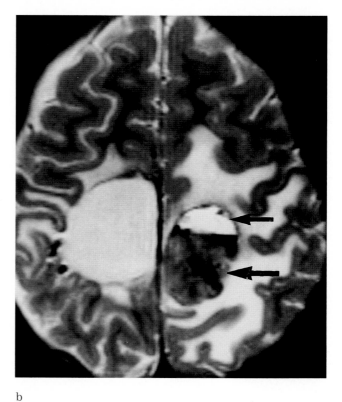

b

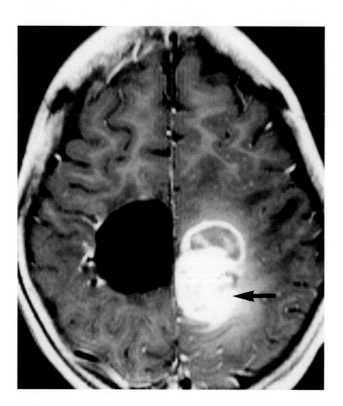

c

Figure 7.20

Recurrent glioma. (a) Proton-density image (SE 3000/22) shows metal artifacts from interstitial seeds (arrowheads) adjacent to right-side surgical defect (straight arrow). There is also an edematous, hemorrhagic mass in the left centrum semiovale with a fluid level (curved arrow). (b) T_2-weighted image (SE 3000/90) through the same level as (a) shows CSF-intensity surgical defect in the right centrum semiovale and hemorrhagic lesion in the left centrum semiovale, with fluid level. The dependent, short-T_2 portion contains deoxyhemoglobin (large arrow), while the nondependent portion contains short-T_1 methemoglobin (small arrow). (c) Gadolinium-enhanced T_1-weighted image (SE 500/15) demonstrates both solid and rim enhancement in recurrent glioma (arrow). (Reprinted with permission from Bradley et al[5].)

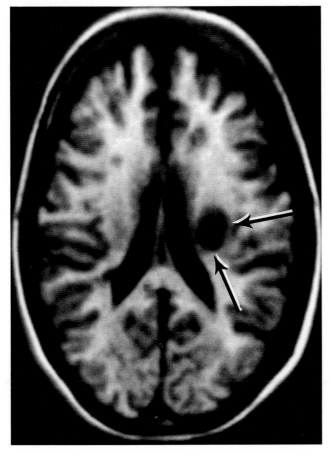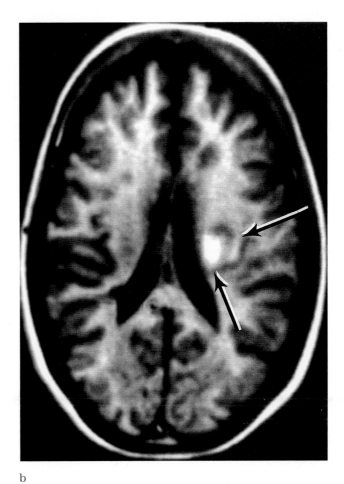

a   b

Figure 7.21

Acute multiple sclerosis. Images (IR 1500/500/44) before (a) and after (b) administration of Gd-DTPA. One lesion (arrows) shows enhancement and mass effect, whereas others do not. (Reprinted with permission from Bydder.[23])

immunodeficiency syndrome) or other immunocompromised states generally do not enhance. The most common fungal infection in AIDS, cryptococcus, enhances only one-third of the time as a basilar meningitis and essentially never as a cryptococcal gel in the perivascular spaces.[31] The most common organism affecting the brain parenchyma in AIDS is the protozoan toxoplasmosis. Like most abscesses, it has a long-T_2 necrotic center and a short-T_2 rim, and is surrounded by long-T_2 vasogenic edema. (The short-T_2 rim is thought by some to represent free radicals at the periphery of the abscess; however, certain forms of hemorrhage would have a similar appearance.) The vascularized rim typically enhances with gadolinium (Fig. 7.22). The rim is typically smooth, which distinguishes an abscess from the less regular enhancing border of a necrotic neoplasm. Prior to frank abscess formation and liquefaction, parenchymal brain infection generally enhances in a solid fashion, reflecting local blood–brain barrier breakdown due to the focal cerebritis.

On the basis of preliminary experience comparing single dose and triple dose gadolinium, it is reasonable to expect the higher-dose gadolinium will be more sensitive in the detection of very early infection than the routine dose. Very early or indolent infections may not enhance at all. Viral infections such as herpes typically do not enhance in the early meningo-encephalitis stage. Bacterial

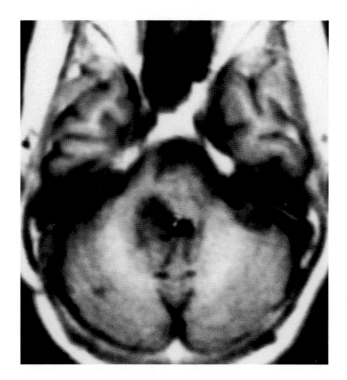

a

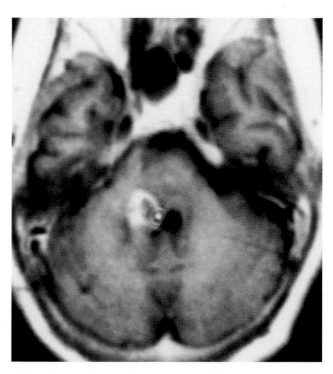

b

Figure 7.22

Abscess. Images (IR 1500/500/44) before (a) and after (b) administration of Gd-DTPA. The abscess displays ring enhancement in (b). (Reprinted with permission from Bradley et al[5].)

cerebritis tends to be more virulent, and enhances at an earlier stage than viral or fungal infections or tuberculosis.

Like cryptococcus, tuberculosis tends to begin as a basilar meningitis, spreading through the perivascular spaces into the brain parenchyma. Unlike cryptococcomas, however, tuberculomas almost always enhance with gadolinium. Similarly, sarcoidosis in the brain begins in the basilar meninges and spreads via the perivascular spaces into the parenchyma.

Infection of the ependymal lining of the ventricles (ventriculitis or ependymitis) can result from preexisting meningitis or contiguous spread from a brain abscess. Subtle ependymal enhancement has been described as a result of cytomegalovirus in AIDS. Bacterial ependymitis (Fig. 7.23) generally enhances with gadolinium, and is often associated with postinflammatory scarring. If such scarring occurs near narrow portions of the ventricular system (i.e. the foramen of Monro or the aqueduct), secondary obstruction can result (Fig. 7.23).

While most infections of the brain are bloodborne, some spread contiguously from adjacent sinusitis, otitis, mastitis or osteomyelitis of the calvarium. Subdural empyemas have an enhancing rim and a nonenhancing center that represents drainable pus. Gadolinium is indicated in the evaluation of such secondary brain abscesses to demonstrate the mature, enhancing capsule of the abscess.

Vascular abnormalities

On unenhanced images, flowing blood generally has low signal intensity (flow void) unless the

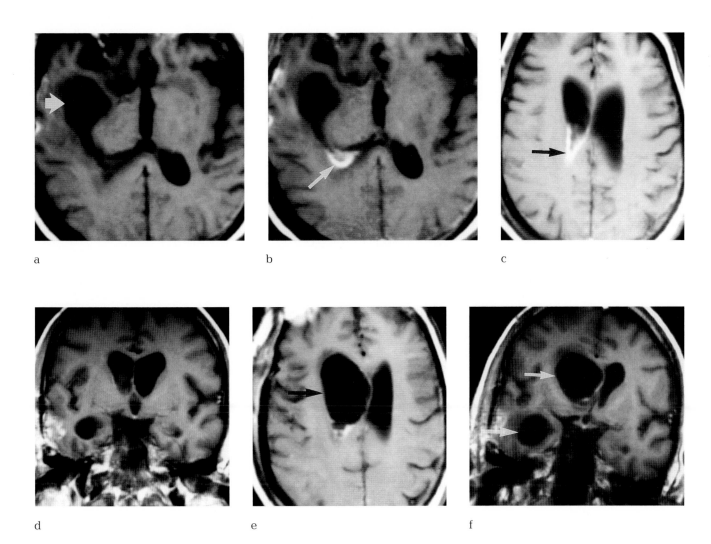

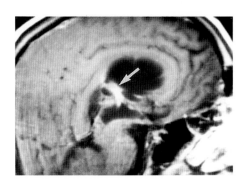

Figure 7.23

Entrapment of the right lateral ventricle secondary to ventriculitis. A 59-year-old man had an abscess drained through his right temporal lobe, and now has secondary ventriculitis. (a) T_1-weighted axial section (SE 800/20) through the right temporal lobe shows the postoperative cavity (arrow). (b) After administration of Gd-DTPA (SE 800/20), there is abnormal enhancement in the right atrium (arrow) secondary to ventriculitis. (c,d) T_1-weighted, enhanced axial and coronal sections (600/20) through the lateral ventricles show abnormal enhancement (arrow in (c)) by asymmetry in the size of the lateral ventricles. (e,f) One week later, T_1-weighted, enhanced axial and coronal sections (SE 600, 800/20) through the same levels as (c) and (d) demonstrate enlargement of the right lateral ventricle (arrows) secondary to obstruction from ventriculitis at the right foramen of Monro. (g) T_1-weighted right parasagittal image (SE 600/20 with Gd-DTPA) shows abnormal enhancement at the foramen of Monro (arrow). (Reprinted with permission from Bradley et al[5].)

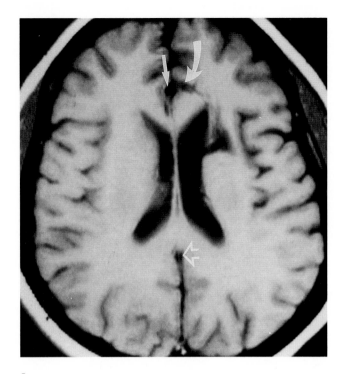

a

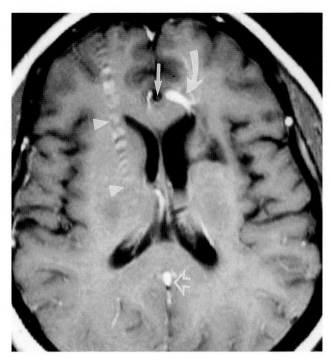

b

Figure 7.24

Venous angioma. (a) Unenhanced T_1-weighted axial section (SE 500/15) through the lateral ventricles shows flow voids in the pericallosal arteries (straight solid arrow), internal cerebral veins (open arrow) and a left frontal venous angioma (curved arrow). (b) After administration of Gd-DTPA, the pericallosal artery still has a flow void (straight solid arrow), but enhancement is now noted in the internal cerebral veins (open arrow) and in the venous angioma (curved arrow). Note also the pulsation artifact (arrowheads) arising from the superior sagittal sinus in this obliquely positioned patient. (Reprinted with permission from Bradley et al[5].)

image is acquired in an entry section, in which case it can have high signal intensity (due to flow-related enhancement). After administration of gadolinium, arterial flow generally continues to have low signal intensity, and venous flow may enhance (Fig. 7.24). Thus gadolinium may cause enhancement of venous angiomas (Fig. 7.24), slowly flowing blood within intracranial aneurysms (Fig. 7.25), and slowly flowing portions of arteriovenous malformations. Unfortunately, the use of gadolinium may also increase flow artifacts, particularly those arising from the dural sinuses.

Although MR angiography is not the principal focus of this chapter, gadolinium chelates may also be used in combination with time-of-flight MR angiography.[27] Gadolinium-enhanced MR angiography can help distinguish totally absent flow from very slow flow by overcoming saturation effects in the latter condition. Gadolinium can also be used in combination with time-of-flight MR angiography to demonstrate the relationship of an enhancing tumor to the intracranial arteries or dural sinuses.

Ischemia and infarction

Infarction can be divided into three stages: acute, subacute and chronic. During the acute stage, there is mass effect (with secondary ablation of cortical sulci) resulting from ischemia and infarction (Figs

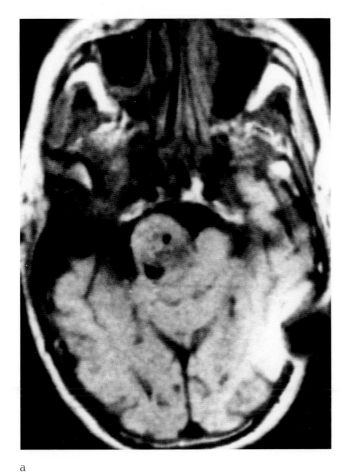

a

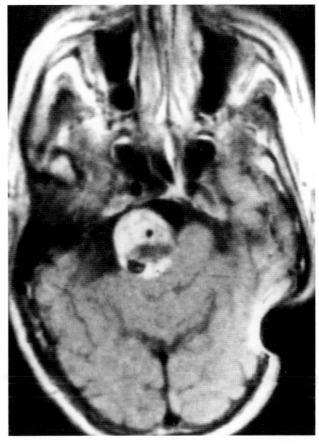

b

Figure 7.25

Giant intracranial aneurysm. Unenhanced (a) and enhanced (b) images (SE 544/44) show enhancing giant intracranial aneurysm. The increased signal intensity reflects both rim enhancement and enhancement of slow flow within the aneurysm. (Reprinted with permission from Bradley et al[5].)

7.26 and 7.27). Ischemia results in reversible cytotoxic edema (with swelling primarily in the gray matter), while infarction results in vasogenic edema. Both forms of edema contribute to the mass effect of an acute infarct. On T_2-weighted images, increased signal intensity may be noted within the gray matter and the subjacent white matter, reflecting increased water content due to vasogenic edema. In some cases of ischemia, however, the long-T_1 ultrafiltrate of cytotoxic edema (Fig. 7.27) may not produce the high signal intensity on T_2-weighted images seen in the transudate of vasogenic edema with its higher protein content and shorter T_1.

Gadolinium has recently found a major new application in the evaluation of acute cerebral infarction.[32-35] It has been noted[31-33] that enhancement of the arteries themselves during acute stroke correlates with a worse prognosis than does a lack of vascular enhancement (Figs 7.26 and 7.27). This finding is similar to the 'dense artery sign' on CT scans[36-38] (Fig. 7.26). Clinical outcome has been correlated with arterial enhancement, with the flow void in the same vessels on unenhanced MR images, and with catheter angiograms, and has been found to correlate more accurately with arterial enhancement than with either of the latter two studies.[32,33] Vascular enhancement with gadolinium was found to be a more sensitive indicator of severe ischemia than was the lack of a flow void on routine MR images or an arterial occlusion or stenosis on angiograms. Thus, when arterial enhancement is seen, it suggests inadequate collateral circulation and a greater degree of ischemia, with a poorer

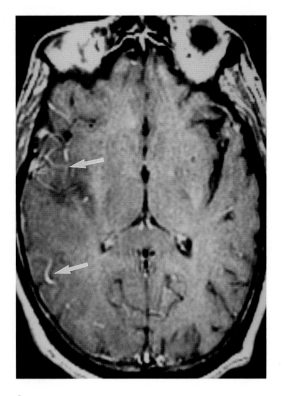

a

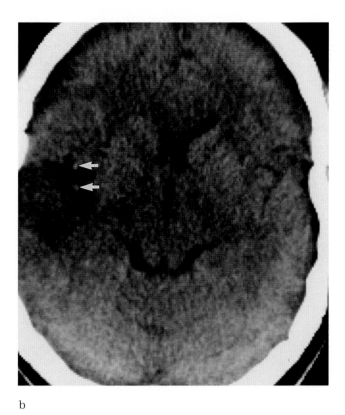

b

Figure 7.26

Comparison of vascular abnormalities depicted by contrast-enhanced MR imaging and CT. (a) Postcontrast axial T_1-weighted image (750/20) obtained three days after onset of symptoms shows abnormal arterial enhancement in distribution of right middle cerebral artery (arrows). Specifically noted is obvious enhancement of distal peripheral small branches.

(b) Axial unenhanced CT scan at the corresponding level of parietal lobes shows 'dense artery sign' (arrows) in region of proximal middle cerebral artery. However, no vascular abnormality in distal arterial branches can be seen. (Reprinted with permission from Crain et al.[33])

clinical prognosis than that for patients in whom there is no vascular enhancement. In patients in whom vascular enhancement is only present during the first day and then resolves, and in those in whom it is never seen, the collateral circulation is considered to be intact and the prognosis is better (i.e. ischemia is milder).

Parenchymal enhancement can be seen in the acute stage of infarction once the blood supply has been reestablished to the region. The cause of this enhancement is unknown, but could represent local hyperemia resulting from the ischemia or even blood–brain barrier breakdown. Such parenchymal enhancement has been noted with mass effect as early as 2 h after 2 min of balloon occlusion of the internal carotid artery (Fig. 7.28). Since parenchymal enhancement implies reestablishment of normal arterial flow, no vascular enhancement is seen (Fig. 7.29). Marked parenchymal enhancement can be noted several days after totally reversible neurologic deficits (i.e. transient ischemic attacks) (Fig. 7.29). In general, the degree of early parenchymal enhancement is inversely correlated with the degree of arterial enhancement and signal abnormality on T_2-weighted images. Such early parenchymal enhancement is also associated with an improved clinical outcome.[32-34]

In the subacute phase of infarction, the mass effect has resolved, and there is generally high signal intensity on T_1-weighted images and low

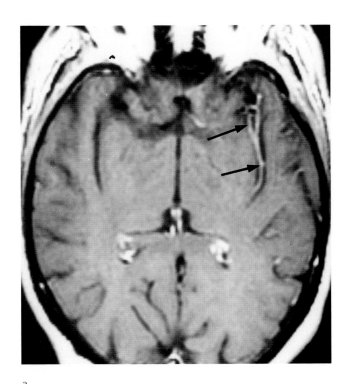

a

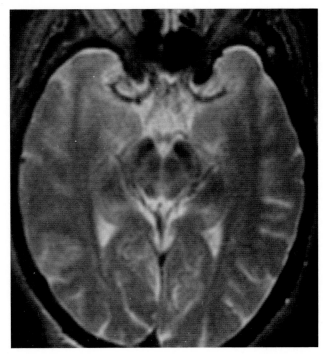

b

Figure 7.27

Early arterial enhancement in cortical infarction.
(a) Postcontrast axial T_1-weighted image (SE 750/20)
shows enhancement in the left middle cerebral artery
(arrows) 2 h after the onset of acute ischemic
symptoms. (b) T_2-weighted axial section (SE 2000/100)
through the same level as (a) shows no evidence of
abnormality. (Reprinted with permission from Crain et
al.[33])

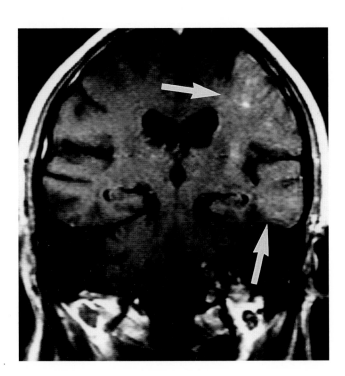

Figure 7.28

A 67-year-old man underwent preoperative balloon
test occlusion of the left internal carotid artery and
developed acute ischemic symptoms after 2 min of
carotid occlusion. After balloon deflation, preservation
of carotid flow was demonstrated angiographically.
Postcontrast coronal T_1-weighted image (583/20)
obtained 2 h after onset shows diffuse parenchymal
enhancement of left crebral hemisphere (arrows).
Parenchymal morphologic changes (swelling) are noted
without evidence of discrete arterial enhancement.
(Reprinted with permission from Yuh et al.[32])

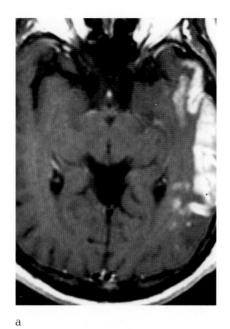

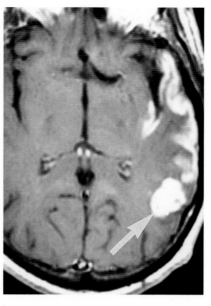

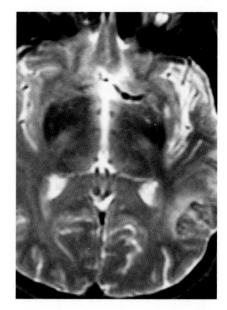

a   b   c

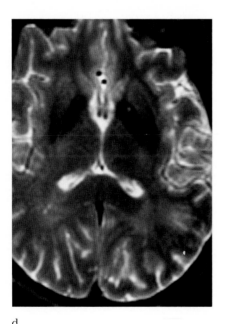

d

Figure 7.29

Example of early, intense parenchymal enhancement in a patient with reversible ischemic neurologic deficit. MR imaging was performed 10 days after transient ischemic episode with right-side weakness and aphasia that resolved almost completely in 2 h. (a,b) Postcontrast axial T_1-weighted images (SE 700/20) show diffuse, intense cortical enhancement in distribution of left middle cerebral artery without evidence of arterial enhancement. (c,d) Corresponding axial T_2-weighted images (SE 2000/100) show a much less extensive area of signal abnormality. The enhancement appears more intense near the watershed zone (arrow in (b)), which may reflect greater availability of contrast material in this region. This case again shows that parenchymal enhancement is inversely related to the appearance of arterial enhancement and signal abnormality on T_2-weighted images. (Reprinted with permission from Yuh et al.[32])

signal intensity on T_2-weighted images, corresponding to petechial hemorrhage (intracellular methemoglobin) (Fig. 7.30). Gyral enhancement is common at this stage because of reestablishment of both parenchymal and collateral circulation and associated blood–brain barrier breakdown. Since the regions of previous ischemia have either progressed to infarction or returned to normal, there is generally no mass effect at this stage. Enhancement with gadolinium is similar to that previously described with iodinated contrast media on CT scans, and reflects not only blood–brain barrier breakdown but also loss of autoregulation and luxury perfusion.[34]

During the chronic stage, encephalomalacia is present with negative mass effect or atrophy. At

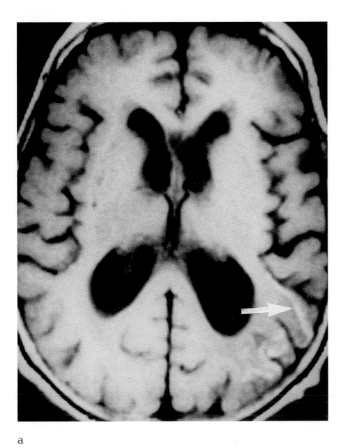

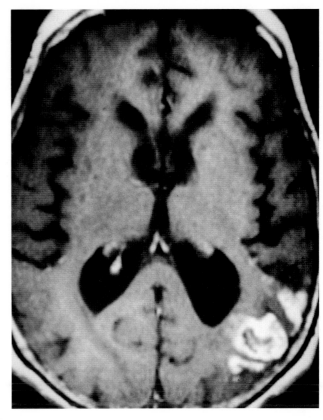

a

b

Figure 7.30

Subacute infarction. (a) Unenhanced T_1-weighted image (SE 500/20) shows gyral hyperintensity (arrow) due to the presence of subacute petechial hemorrhage (methemoglobin). Note the lack of mass effect.
(b) After administration of Gd-DTPA (SE 500/20), there is dense gyral enhancement due to the combination of luxury perfusion, loss of autoregulation and blood–brain barrier breakdown. (Reprinted with permission from Bradley et al[5].)

this stage (6–8 weeks after the acute infarct), there is generally no evidence of gyral enhancement or blood–brain barrier defect.

Conclusions

Lesion detectability in the brain depends on size, contrast (L/B), location (background) and type. Large lesions, even those with low contrast, can be detected with MR imaging without administration of contrast media. The detection of small, enhancing intraparenchymal lesions, such as early metastases, requires high lesion contrast. Increased lesion contrast can be achieved by either delayed imaging, or, to a greater extent, by increased doses of contrast media.[17] Unfortunately while higher doses of gadolinium can be justified from a clinical or imaging standpoint, they may not be allowed from an economic standpoint, particularly in these days of increasingly managed care. Recent studies using magnetization transfer (MT) background suppression and single doses of gadolinium have shown similar contrast to that previously reported for high-dose gadolinium without MT.[39] The delineation of gliomas can also be improved with high-dose studies, which frequently demonstrate enhancement extending beyond the region of apparent abnormality on T_2-weighted images. In pituitary adenomas (negative contrast), a high-dose technique or delayed imaging may reduce lesion contrast. The use of fractional doses of gadolinium and immediate imaging should provide better lesion contrast. Fractional-dose studies may also be useful in enhancing lesions surrounded by low-signal-intensity background, such as those found in the region of the IAC and CPA, where sufficiently high lesion contrast can be obtained.

References

1. Bydder GM, Clinical application of gadolinium-DTPA. In: *Magnetic resonance imaging* (ed DD Stark, WG Bradley) 182–200. Mosby-Year Book, St Louis, 1988.

2. Bradley WG, Waluch V, Yadley RA, Wycoff RR, Comparison of CT and MR in 400 patients with suspected disease of the brain and cervical spinal cord. *Radiology* 1984; **152:** 695–702.

3. Palmer FJ, The RACR survey of intravenous contrast media reaction: final report. *Aust Radiol* 1988; **32:** 426–8.

4. Caro JJ, Trindade E, McGregor M, Risks of death and of severe nonfatal reactions with high- vs low-osmolality contrast media: a meta-analysis. *AJR* 1991; **156:** 825–32.

5. Bradley WG, Yuh WTC, Bydder GM, Use of MR imaging contrast agents in the brain. *J Magn Reson Imaging* 1993; **3:** 199–218.

6. Yuh WTC, Fisher DJ, Engleken JD et al, MR evaluation of CNS tumors: dose comparison study with gadopentetate dimeglumine and gadoteridol. *Radiology* 1991; **180:** 485–91.

7. Runge VM, Gelblum DY, Pacetti ML et al, Gd-HP-DO3A in clinical MR imaging of the brain. *Radiology* 1990; **177:** 393–400.

8. Niendorf HP, Laniado M, Semmler W et al, Dose administration of gadolinium-DTPA in MR imaging of intracranial tumors. *AJNR* 1987; **8:** 803–15.

9. Graif M, Bydder GM, Steiner RE et al, Contrast-enhanced MR imaging of malignant brain tumors. *AJNR* 1985; **6:** 855–62.

10. Schorner W, Laniado M, Niendorf HP et al, Time-dependent changes in image contrast in brain tumors after gadolinium-DTPA. *AJNR* 1986; **7:** 1013–20.

11. Bydder GM, Kingsley PE, Brown J et al, MR imaging of meningiomas including studies with and without gadolinium-DTPA. *J Comput Assist Tomogr* 1985; **9:** 690–7.

12. Strich G, Hagan PL, Gerber KH, Slutsky RA, Tissue distribution and magnetic resonance spin lattice relaxation effects of gadolinium-DTPA. *Radiology* 1985; **154:** 723–6.

13. Runge VM, Kaufman DM, Wood ML et al, Experimental trials with Gd(DO3A)—a nonionic magnetic resonance contrast agent. *Nucl Med Biol* 1989; **16:** 561–7.

14. Tweedle MF, Eaton SM, Eckelman WC et al, Comparative chemical structure and pharmacokinetics of MRI contrast agents. *Invest Radiol* 1988; **23**(supp 1): S236–9.

15. Elster AD, DiPersio DA, Cranial postoperative site: assessment with contrast-enhanced MR imaging. *Radiology* 1990; **174:** 93–8.

16. Burke JW, Podrasky AE, Bradley WG, Meninges: benign postoperative enhancement on MR images. *Radiology* 1990; **174:** 99–102.

17. Yuh WTC, Engelken JD, Muhonen MG et al, Experience with high dose gadolinium MR imaging in the evaluation of brain metastases. *AJNR* 1992; **13:** 335–45.

18. Haustein J, Bauer W, Milbertz T et al, Dosing of Gd-DTPA in MRI imaging of intracranial tumors: a randomized double-blind multicenter study in 90 cases. *Abstracts Ann Mtg Soc Magn Reson Med, Berkeley, CA, 1990*, 259.

19. Sze G, Milano E, Johnson C, Heier L, Detection of brain metastases: comparison of contrast-enhanced MR with unenhanced MR and enhanced CT. *AJNR* 1990; **11:** 785–91.

20. Yuh WTC, Fisher DJ, Nguyen HD et al, The application of contrast agents in the evaluation of neoplasms of the central nervous system. *Top Magn Reson Imaging* 1992; **4:** 1–6.

21. Nelson DR, Yuh WTC, Waziri MH et al, MR imaging of Hippel–Lindau disease: value of gadopentetate dimeglumine. *J Magn Reson Imaging* 1991; **1:** 469–76.

22. Hasso AN, Kortman KE, Bradley WG, Supratentorial neoplasm. In: *Magnetic resonance imaging*, 2nd edn (ed DD Stark, WG Bradley) Chap 25. Mosby-Year Book, St Louis, 1992.

23. Bydder GM, Use of gadolinium-DTPA. In: *MRI atlas of the brain* (ed WG Bradley, GM Bydder) Chap 9. Martin Dunitz, London, 1990.

24. Goldsher D, Litt AW, Pinto RS et al, Dural 'tail' associated with meningiomas on Gd-DTPA-enhanced MR images: characteristics, differential diagnostic value, and possible implications for treatment. *Radiology* 1990; **176:** 447–50.

25. Bradley WG, Widoff BE, Yan K et al, Comparison of routine and gadodiamide-enhanced 3D time-of-flight MR angiography in the brain. *Radiology* 1992; **185(P):** 121(abst).

26. Davis PC, Gokhale KA, Joseph GJ et al, Pituitary adenoma: correlation of half-dose gadolinium-enhanced MR imaging with surgical findings in 16 patients. *Radiology* 1991; **180:** 779–84.

27. Hasso AN, Hinshaw SB, Kief-Garcia ML, Neoplasms of the cranial nerves and skull base. In: *Magnetic resonance imaging*, 2nd edn (ed DD Stark, WG Bradley) Chap 27. Mosby-Year Book. St Louis, 1992.

28. Oger J, O'Gorman M, Willoughby E, Li D, Paty DW, Changes in immune function in relapsing multiple sclerosis correlate with disease activity as assessed by magnetic resonance imaging. *Ann NY Acad Sci* 1988; **540:** 597–601.

29. Grossman RI, Gonzalez-Scarano F, Atlas SW et al, Multiple sclerosis: gadolinium enhancement in MR imaging. *Radiology* 1986: **161:** 721–5.

30. Hashemi RH, Bradley WG, Chen D-Y et al, Suspected multiple sclerosis: MR imaging with a thin-section fast FLAIR pulse sequence. *Radiology* 1995; **196:** 505–10.

31. Wehn SM, Heinz ER, Burger PC et al, Dilated Virchow–Robin spaces in cryptococcal meningitis associated with AIDS: CT and MR findings. *J Comput Assist Tomogr* 1989; **13:** 756–62.

32. Yuh WTC, Crain MR, Loes DJ et al, MR imaging of cerebral ischemia: findings in the first 24 hours. *AJNR* 1991; **12:** 621–9.

33. Crain MR, Yuh WTC, Greene GM et al, Cerebral ischemia: evaluation with contrast-enhanced MR imaging. *AJNR* 1991; **12:** 631–9.

34. Yuh WTC, Crain MR, Magnetic resonance imaging of acute cerebral ischemia. *Stroke* 1992; **2:** 421–39.

35. Elster AD, Moody DM, Early cerebral infarction: gadopentate dimeglumine enhancement. *Radiology* 1990; **177:** 627–32.

36. Pressman BD, Tourje EJ, Thompson JR, An early CT sign of ischemic infarction: increased density in a cerebral artery. *AJNR* 1987; **8:** 645–8.

37. Tomsick TA, Brott TG, Chambers AA et al, Hyperdense middle cerebral artery sign on CT: efficacy in detecting middle cerebral artery thrombosis. *AJNR* 1990; **11:** 473–7.

38. Schuknecht B, Ratzka M, Hofmann E, The 'dense artery sign': major cerebral artery thromboembolism demonstrated by computed tomography. *Neuroradiology* 1990; **32:** 98–103.

39. Elster AD, King JC, Mathews VP, Hamilton CA, Cranial tissues: appearance at gadolinium-enhanced and nonenhanced MR imaging with magnetization transfer contrast. *Radiology* 1994; **190:** 541.

8

Contrast mechanisms in functional MRI of the brain

Joseph V Hajnal, Ian R Young and Graeme M Bydder

Introduction

In most functional MRI (fMRI) studies, image sets are repeatedly acquired from the same location while the subject is alternatively in an active and a control state. These images are then processed to extract the part that correlates with the stimulus paradigm. Using approaches of this type, numerous groups have shown brain signals that are clearly correlated with the task being performed.[1-5]

In the initial studies, the detection of stimulus-correlated signals was so striking that the intellectual step from observing these signals to inferring that their source was physiological activation of the brain seemed small and well justified. Like many others, we were impressed and set to work to reproduce and extend the scope of these studies. Like most other groups, we found that startling results could be produced, but there was also a disconcerting variability. Some subjects consistently showed marked changes, others showed little or no effect, and a third group displayed quite variable results.

Another cause for concern soon emerged. The basic mechanism for detecting activation through changes in blood oxygenation (the blood oxygen-level, dependent or 'BOLD' effect; see Table 8.1) is expected to be field-dependent, with larger effects detectable on scanners operated at higher field strength B_0. Yet we found that 'activation', as defined by the presence of stimulus correlated signals, could be detected without particular difficulty at the low field of 0.15 T (Fig. 8.1).[6]

Table 8.1 Types of image contrast in fMRI

BOLD	*Blood Oxygen Level Dependent:* Proposed mechanism for contrast in activation studies based on animal work. Depletion of oxygen increases the proportion of deoxyhemoglobin, which is paramagnetic. This produces dephasing effects, resulting in a loss of signal, which is manifest as a reduction in $T_2{}^*$. In human activation experiments, increased blood supply is implicated in the reduction of the proportion of deoxyhemoglobin, reduction of dephasing and production of an increase in signal.
b-FOLD	*blood FlOw Level Dependent:* Proposed mechanism for contrast due to increased local blood flow associated with activation.
c-FOLD	*cSF FlOw Level Dependent:* Contrast produced by motion of CSF.
MOLD	*MOtion Level Dependent:* Changes in signal intensity produced by stimulus correlated motion of the brain and other forms of brain motion.
COLD	*CSF Oxygen Level Dependent:* Change in signal intensity in CSF produced by inhaled oxygen and attributed to a reduction in CSF T_1.

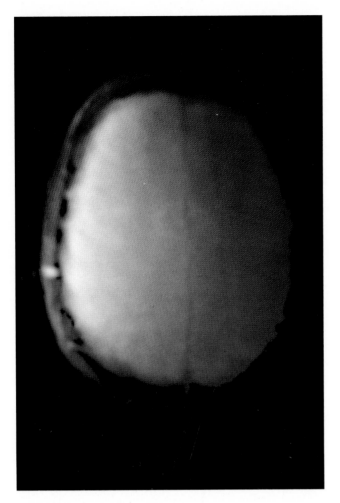
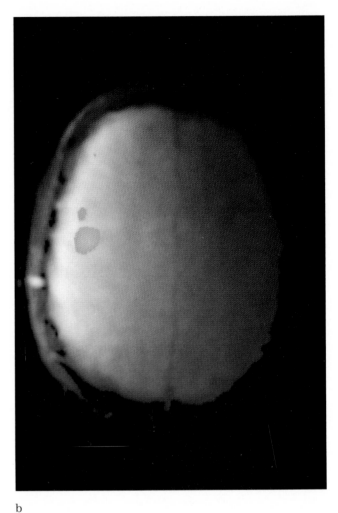

a   b

Figure 8.1

Control (a) and activated image (b) obtained at 0.15 T with subject observing a home movie using a surface coil for signal reception and a FLAIR sequence. Subtraction produces an increase in signal intensity in the appropriate location (frontal eye fields), which is superimposed on the anatomical image. This experiment does not distinguish brain activation from stimulus correlated motion.

The observed signals might have been attributed to flow effects—had the FLAIR sequence employed not been flow-insensitive by virtue of its use of spatially unselective inversion pulses provided by a whole body transmit coil.

It was tempting to dismiss the low-field results as artifacts. However, this only raised a more fundamental problem. If signals that correlate with the stimulus protocol and show a positive change with activation in an appropriate location in the brain are not markers of brain activation when B_0 is low then why should signals with exactly the same characteristics be regarded as true activation when B_0 is higher? Also, if the low-field results were not due to brain activation, what were they due to? The most obvious possibility was subject motion.

Stimulus correlated motion: motion-level-dependent (MOLD) contrast

Most fMRI studies employ sequences of images acquired at a fixed spatial location relative to the scanner. Changes in subject position within the scanner may therefore change the composition of the anatomy in the fixed voxel or voxels of interest, and thus change the signal intensity even when no physiological change has occurred in the brain. This is manifested most clearly as a difference on a subtraction image. These displacement-induced changes in voxel signal intensity are different from conventional motion artifacts, and can be highly localized.

To explore the possible contribution of movement to stimulus correlated signals, we performed a series of motor and visual activation experiments on a Picker HPQ system operating at 1.0 T using a conventional long-TE gradient echo sequence to image a single slice repeatedly at a rate of one image every 20 s.[7] This approach is similar to that used by a number of other groups, and is sensitive to both the BOLD effect and flow effects. An example of a motor study is shown in Fig. 8.2. The protocol consisted of finger-to-thumb touching with the right hand for the duration of five images, followed by exercising with the left hand for the next five images, reverting to the right hand for the next five, and so on for a total of 40 images. The image slice was coronal (as illustrated in Fig. 8.2a), and a mean difference image (right-hand action minus left-hand action) is shown in Fig. 8.2(b). The result (Fig. 8.2b) was a focal signal change of about 6% on the left side of the brain at the expected location for the motor cortex. It seemed likely to represent true brain activation.

To detect the presence of subject motion during the study, we used image registration as originally developed by Woods et al[8] to determine the translations and rotations required to retrospectively match for position one image to each of the other 39 images. The resulting history of displacements is shown in graphical form in Fig. 8.2(c). The registration procedure detected tiny displacements, with maximum left–right and head–foot shifts of 0.5 mm and maximum in-plane rotations of 0.3°. These displacement histories contained motion that correlated with the stimulus protocol, with a predominance of small changes in position that occurred as the hand being exercised was changed (i.e., at multiples of five images; see Fig. 8.2c). To

confirm this finding, the motion data were analyzed to derive power spectra that were found to contain dominant contributions at exactly the period of the cyclic stimulus protocol.

This showed that stimulus correlated motion was present. To determine the effects of this motion on images, comparison was made between the ostensibly real functional image shown in Fig. 8.2(b) and a second difference image (Fig. 8.2d) created by replacing each image in the original series of 40 field echo images with a copy of the reference image shifted according to the displacement information shown in Fig. 8.2(c). Figure 8.2(d) gives a direct visualization of the effect of the stimulus correlated motion. It produced a highly focal response in the expected location, and replicated the features that had been ascribed to brain activation in Fig. 8.2(b). This showed that stimulus-correlated motion could generate signals that satisfy the criteria normally used for brain activation.

This produced a perplexing scenario. A subject performs a task, makes tiny movements of his or her head, and produces signal changes in just the expected places to mimic localized brain activation. Surely this is so unlikely that it can be ignored? The example in Fig. 8.2 shows that this does indeed occur, and also gives clues as to why it may be much less improbable than might at first appear. An important factor is the limited coverage of most fMRI experiments. Collecting data from a single slice or a very few adjacent slices and/or the use of surface coils to locally enhance the signal-to-noise ratio may serve to hide remote signal changes. An essential step in any experiment that offers only limited spatial coverage is to choose the region of study. This choice is made for each individual subject and is guided by anatomical landmarks, but the final selection is influenced by the detection of appropriate signals. This allows great freedom and may result in unconscious selection of erroneous signals.

The general belief that activation signals are positive means that negative signal changes are easily ignored or are suppressed during data processing. Many published functional images show both positive and negative changes, and it is not uncommon to select one region for comment when others are present and equally prominent. The use of thresholds and presentation of positive signals against a dark background preclude detection of negative regions. The common practice of overlaying extracted functional data on anatomical images acquired with different parameters or pulse sequences also makes it difficult to assess the true nature of the signals presented.

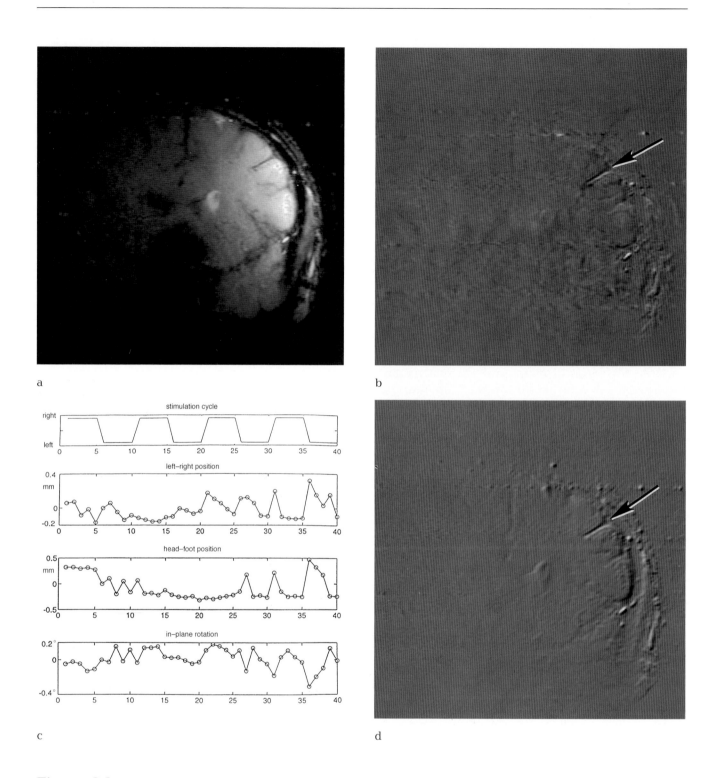

Figure 8.2

Coronal gradient echo image ($TR = 150$ ms, $TE = 100$ ms, flip angle $65°$) taken from a series of 40 images of the same slice acquired with a surface coil during a motor activation study (a). The mean difference image (right-hand activation minus left-hand activation) shows a focal signal change in an appropriate anatomical location (b) (arrow). Using image registration, the head position can be tracked from image to image in the series. The resulting left–right and head–foot displacements and in-plane rotations are plotted against image number (time) in (c). By combining this displacement information with the anatomical content in (a), the signal changes associated with stimulus correlated motion can be determined (d). The correspondence between the putative activation signals in (b) and the displacement-induced signals in (d) is striking.

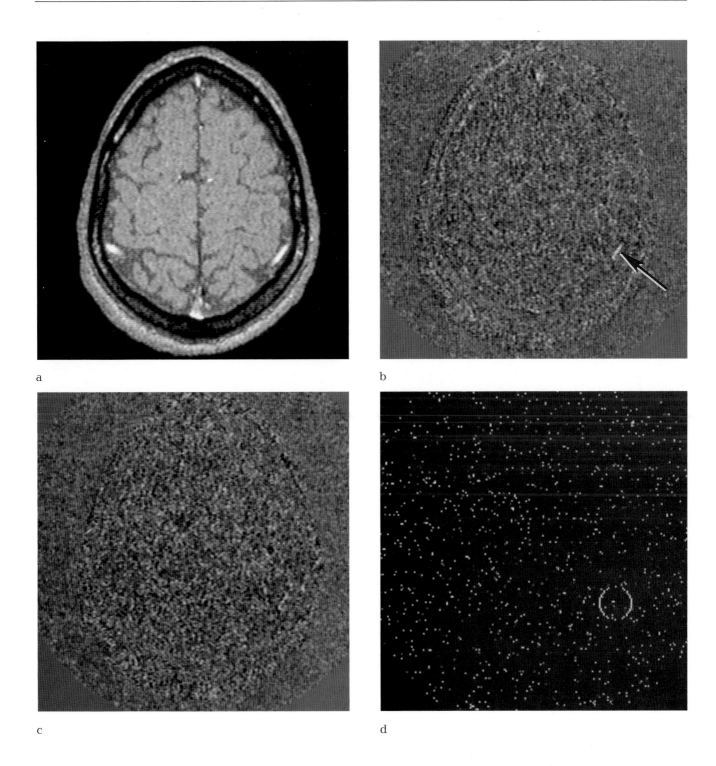

a

b

c

d

Figure 8.3

Motor stimulation study using a 3D inflow sensitive sequence ($TR = 40$ ms, $TE = 8$ ms, 20° flip angle, 190 × 180 × 40 matrix, 1 mm partitions) and an enveloping coil for signal reception. The anatomical image (a) shows two prominent draining vessels, and the mean difference image (right-hand activation minus left-hand activation) shows a signal change in the left-hand vessel with little evidence of misregistration (b) (arrow). However, after image registration, differences between right-hand and left-hand activation have been reduced to the noise level (c). A possible signal change is just discernible amidst the noise (c) but a paired t-test map showed that this was not significant at the 5% level (d) (circled region). The speckled appearance in (d) results from random isolated voxels that exceed the threshold of significance by chance.

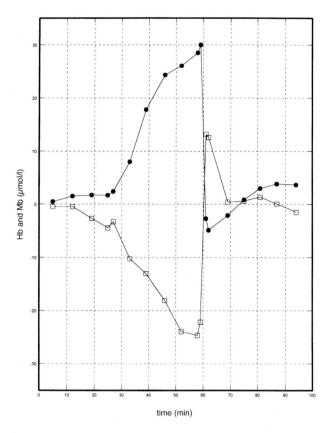

a

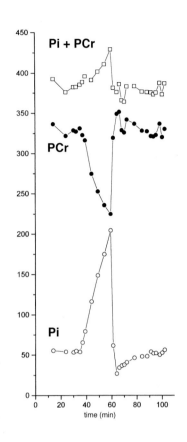

b

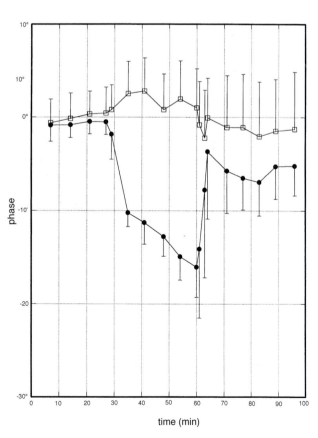

c

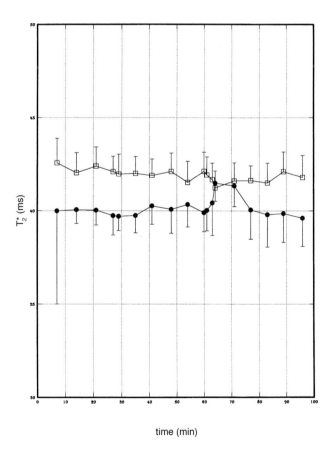

d

Figure 8.4

Human leg ischemia study. (a) Oxy- (□) and deoxy-
(●) hemoglobin and myoglobin concentrations versus
time: near-infrared data acquired before, during and
after 30 min of ischemia. There is a profound
reduction in the oxy- forms and an increase in the
deoxy- forms of hemoglobin and myoglobin.

(b) MR spectroscopy. Time course of PCr, Pi and
PCr + Pi. There is a decrease in PCr and an increase
in Pi during the ischemic phase.

(c) Means of region-of-interest measurements of MRI
phase difference plotted against time for the muscle of
the leg with the cuff (●) and the leg without a cuff
(□). Phase changes are seen in the ischemic leg.

(d) Plot of T_2^* versus time for leg with the cuff
(ischemia) (●) and leg without a cuff (□). Neither leg
shows a significant change during the ischemic period.
A small change in T_2^* is seen during the subsequent
hyperemia in the ischemic limb following release of
the cuff at 60 min.

Having shown that stimulus correlated motion
was present and that it could produce localized
effects that simulated brain activation, the next
question was whether its effects could be avoided
or removed. Since it is impractical in most
instances to hold the subject's head in a fixed
position to within a fraction of a millimeter, it was
necessary to realign the images acquired during
an activation experiment to correct for small
changes in position.

To shift images though fractions of a voxel,
intensity values must be generated using values
from the voxel of interest and its neighbors in a
process known as interpolation. This process may
corrupt voxel signal intensity values if it is not
performed in a way that preserves the integrity of
the data. The data acquisition must also be appropriate for the registration process.

Registration techniques are now beginning to be
applied to fMRI data, but in most cases only partial
correction of stimulus-correlated motion is possible. The reasons for this are numerous. Edge
detection or feature detection methods are easy to
use, but they are usually only accurate to the
nearest voxel and thus do not provide subvoxel
accuracy. The influence of extraneous changes in
extracerebral soft tissues needs to be excluded.
Linear interpolation is frequently employed, but
this introduces errors—particularly at boundaries.
2D (multislice) rather than 3D acquisitions are
generally used, but these result in inaccurate
through-plane corrections.

Even with the best attainable registration procedure and matched data acquisition, there are
changes that may not be correctable by rigid-body
translation and rotation. These include some
susceptibility effects,[12] changes in the shape of the
brain with differences in position, as well as some
flow effects. And, ultimately, the process of registration is signal-to-noise (and artifact) limited.

In spite of these difficulties, it is possible to apply
forms of registration that address the issues
described above and provide accurate and robust
subvoxel registration in three dimensions.[9–11] What
happens if registration of this type is used? To find
out, we performed an activation experiment using
a flow-sensitive sequence and a susceptibility-
sensitive (T_2^*-weighted) sequence.

Registration of functional magnetic resonance images

At a high-contrast boundary, such as that
frequently found between brain and CSF,
misalignment between images of a tenth of a voxel
(typically 0.1 mm) may produce as much as a 5%
change in signal. Since in fMRI we are often
seeking changes of this order or less, image alignment must be to within a small fraction of a
voxel.[9–11]

Activation experiment using blood flow-level-dependent (b-FOLD) contrast

Changes in blood flow are thought to be an essential feature of brain activation. An example of a
flow-sensitive study involving motor stimulation is
shown in Fig. 8.3. A representative anatomical
slice is shown in Fig. 8.3(a), with a prominent
vessel on each side of the brain.

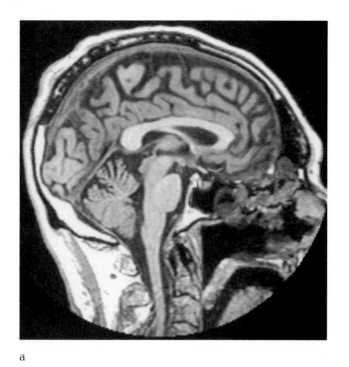

a

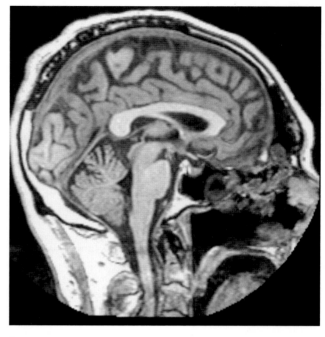

b

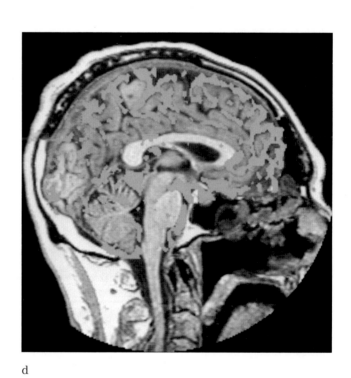

c   d

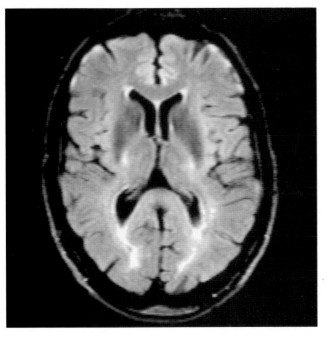

e

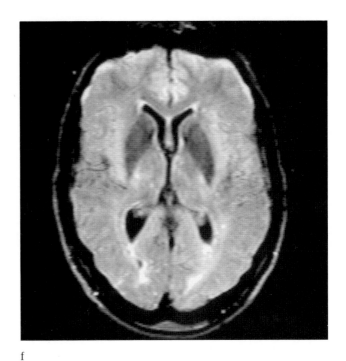

f

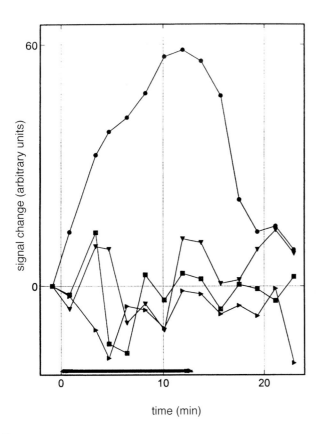

time (min)

g

Figure 8.5

Inhalation of air and 100% oxygen: T_1-weighted 3D scans (TE = 21 ms, TE = 6 ms, 35° flip angle, 152 × 456 × 114, 2 NEX, 1.6 mm sections) of a normal male aged 63 years, showing air image (a), oxygen image (b), subtraction of air from oxygen (c), and subtraction of air from oxygen (yellow) superimposed on (a) (d). There is an increase in the signal in the sulci and basal cisterns in (c) and (d) although no significant change is seen in the ventricles. Transverse FLAIR sequences (IR600/160/2100 ms) before (e) and during oxygen inhalation (f) are also shown. There is an increase in the signal of the extracerebral CSF during inhalation of oxygen. As a result, numerous sulci seen in (e) appear effaced in (f). No change is seen in the lateral or third ventricles. The time course of these changes is shown in (g): ●, extraventricular CSF; ■, ventricular CSF; ▶, sagittal sinus; ▼, cortex; ▬▬, 100% oxygen. The signal from the extraventricular CSF increases over about 10 min, while that from the ventricular CSF, sagittal sinus and cortex shows no significant change.

The unregistered difference image (right-hand activation minus left-hand activation; see Fig. 8.3b) shows little evidence of misregistration, and reveals an apparent unilateral change in the left-side vessel (arrow), which would be appropriate for increased flow on the contralateral side associated with right-hand activation. However, after image registration, the differences were reduced to the noise level of the scan, with just the hint of a residual difference at the edge of the vessel (Fig. 8.3c) This putative difference signal did not correspond with the full shape of the vessel, and was not found to be statistically significant at the 5% level (Fig. 8.3d, circled region). In each of 10 studies performed with either an enveloping coil or a surface coil, no significant vascular changes were observed. With the signal-to-noise ratio available in these studies, this implied that any functionally induced changes were less than 5% of the vessel signals. This was disappointing, but the protocol only tested the flow mechanism (b-FOLD) for activation, and it is possible that the BOLD mechanism might have resulted in detectable changes.

We therefore decided to look more closely at the BOLD mechanism.

Activation experiment using blood oxygen-level-dependent (BOLD) contrast

We performed a similar motor study at 1.5 T using a T_2^*-weighted volume sequence ($TR = 44$ ms, $TE = 35$ ms, flip angle 10°). This time we required that the result be obtained on two occasions, and used registration to align the two sets of images. One volunteer showed no change, a second showed a marginal result and a third showed a correlated response. Although this response was in the appropriate general region, it was outside the brain. We are uncertain of the significance of these results.

Blood oxygen-level-dependent (BOLD) contrast: ischemic experiment

The BOLD mechanism relies on the paramagnetic properties of deoxygenated hemoglobin, so we studied the effect of drastically reducing the saturation level. Since it is not realistic to stop the blood supply to the brain in humans, we performed our experiment on depletion of oxygen using a standard ischemia protocol. We applied a pressure cuff at 300 Torr for 30 min to a human leg, cutting off all arterial and venous blood supply (and flow) and monitored the oxy- and deoxy-hemoglobin and myoglobin concentrations within the leg with near-infrared spectroscopy as well as observing T_2^* and phase changes using MRI at 1.0 T and performing ^{31}P spectroscopy at 1.5 T. From the near-infrared data, we found that the oxy-hemoglobin and oxymyoglobin were rapidly depleted, and deoxyhemoglobin and deoxymyo-globin were markedly increased (Fig. 8.4a). The MRI phase of the muscle also changed (Fig. 8.4b), and so did the level of PCr (down) and Pi (up), but a most surprising result was the fact that the T_2^* of ischemic muscle remained virtually unchanged throughout this drastic insult, and showed only a small change during the subsequent hyperemia (Fig. 8.4c).

According to the BOLD hypothesis, the large increase in deoxyhemoglobin and deoxymyoglobin (which are both paramagnetic) should have resulted in dephasing of the signal and a marked reduction in T_2^*. Most fundamental BOLD experiments have been performed at high fields (e.g. 7.1 T) on small animals, and it is possible that this effect is much less in humans at lower, conventional imaging fields.

Having seen that extreme reduction in oxygen produced little or no change in the T_2^* of muscle, the next question was what would happen if the oxygen level was increased?

CSF oxygen-level-dependent (COLD) contrast

Normal volunteers were imaged breathing normal air then 100% oxygen and then air again. We then accurately registered the separate sets of images of their brains, and obtained difference images. We also performed FLAIR scans (Fig. 8.5). We found no change in the brain. However, there was a well-defined change in the extracerebral CSF (28 ± 14%) with little or no change in the intra-ventricular CSF.[13] It is probable that the change in extracerebral CSF was due to the paramagnetic effect of molecular oxygen shortening the T_1 of CSF. Previous studies of this type have described increased signal in the brain with inhalation of 100% oxygen, without commenting on changes in the CSF, whether extracerebral or intraventricular.[14-16]

The time course of these changes was similar to that previously described for increase in the CSF P_{O_2} level in animals and humans.[17-22]

Perfusion and CSF flow-level-dependent (c-FOLD) contrast

We have attempted to use spin inversion as a marker of cerebral perfusion as described by others.[22-24] However, we have found that results are readily confounded by CSF inflow effects, and that designing, implementing and validating sequences that are immune to this problem is not an easy task. We have had some results of interest, but as yet none that unequivocally separate the two effects.

Conclusions

On each occasion we have sought to extend the scope of the activation experiment, we have found unexpected results that have raised fundamental questions about the mechanisms underlying studies of this type. The detection of stimulus-correlated signals at low field led us into determining the role of subject motion in fMRI. The presence of stimulus correlated motion in fMRI has only recently been accepted, and implementation of techniques designed to correct for its effects is just beginning.[25-29]

Our study combining a sequence designed to detect flow with accurate image registration produced negative results. The results obtained with T_2^*-weighted sequences were only slightly more promising.

We were surprised to find that gross hypoxia failed to produce significant change in T_2^* of muscle, and this raised questions about the relevance of the BOLD mechanism to human activation studies. In tests of hyperoxia, we found that, contrary to previous reports, the brain did not change, but the extracerebral CSF did.

We are investigating effects of inversion labelling, but have found that the results are readily confounded by CSF flow effects.

In summary, we have found that the generally accepted mechanisms of fMRI (BOLD and blood flow) produce little or no change, but that other mechanisms that have not previously been recognized in this context (stimulus correlated motion, CSF oxygenation and CSF flow) readily produce changes.

We remain committed to identifying the problems with fMRI and resolving them as far as possible, in the belief that this is the most certain way of placing this application of MRI on a firm foundation.

Acknowledgements

We wish to thank the Medical Research Council, The Wellcome Trust, Picker International and Nycomed for their continued support.

References

1. Kwong KK, Belliveau JW, Chesler DA et al, Dynamic magnetic resonance imaging of human brain activity during primary sensory stimulation. *Proc Natl Acad Sci USA* 1992; **89**: 5675–9.

2. Ogawa S, Tank DW, Menon R et al, Intrinsic signal changes accompanying sensory stimulation: functional brain mapping with magnetic resonance imaging. *Proc Natl Acad Sci. USA* 1992; **89**: 5951–5.

3. Bandettini PA, Wong EC, Hinks RS et al, Time course EPI of human brain function during task activation. *Magn Reson Med* 1992; **25**: 390–7.

4. Kim S-G, Ashe J, Hendrich K et al, Functional magnetic resonance imaging of the motor cortex: hemispheric asymmetry and handedness. *Science* 1993; **261**: 615–17.

5. Frahm J, Merboldt KD, Hanicke W, Functional MRI of human brain activation at high spatial resolution. *Magn Reson Med* 1993; **29**: 139–44.

6. Hajnal JV, Collins AG, White SJ et al, Imaging of human brain activity at 0.15 T using fluid attenuated inversion recovery (FLAIR) pulse sequences. *Magn Reson Med* 1993; **30**: 650–4.

7. Hajnal JV, Myers R, Oatridge A et al, Artifacts due to stimulus correlated motion in functional imaging of the brain. *Magn Reson Med* 1994; **31**: 283–91.

8. Woods RP, Cherry SR, Mazziota JC, Rapid automated algorithm for aligning and reslicing PET images. *J Comput Assist Tomogr* 1992; **16**: 620–33.

9. Hajnal JV, Saeed N, Soar EJ et al, A registration and interpolation procedure for subvoxel matching of serially acquired MR images. *J Comput Assist Tomogr* 1995; **19**: 289–96.

10. Hajnal JV, Saeed N, Oatridge A et al, Detection of subtle brain changes using subvoxel registration and subtraction of serial MR images. *J Comput Assist Tomogr* 1995; **19**: 677–91.

11. Bydder GM, Detection of small changes to the brain with serial MRI. *Br J Radiol* 1995; **68**: 1271–95.

12. Wu DH, Lewis JS, Duerk JL, Inadequacy of motion correction algorithms in functional MR: role of susceptibility induced artifacts. *Proc 3rd Ann Mtg Soc Magn Reson, Nice, 19–25 August 1995*, p 821. SMR, Berkeley, 1995.

13. Hajnal JV, Oatridge A, Saeed N et al, Detection of changes followed by inhalation of pure oxygen and carbogen using $3T_1$-weighted brain imaging. *Proc 3rd Ann Mtg Soc Magn Reson, Nice, 19–25 August 1995*, p 769. SMR, Berkeley, 1995.

14. Rostrop LS, Larson HBW, Toft PB et al, Signal changes in gradient echo images of human brain induced by hypo- and hyperoxia. *NMR Biomed* 1995; **8**: 41–7.

15. Kwong KK, Hanke I, Donahue K et al, EPI imaging of global increase of brain MR signal with breath-hold preceeded by breathing O_2. *Magn Reson Med* 1995; **33**: 448–52.

16. Berthezene Y, Tourmet P, Turjman F et al, Inhaled oxygen: a brain MR contrast agent. *AJNR* 1995; **16**: 2010–12.

17. Bloor BM, Fricker J, Hellinger F, McCutchen J, A study of cerebrospinal fluid oxygen tension. *Arch Neurol* 1961; **4**: 37–46

18. Dunkin RS, Bondurant S, The determinants of cerebrospinal fluid pO_2. *Ann Int Med* 1966; **64**: 71–80.

19. Jarnum S, Lorenzen I, Skinhoj E, Cisternal fluid oxygen tension in man. *Neurology* 1964; **14**: 703–7.

20. Rossanda M, Gordon E, The oxygen tension of cerebrospinal fluid in patients with brain lesions. *Acta Anaesth Scandinav* 1970; **14**: 173–81.

21. Halmagyi DFJ, Gillett DJ, Cerebrospinal fluid oxygen tension at different levels of oxygenation. *Respir Physiol* 1967; **2**: 207–12.

22. Edelman RR, Siewert O, Darby DG et al, Qualitative mapping of cerebral blood flow and functional localisation with echo-planar MR imaging and signal targetting with calibrating radiofrequency. *Radiology* 1994; **192**: 513–20.

23. Kim SG, Quantification of relative cerebral blood flow change by flow sensitive alternating inversion recovery (FLAIR) techniques. Application to function mapping. *Magn Reson Med* 1995; **34**: 293–301.

24. Kwong K, Chester DA, Weisskoff RM et al, MR perfusion studies with T_1-weighted echo planar imaging. *Magn Reson Med* 1995; **34**: 878–87.

25. Hill DLG, Simmons A, Studholme C et al, Removal of stimulus correlated motion from echo planar fMRI studies. *Proc 3rd Ann Mtg Soc Magn Reson, Nice, 19–25 August 1995*, p 840. SMR, Berkeley, 1995.

26. Wowk B, McIntyre MC, Scorth G et al, Image registration for high resolution fMRI: Experience with a Fourier Algorithm. *Proc 3rd Ann Mtg Soc Magn Reson, Nice, 19–25 August 1995*, p 845. SMR, Berkeley, 1995.

27. Mock BJ, Lowe MJ, Wang X et al, In-plane motion correction of EPI functional magnetic resonance images (fMRI) via one-dimensional cross-correlation. *Proc 3rd Ann Mtg Soc Magn*

Reson, Nice, 19–25 August 1995, p 841. SMR, Berkeley, 1995.

28. Biswak B, Hyde JS, Processing strategies to differentiate between task-activated and head motion-induced signal variations. *Proc 3rd*

Ann Mtg Soc Magn Reson, Nice, 19–25 August 1995, p 835. SMR, Berkeley, 1995.

29. Friston KJ, Williams S, Havard R et al, Movement-related effects in fMRI time-series. *Magn Reson Med* 1996; **35**: 346–55.

9

Cerebrospinal fluid velocity imaging

William G Bradley

Hydrocephalus

Cerebrospinal fluid (CSF) is produced by the choroid plexus within the ventricles of the brain at a rate of 500 ml/day. It flows down through the foramen of Monro, down through the aqueduct of Sylvius, and out through the foramina of Lushka and Magendie in the fourth ventricle. Some of the CSF flows down around the spinal cord; most of it, however, flows up through the basal cisterns and over the cerebral convexities, eventually to be absorbed by the arachnoidal villi on either side of the superior sagittal sinus.[1] Superimposed on this slow, steady egress of CSF from the ventricular system is a much more prominent to-and-fro motion due to cardiac pulsations, i.e. the systolic expansion and diastolic contraction of the brain. When the local CSF velocity is sufficiently high (e.g. through the narrow aqueduct of Sylvius), a 'CSF flow void'[2,3] is normally produced, similar to that seen with rapidly flowing blood.[4] When there is obstruction to CSF flow, the flow void is not observed (e.g. in aqueductal stenosis).[3]

Obstruction proximal to the outlet foramina of the fourth ventricle is termed 'obstructive hydrocephalus'; obstruction between the outlet foramina of the fourth ventricle and the arachnoidal villi is termed 'communicating hydrocephalus' or 'extra-ventricular obstructive hydrocephalus'. Obstructive hydrocephalus most often results from a tumor or inflammation blocking the narrowest parts of the ventricular system: the foramen of Monro, the aqueduct and, occasionally, the fourth ventricle itself. Communicating hydrocephalus most often follows subarachnoid hemorrhage or meningitis, owing to blockage of the arachnoidal villi or the basal cisterns. Occasionally, elderly patients may present with a radiographic pattern of communicating hydrocephalus without a history of either of these preceding events. Such hydrocephalus is termed 'occult' or 'idiopathic'.[5,6] Since the mean intraventricular pressure is normal, it has also been called 'normal-pressure hydrocephalus (NPH)'. Rarely, hydrocephalus results from overproduction of CSF (e.g. with choroid plexus papillomas).

Normal-pressure hydrocephalus (NPH)

Classically, NPH patients present with a clinical triad of gait apraxia, dementia and incontinence.[5-7] Although the mean intraventricular pressure is normal in these patients, the pulse pressure, i.e. the change in CSF pressure over the cardiac cycle, is much greater than normal. A 'waterhammer' pulse has been described in such patients when their intraventricular pressure is monitored.[8,9] Until now, the diagnosis of NPH has been based on the clinical presentation and the radiographic pattern of ventricles enlarged out of proportion to any cortical sulcal enlargement (to distinguish NPH from atrophy).

Prior to the advent of MRI, this radiographic picture and the appropriate clinical triad alone were not sufficient to predict which patients would respond to the primary treatment for NPH, namely ventriculoperitoneal (VP) shunting. Recently, the magnitude of the aqueductal CSF flow void (Fig. 9.1) has been used to predict which patients with

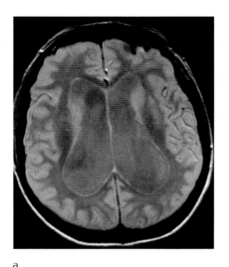 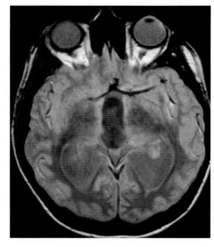 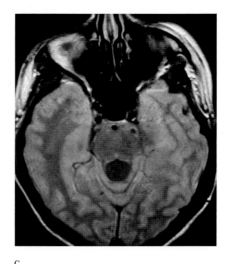

a   b   c

Figure 9.1

CSF flow void in normal-pressure hydrocephalus. Proton-density-weighted axial images demonstrate marked ventriculomegaly and CSF flow void.

(a) Lateral ventricle. (b) Third ventricle. (c) Fourth ventricle.

clinical NPH will respond to shunting.[10] The CSF flow void is a normal phenomenon, resulting from the pulsatile motion of CSF back and forth through the ventricular system during the cardiac cycle.[11] In the normal patient, there is space over the cerebral convexities occupied by the cortical veins and the CSF in the subarachnoid space (Fig. 9.2). When the brain expands during systole, it expands outward, compressing the cortical veins (leading to subsequent venous outflow), and it expands inward, compressing the lateral ventricles (leading to outflow or CSF through the aqueduct that produces the normal flow void).[10] In communicating hydrocephalus, the brain has already expanded against the inner table of the calvarium, so further outward expansion is not possible. Thus, during systole, all cerebral expansion is directed inward, compressing the lateral and third ventricles, leading to increased outflow of CSF through the aqueduct. This is the etiology for the increased CSF flow void[10] in patients with communicating hydrocephalus and normal cerebral blood flow (Fig. 9.2). When the blood supply to the brain decreases owing to atrophy, the main force behind the CSF pump decreases and the CSF flow void is consequently also reduced.

A significant correlation has been demonstrated between an increased CSF flow void, i.e. one extending from the third ventricle through the obex of the fourth ventricle, and a successful response to ventriculoperitoneal shunting.[10] Patients with clinical NPH who did *not* have a hyperdynamic flow void, on the other hand, failed to respond to shunting. This association was significant at the $p < 0.003$ level.[10] Thus, in the setting of an appropriate clinical triad for NPH and ventricular enlargement out of proportion to cortical sulcal dilatation, the presence of an increased aqueductal CSF flow void on MRI should prompt the neurosurgeon to perform a VP shunt. It should be emphasized, however, that younger patients with communicating hydrocephalus and normal cerebral blood flow may also have hyperdynamic CSF flow. Thus the sign is not specific for NPH.

Since NPH is a disease of elderly patients, it appears that symptoms result from a *combined* insult related both to the ventricular enlargement (and 'barotrauma' of the waterhammer pulse) and to the decreased perfusion of the periventricular region, i.e. the same process that leads to deep white matter ischemia and infarction.[12] It was originally postulated by Hakim that tangential shearing forces involving the periventricular (corona radiata) fibers led initially to the gait disturbance.[7] Later, with continued ventricular enlargement, radial shearing forces involving the cortical gray matter led to the dementia.[7]

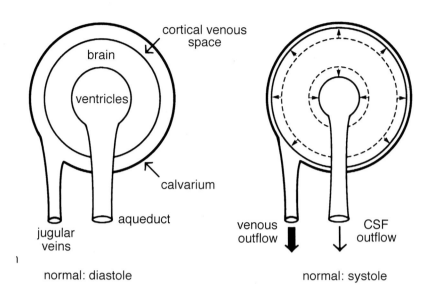

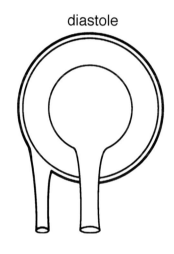

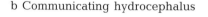

a Normal

b Communicating hydrocephalus

Figure 9.2

Schematic representation of CSF flow mechanism. (a) In normal patients, systolic expansion of cerebral hemispheres occurs outward, compressing cortical veins, and, to a lesser extent, inward, compressing the lateral ventricles. (b) In communicating hydrocephalus, the brain has already expanded against·the inner table of the calvarium. Since outward expansion of the brain is no longer possible, the entire increase in volume due to systolic expansion is directed inward, towards the lateral ventricles. The combination of this greater inward displacement and the mild aqueductal enlargement that accompanies communicating hydrocephalus leads to hyperdynamic CSF flow.

MR techniques used to measure CSF flow

A number of MR observations and techniques have been employed to take advantage of signal changes associated with CSF flow. The aqueductal CSF flow void (Fig. 9.1) noted on routine MR images was the first indication of CSF motion.[2,3] Subsequently, the CSF flow void was shown to be related to the cardiac cycle.[13] Although a CSF flow void may be appreciated on routine spin echo and gradient echo MR images, the degree of signal loss is not consistent, nor does it change in a linear fashion with velocity.[1] Thus, by using the CSF flow void sign alone, it may be difficult to appreciate when CSF flow is mildly abnormal. When a CSF flow void is not visualized at all in areas where it it normally expected (e.g. the aqueduct), however, inferences can be made concerning obstruction.[3] Axial single-slice gradient echo techniques that maximize flow-related enhancement[4] (entry phenomenon) have also been used[14] to evaluate aqueductal patency. However, the best observations of CSF flow have been obtained using dedicated techniques, gated to the cardiac cycle.

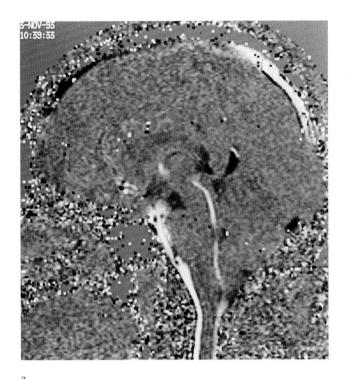

a

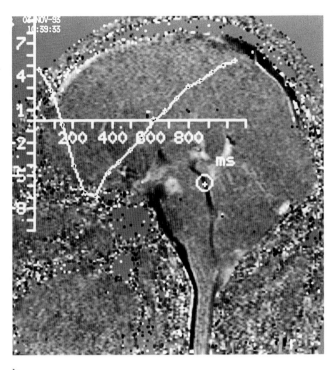

b

Figure 9.3

Sagittal phase-contrast technique. (a) During systole, CSF flow is down (craniocaudad), indicated by shades of white. (During diastole, CSF flow is up [caudocraniad], indicated by shades of black). (b) By placing a cursor over any point in the image, the velocity can be obtained as a function of the cardiac cycle.

In 1985, Feinberg and Mark used MR 'velocity density imaging'[15,16] to measure the velocity of CSF through the aqueduct as a function of the cardiac cycle. Subsequently, Edelman et al[17] used saturation pulses and bolus tracking techniques while Axel et al[18] used spatial modulation magnetization (SPAMM) to measure CSF velocity. Today, most investigators are using phase-contrast techniques.[19-21]

The phase-contrast CSF velocity imaging techniques[19-21] can be divided on the basis of the form of cardiac gating used, i.e. prospective or retrospective,[22] and on the basis of background phase determination.[23] Most investigators[19,20] determine the background phase from an additional acquisition. This approach necessitates obtaining two interleaved acquisitions and then subtracting them. We make the assumption of zero net flow[21] over the cardiac cycle, and calculate the background phase (which entails a single acquisition in one-half the time).

The relationship between the phase shift θ and velocity v is given by the equation

$$\theta = \gamma \int_0^t G(t)\, vt\, dt,$$

where γ is the gyromagnetic ratio, $G(t)$ is the gradient strength as a function of time, and t is the elapsed time.[24] Thus, for an appropriate gradient pulse of strength G and duration t, a linear relationship should exist between the phase shift (from zero to $\pm 180°$, depending on the direction of flow) and the actual CSF velocity. A new parameter, V_{enc}, is the aliasing or 'encoding' velocity, which leads to a 180° phase shift for flow in either direction.

There are two ways to do cardiac gating: prospectively and retrospectively. Prospective cardiac gating is the most commonly used, and is also called 'EKG triggering' (although it also includes triggering from a finger plethysmograph).

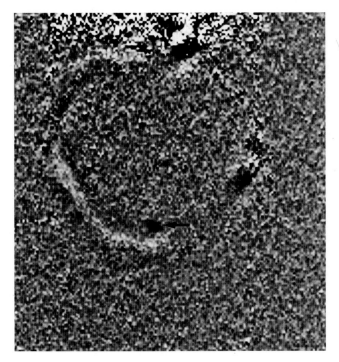

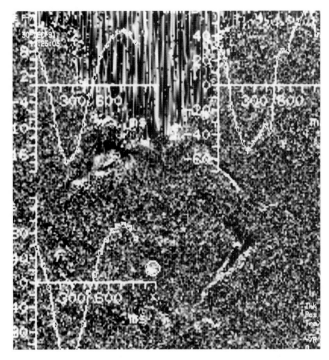

a

b

Figure 9.4

Axial phase-contrast technique. (a) High-resolution axial image obtained during diastole indicates flow up (black) in the aqueduct (arrow). (During systole, flow is down [white]). (b) The mean velocity (left upper), peak velocity (right upper), and volumetric flow rates (left lower) through the aqueduct are shown as a function of the cardiac cycle.

With prospective cardiac gating, acquisition starts at a predetermined time interval after the R-wave, and continues at approximately 50–75 ms intervals to within about 200 ms of the next R-wave (to allow for respiratory variation).[19] The R-wave can be determined electrically (from the EKG) or mechanically (from the finger plethysmograph). Since there is no sampling of CSF motion during the final 100 or 200 ms of the R–R interval (when flow is in a rostral or retrograde direction), there appears to be a large net flow of CSF in the systolic direction (i.e. craniocaudal) over this partially sampled cardiac cycle.[21]

With retrospective cardiac gating or 'cine-PC',[22] the computer keeps track of the R-wave (defined electrically or mechanically), and data are acquired throughout the cardiac cycle and then retrospectively 'binned' into a predetermined number of cine frames.[22] The entire cardiac cycle is sampled; therefore there is no time for eddy currents to build up, as they do during the 200 ms dead time when prospective cardiac gating is used.[21]

We routinely use two retrospective cardiac gated techniques:[21] a 'routine resolution' sagittal acquisition in the midline (Fig. 9.3) and a 'high-resolution' axial acquisition through the aqueduct (Fig. 9.4). In the sagittal technique, a 4 mm slice is acquired in the midsagittal plane (Fig. 9.3), with velocity sensitization along the readout axis (which is also the craniocaudal axis of the patient). (It is better to perform cardiac gating with EKG leads rather than using finger plethysmography, since the systolic motion of the brain may actually precede the systolic pulse in the finger.[21]) The basic MR technique is a flow-compensated, 2D FISP (on our Siemens unit) or a 2D GRASS with cine-PC (on our GE) with a TR of 70 ms, a TE of 13 ms and a 15° flip angle (Fig. 9.3). A 192 × 256 matrix is acquired over a 25 cm field of view, providing in-plane spatial resolution of approximately 1 mm. The aliasing velocity is set to 100 mm/s. Such images

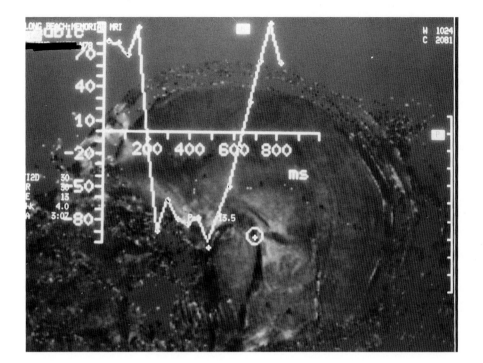

Figure 9.5

Normal pressure hydrocephalus.
In this 78-year-old man with
clinical NPH, hyperdynamic flow
is demonstrated through the
aqueduct.

are used routinely in the head to document
midsagittal CSF flow. Using a single excitation and
taking 32 acquisitions before advancing the phase,
this technique takes about 7 min. When a
computer cursor is placed over any point on the
phase-contrast velocity image on the monitor,
craniocaudal CSF velocities can be measured and
plotted versus phase of the cardiac cycle. This
allows comparison of phase relationships of CSF
motion at different points in the midline ventricular system, basal cistern and cervical subarachnoid
space[21] (Fig. 9.3).

The measured velocity through the aqueduct on
this sagittal acquisition unfortunately also reflects
the stationary tissue in the midbrain on either side
of the aqueduct in a 4 mm thick slice. Therefore
the measured velocity is artifactually reduced
owing to partial volume effects.[21] To circumvent
these effects, the high-resolution axial technique
was developed.[21] In this technique, an angled axial
slice is positioned perpendicular to the aqueduct
so that the CSF is viewed *en face*, without inclusion of adjacent stationary tissue (Fig. 9.4). Velocity sensitization is provided by the slice-selection
gradient, i.e. for through-plane flow. We currently
use a 512 × 512 matrix (half Fourier with 16 lines
of over-sampling) over a 16 cm field-of-view,
providing pixels 0.3 mm on a side. Thirty such

pixels can be placed in an average 2 mm diameter aqueduct. Like the sagittal technique, this is a
modified 2D FISP/GRASS technique with a 15° flip
angle, a *TR* of 100 ms and a *TE* of 16 ms. With a
single excitation and 32 acquisitions per phase
step, it takes about 14 min.[21] An aliasing velocity
of 200 mm/s is routinely used. Integrating the
volumetric flow rate over the cardiac cycle, an
aqueductal CSF 'stroke volume' can be calculated.[21] Using a pulsatile flow phantom, velocity
and volumetric flow measurements have recently
been validated.[25]

Normal CSF flow in the brain

In normals, the maximal downward wave of CSF
movement through the aqueduct occurs 175–200
ms after the R-wave, however, it is usually
preceded by CSF flow out of the fourth ventricle
through the foramen of Magendie.[20] Mixing occurs
in the mid fourth ventricle, resulting in turbulence.[21] Midway through the cardiac cycle, a
diastolic cephalad (retrograde) wave of CSF can be

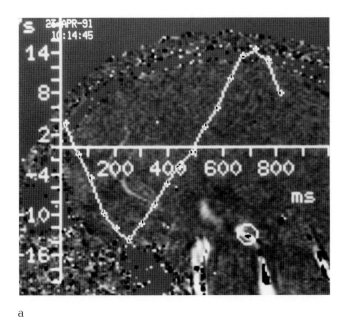

a

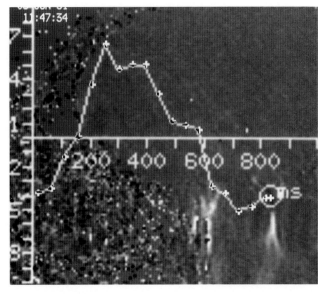

b

Figure 9.6

Shunt malfunction in NPH. (a) A 73-year-old man shunted initially for NPH one year previously now presents with recurrent symptoms and 'normal' flow pattern through the aqueduct. (b) Two months later, when the shunt has been revised and the patient is again asymptomatic, the CSF flow pattern through the aqueduct is reversed (as expected with normal shunt function).

seen rising through the aqueduct.[20] Variable degrees of CSF flow within the posterior third ventricle are observed, and occasionally flow at the level of the foramen of Monro is also seen in normals. Flow is less often observed in the lateral ventricles, however, because of the larger diameters involved. As a result of volume changes in the brain over the cardiac cycle, CSF also flows to and fro in the basal cisterns.[21]

Flow out of the inferior portion of the fourth ventricle through the foramen of Magendie is not simply a continuation of the flow coming down from the aqueduct. Such asynchrony may result from pulsations of the choroid plexus of the fourth ventricle.[20] In fact, the caudally directed CSF pulse wave is observed to start first in the fourth ventricle, followed approximately 100 ms later by caudal flow in the aqueduct.[20] Cranial flow of CSF back through the aqueduct may still be occurring when the first downward motion through the foramen of Magendie is seen. Clearly, therefore, this cephalad aqueductal CSF flow is not simply the result of retrograde flow from the basal cisterns

into the fourth ventricle and upwards.[20] There are a number of probable reasons for these normal variations, but they most likely relate to the size of the nearby vascular structures, the compliance of surrounding brain and spinal cord, the anatomy of the CSF spaces, the volume and vascularity of the choroid plexus, and the resulting systemic hydrodynamics.[20]

Abnormal CSF flow in the brain

Using phase-contrast CSF velocity imaging, the hyperdynamic CSF flow of NPH (Fig. 9.5) can be distinguished from normal flow or from the decreased flow of atrophy. The high-resolution axial technique provides a reliable, quantitative

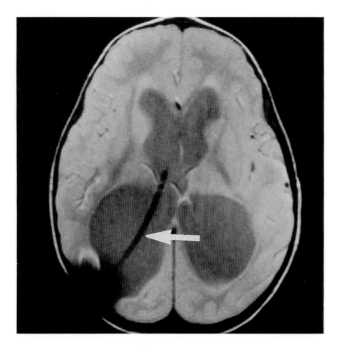

a

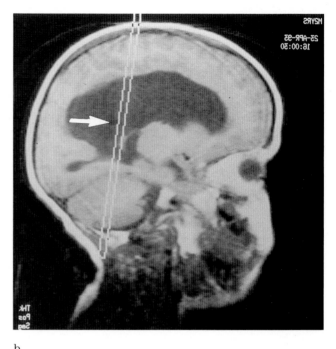

b

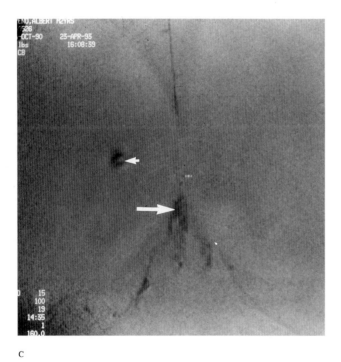

c

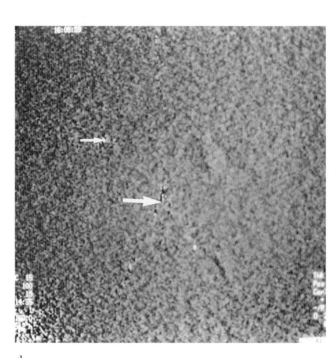

d

Figure 9.7

Normal shunt function. (a) Shunt tube (arrow) is noted in a two-year-old boy with obstructive hydrocephalus. (b) Right parasagittal section demonstrates prescribed position of CSF flow study acquisition plane perpendicular to dark shunt tube (arrow). (c) 'Magnitude' image from high-resolution coronal acquisition, angled perpendicular to shunt tube (small arrow), also demonstrates quadrigeminal plate cistern (large arrow). (d) Phase-contrast image again demonstrates quadrigeminal plate cistern (large arrow) and high signal intensity (small arrow) in shunt, corresponding to forward flow.

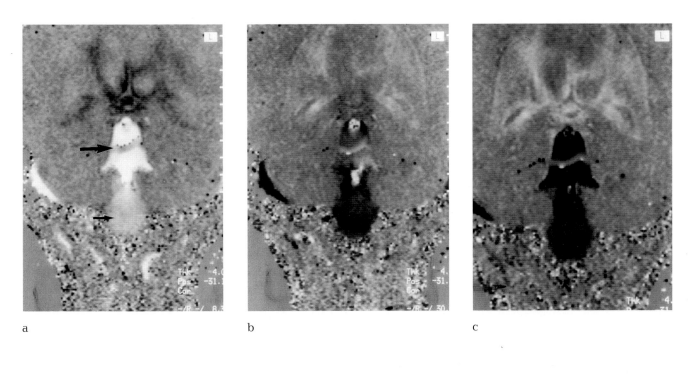

a   b   c

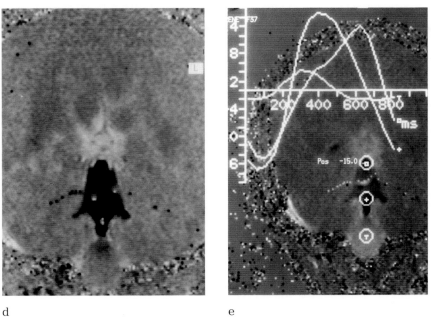

d   e

Figure 9.8

'Rebound sign' in arachnoid cyst. The qualitative (sagittal) technique has been rotated into the coronal plane, with velocity encoding along the craniocaudal readout axis. White is flow down and black is flow up (zero flow is gray). (a) During systole, flow in the fourth ventricle (large arrow) is down, while flow in the arachnoid cyst (small arrow) has stopped owing to maximal deformation by the surrounding CSF. (b) 200 ms later, flow in the fourth ventricle has stopped (turning gray), while flow in the cyst has already started heading up (turning black). (c) 200 ms later, CSF flows both in the cyst and the fourth ventricle are up. (d) 100 ms later, the cyst has become maximally deformed and has stopped flowing (turning gray), while flow continues in the caudocraniad direction in the fourth ventricle. (e) By placing cursors on the fourth ventricle and the cyst, motion in the cyst is seen to be of lower amplitude and 90° phase-advanced relative to flow within the fourth ventricle.

measurement of the aqueductal CSF stroke volume. In a recent study of 18 patients with clinically suspected NPH, 12 were found to have hyperdynamic CSF flow, i.e. stroke volumes greater than 42 µl, while six were found to have hypodynamic flow.[26] All 12 of the patients with hyperdynamic flow responded favorably to ventriculoperitoneal shunting. Thus, in this series, this technique had a positive predictive value of 100%. Of the six patients who had stroke volumes less than or equal to 42 µl, three responded to shunting and three did not, probably reflecting the presence of concomitant atrophy in these patients. Interestingly, of the 12 patients with hyperdynamic flow (as determined by the measured stroke volume), only six (50%) had hyperdynamic CSF flow voids on their routine MR images. This most likely reflects the current widespread use of first-order flow compensation on the proton-density-weighted images, which was not available when the earlier study was performed.[10] Thus quantitative CSF velocity imaging is an even better technique than routine MRI to determine the presence of *shunt-responsive* normal pressure hydrocephalus.

CSF velocity imaging is also useful in the evaluation of potential shunt malfunction.[27] In patients who have been shunted for communicating hydrocephalus, the normal pattern of CSF flow through the aqueduct is exactly 180° out of phase with normal with respect to the cardiac cycle, i.e. CSF flows caudocraniad during systole and craniocaudad during diastole (Fig. 9.6). This probably reflects the fact that the shunt tube is the lowest-resistance pathway to outflow of CSF following systolic expansion of both the cerebrum and the cerebellum. (It should also be noted that the phase relationship between CSF flow and the cardiac cycle depends on how the R-wave is acquired. Since the R-wave reaches the finger approximately 400 ms after electrical systole, the use of finger plethysmography may give the false appearance of expected flow reversal through the aqueduct when the shunt is, in fact, nonfunctional.)

In patients with either obstructive or communicating hydrocephalus, the high-resolution axial technique can also be used to assess flow through the shunt tube itself (Fig. 9.7). In cases of normal shunt function, CSF motion tends to be intermittent and unidirectional, rather than sinusoidal (as is normally seen through the aqueduct), reflecting the presence of the one-way valve.

Since the plane and position of both CSF velocity imaging techniques can be modified, they can also be used to distinguish cysts from enlarged CSF spaces. Within the cyst, the motion of CSF appears to rebound against the flowing CSF around it. This 'cyst rebound sign'[28] is the finding of decreased CSF velocity (within the cyst) 90° phase-advanced relative to the motion of the surrounding CSF (Fig. 9.8).

References

1. Bradley WG, Quencer RM, Hydrocephalus, atrophy, and intracranial CSF flow. In: *Magnetic resonance imaging*, 2nd edn (ed DD Stark, WG Bradley). Mosby-Year Book, St Louis, MO, 1992.

2. Bradley WG, Kortman KE, Burgoyne B, Flowing cerebrospinal fluid in normal and hydrocephalic states: appearance on MR images. *Radiology* 1986; **159**: 611–16.

3. Sherman JL, Citrin CM, Magnetic resonance demonstration of normal CSF flow. *AJNR* 1986; **7**: 3–6.

4. Bradley WG, Waluch V, Blood flow: magnetic resonance imaging. *Radiology* 1985; **154**: 443–50.

5. Hakim S, Some observations on CSF pressure: hydrocephalic syndrome in adults with 'normal' CSF pressure. Thesis 957, Javerian University School of Medicine, Bogota, Columbia, 1964.

6. Adams RD, Fisher CM, Hakim S et al, Symptomatic occult hydrocephalus with 'normal' cerebrospinal fluid pressure: a treatable syndrome. *N Engl J Med* 1965; **273**: 117–26.

7. Hakim S, Venegas JG, Burton JD, The physics of the cranial cavity hydrocephalus and normal pressure hydrocephalus: mechanical interpretation and mathematical role. *Surg Neurol* 1970; **5**: 187–209.

8. Ekstedt J, Friden H, CSF hydrodynamics of the study of the adult hydrocephalus syndrome. In: *Hydrocephalus* (ed K Shapiro, A Marmarou, H Portnoy). Raven Press, New York, 1984.

9. Foltz EL, Hydrocephalus and CSF pulsatility: clinical and laboratory studies. In: *Hydrocephalus* (ed K Shapiro, A Marmarou, H Portnoy). Raven Press, New York, 1984.

10. Bradley WG, Whittemore AR, Kortman KE et al, Marked cerebrospinal fluid void: indicator of successful shunt in patients with suspected normal pressure hydrocephalus. *Radiology* 1991; **178**: 459–66.

11. DuBoulay GH, Pulsatile movements in the CSF pathways. *Br J Radiol* 1966; **39**: 255–62.

12. Bradley WG, Whittemore AR, Watanabe AS et al, Association of deep white matter infarction with chronic communicating hydrocephalus: implications regarding the possible origin of normal pressure hydrocephalus. *AJNR* 1991: **12**: 31–9.

13. Citrin CM, Sherman JL, Gangarosa RE et al, Physiology of the CSF flow-void sign: modification by cardiac gating. *AJNR* 1986; **7**: 1021–4.

14. Atlas SW, Mark AS, Fram EK, Aqueductal stenosis: evaluation with gradient-echo rapid MR imaging. *Radiology* 1988; **169**: 449–56.

15. Feinberg DA, Crooks LE, Sheldon P et al, Magnetic resonance imaging in the velocity vector components of fluid flow. *Magn Reson Med* 1985; **2**: 555–6.

16. Feinberg DA, Mark AS, Human brain motion and cerebrospinal fluid circulation demonstrated with MR velocity imaging. *Radiology* 1985; **154**: 443–50.

17. Edelman RR, Mattle HP, Kleefield J, Silver MS, Quantification of blood flow with dynamic MR imaging and presaturation bolus tracking. *Radiology* 1989; **171**: 551–6.

18. Axel L, Dougherty L, MR imaging of motion with spatial modulation of magnetization. *Radiology* 1989; **171**: 841.

19. Quencer RM, Donovan Post MJ, Hinks RS, Cine MR in the evaluation of normal and abnormal CSF flow: intracranial and intraspinal studies. *Neuroradiology* 1990; **32**: 371–91.

20. Enzmann DR, Pelc NJ. Normal flow patterns of intracranial and spinal cerebrospinal fluid defined by phase-contrast Cine MR imaging. *Radiology* 1991; **178**: 467–77.

21. Nitz WR, Bradley WG Jr, Watanabe AS et al, Flow dynamics of CSF: assessment with phase contrast velocity MR imaging performed with retrospective cardiac gating. *Radiology* 1992; **183**: 1–12.

22. Spraggins TA. Wireless retrospective gating application to Cine cardiac imaging. *Mag Res Med* 1990; **8**: 676–81.

23. Firmin DN, Nayler GL, Kilner PJ, Longmore DB. The application of phase shifts in NMR for flow measurement. *Magn Res Med* 1990; **14**: 230–41.

24. Moran PR. Flow velocity zeugmatographic interlace for NMR imaging in humans. *Magn Reson Imaging* 1982; **1**: 197–203.

25. Mullin WJ, Atkinson D, Hashemi R, Yu J, Bradley WG. Cerebrospinal fluid flow quantitation: pulsatile flow phantom comparison of three measurement methods. *JMRI* 1993; **3(P)**: 55.

26. Bradley WG, Scalzo D, Queralt J, Nitz WN, Atkinson DJ, Wong P. Normal-pressure hydrocephalus: evaluation with cerebrospinal fluid flow measurements at MR imaging. *Radiology* 1996; **198**: 523–9.

27. Bradley WG, Atkinson D, Chen D-Y, Nitz WR, Mullin WJ. Evaluation of ventriculoperitoneal shunt status with cerebrospinal fluid velocity imaging. *Radiology* 1993; **189(P)**: 223.

28. Herbst MD, Bradley WG, Nitz WR, Burgoyne B, Lee RR, O'Sullivan RM. Reproduction of the arachnoid cyst rebound sign in a cerebrospinal fluid flow phantom. *Radiology* 1991; **181(P)**: 287.

10

Registration and subtraction of serial magnetic resonance images Part 1: Technique

Joseph V Hajnal and Graeme M Bydder

Introduction

Detection of small changes to the brain on serial imaging examinations is a common and important problem. Image subtraction is often used in this situation but differences in the angle and position at which the images are acquired usually result in misregistration artifacts, which are often greater than the changes being sought. Numerous attempts have been made to improve the alignment of image sets obtained on serial examination, such as the use of standardized positioning, patient fixation devices and image processing techniques. Even with these techniques, positional matches between image sets are usually to no better than 1–2 voxels (typically 1–2 mm). As a result, recognition of small differences in signal intensity at or near boundaries is problematic, and detection of changes in brain site, shape or size of the order of 1–2 mm is difficult or impossible.

It is possible to obtain much more accurately matched brain images using serial three-dimensional (3D) magnetic resonance imaging (MRI), image segmentation, rigid-body translation and rotation with sinc interpolation and a least squares optimization procedure. This can produce alignment of images to a fraction of a voxel (typically less than 0.01 mm in each linear dimension) whilst preserving the integrity of voxel signal intensity values, so that accurate comparison can be made between images acquired at different times.[1]

In this chapter we describe this technique and how it has been validated. Chapter 10 discusses methods of image interpretation, which are required to make use of the registered images in radiological applications. Finally Chapter 11 presents examples of some of the many possible applications where the capability to make precise comparisons over time, from one examination to the next, can substantially improve diagnosis and monitoring of disease progression.

Theory

Subvoxel shifts

A distinction needs to be drawn between the resolution of an image of an object and the information that image contains about where that object is in space. Image resolution is a measure of the smallest feature of the object that can be resolved on the image, and for most magnetic resonance (MR) images is approximately the field of view (FOV) divided by the number of phase- (or frequency-) encoded steps used to acquire the image. The linear dimensions of the image voxels are generally equal to or, if the data was zero-filled prior to image reconstruction, slightly smaller than, a resolution element.

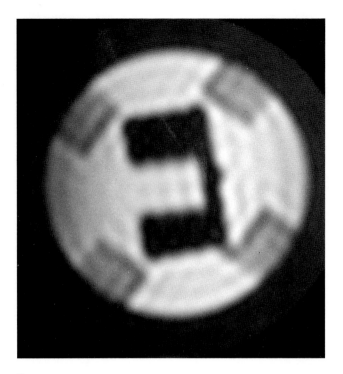

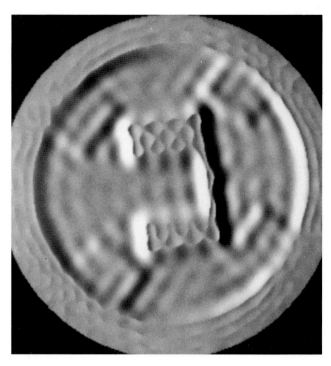

a

b

Figure 10.1

A subvoxel shift. (a) Low-resolution spin echo image of a phantom acquired with a FOV of 25 cm and 32 phase-encoding steps (TR = 300 ms, TE = 20 ms, 5 mm slice thickness, data zero-filled to a 256 × 256 matrix). The difference produced by subtracting the image in (a) from a second identical acquisition horizontally offset by 0.2 mm is shown in (b). A clear difference signal is seen, even though the images are misregistered by only 1/39 of the nominal resolution element of the scans. These effects are most obvious at the boundaries of the phantom, with an increase in signal intensity at the external surface (light area) on the side to which the phantom was displaced and a decrease on the opposite side.

Location of an object's position in space on the image is a separate issue. This is determined by the distribution of voxel intensity values. Differences in object position of much less than the dimension of a voxel can be detected on serial images. This is illustrated in Fig. 10.1(a), which shows a phantom imaged with an FOV of 25 cm and 32 phase-encoding steps. The nominal resolution of the image is 7.8 mm. Figure 10.1(b) shows a difference image obtained by subtracting the image in Fig. 10.1(a) from a second image of the phantom obtained with the same resolution, but acquired with a shift of 0.2 mm or 1/39th of a resolution element.

The difference image shows spatially coherent signals that reveal the change in the position of the phantom even though the displacement is only a small fraction of the voxel size.

Figure 10.2 shows the same result in diagrammatic form. Figure 10.2(a) shows the profile of an object with voxel intensity values represented by the height of the vertical bars. The object has been displaced 0.4 of a voxel to the right in Fig. 10.2(b), and a subtraction between Fig. 10.2(a) and Fig. 10.2(b) has been performed in Fig. 10.2(c). The subtraction profile reveals a pattern of voxel intensity differences that reflects the change in position.

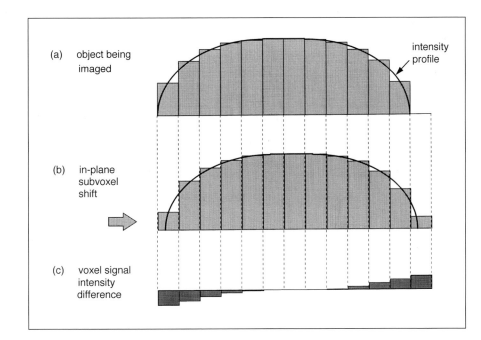

(a)   object being
      imaged

      intensity
      profile

(b)   in-plane
      subvoxel
      shift

(c)   voxel signal
      intensity
      difference

Figure 10.2

Changes in image voxel signal intensities as a result of a subvoxel shift. (a) Signal profile of an object with voxel intensity values (vertical bars), reflecting the structure of the object being imaged. (b) If the object is shifted in plane to the right by a fraction of a voxel (in this case 0.4 units), the pattern of intensity values changes. (c) Subtraction of (a) from (b) reveals a coherent pattern of voxel signal intensity differences that reflects the change in the position of the object. Changes are greatest at the boundaries and least in the central high-signal-intensity region of the object.

Difference signals such as those depicted in Figs 10.1(b) and 10.2(c) (which depend both on signal intensity gradients within the object and on the size of the displacement) must be detected against a background of image noise and artifacts. For the images acquired in this study, the signal-to-noise ratio for brain was typically 20:1. With this ratio, shifts of a few percent of a voxel can be detected at steep boundaries such as that which may be seen between brain and CSF. This has two consequences. Firstly, serial images must be aligned to a very small part of a voxel if misregistration errors are to be kept below the image noise level. Secondly, if images are aligned to this degree of accuracy then small changes in signal intensity and subvoxel shifts of the order of a few percent of a voxel produced by genuine changes in the brain site, shape or size may be detected as a result of the signal changes they produce on accurately registered difference images.

Correction of shifts by translation, rotation and interpolation of voxel signal intensity values

The above considerations place a premium on developing methods that produce very accurate

registration of serial images. If the second image is displaced a whole number of voxels, n, away from the first in the row, column or slice direction of the image matrix, registration simply consists of replacing the value of the ith voxel by that of the $(i + n)$th voxel. This is a translation in one direction, and provides a precise correction for the shift. This maneuver can be performed in two or three directions, but difficulties arise when the displacement required is not a whole number of voxels and/or a rotation is needed, since both of these corrections require shifts of a fraction of a voxel. In these circumstances it is necessary to estimate what the voxel values should be using information from neighboring voxels. This process is called image interpolation. One of its simplest forms is linear interpolation. For example, in Fig. 10.2, where the image was displaced 0.4 voxels to the right, linear interpolation of the ith voxel would give 0.6 of the value of the existing voxel plus 0.4 of the value of the $(i + 1)$th value. While this procedure is rapid, it introduces errors, particularly at boundaries. For example, in Fig. 10.2, using linear interpolation, the curved intensity profile of the object would be approximated by a straight line, which introduces an error (Fig. 10.3).

To achieve fractional voxel shifts without distortion, it is necessary to use an interpolation function appropriate to the nature of the image data, and in this regard the sinc function, sin x = (sin x)/x is particularly suitable for MR images.

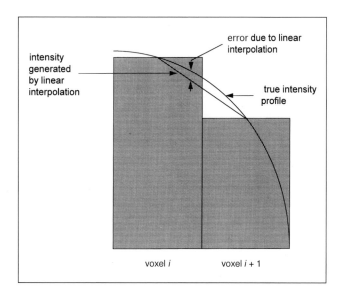

Figure 10.3

Interpolation. To correct for the change in position in Fig. 10.2(b), new intensity values must be calculated for each voxel (which remains in the same location). This requires interpolation, in which information from neighboring voxels is used to synthesize a new voxel value. In the case of linear interpolation, only the nearest neighbors are used, and the intensities are added in inverse proportion to the distance required to correct for the initial shift (i.e. 0.4 units in this case). This generates a linear change in signal intensity, which differs from the curved true intensity profile by the error shown in the diagram.

Sinc interpolation

Since MR images are acquired in the Fourier domain with data obtained over a bounded region of k-space, their frequency content is strictly band-limited. The inplane point spread function for MR images is thus the sinc function.[2] For this reason, sinc interpolation can, in principle, be used to generate interstitial data values without introducing errors (Fig. 10.4).

In the through-plane (slice) direction of a two-dimensional (2D) image, the point spread function depends on the details of the method of slice selection, and this does not generally result in a sinc function. Even the ideal slice profile (which has uniform sensitivity in the slice and zero elsewhere) is not amenable to error-free interpolation, because each slice is represented by an isolated set of data points. The consequences of using linear interpolation on idealized multislice data are illustrated in Fig. 10.5. Instead of the desired effect of shifting the slice (Figs 10.5a,b), the process of combining information from two slices simply distorts the slice profile (Fig. 10.5c). The modified slice profile can incorporate new, unrelated anatomic structures into the interpolated image. Because these structures were not represented in the original image, their inclusion can produce apparently unpredictable results that may be difficult to detect by visual assessment of the final image content.

True three-dimensional (3D) acquisitions (in which phase encoding is employed in the slice direction as well as one in-plane direction) are band-limited in all directions, and can therefore be interpolated faithfully using the sinc function. The spatial spread of the sinc point spread function allows data from nearby slices to be combined in a way that precisely preserves the integrity of the slice profile when it is displaced.

To express the process of sinc interpolation in more formal terms, consider an image data set consisting of a 3D matrix of voxels with intensities $\mathbf{I}(X, Y, Z)$ identified by integer position coordinates (X, Y, Z). We wish to calculate the intensity $\mathbf{I}(x, y, z)$ associated with an interstitial point defined by non-integer coordinates (x, y, z). For band-limited MR images, this can be achieved without error by forming the triple sum

$$I(x, y, z) = \sum_{X}\sum_{Y}\sum_{Z} \mathbf{I}(X, Y, Z) \, \text{sinc} \, [\pi(x - X)]$$
$$\times \, \text{sinc} \, [\pi(y - Y)] \, \text{sinc} \, [\pi(z - Z)], \quad (1)$$

where

$$\text{sinc} \, \pi\alpha = \frac{\sin \pi\alpha}{\pi\alpha}. \quad (2)$$

The sinc function takes both positive and negative values (Fig. 10.4a). As a result, when a real positive object is convolved with it, both positive and negative intensity values can be produced. The process of constructing magnitude images reverses the sign of the negative intensity values. These sign-reversed voxel values introduce errors into the interpolation process, so that magnitude data may not be suitable for error-free image shifting. In practice, negative voxel values only occur on the dark side of sharp edges. This can be problematic in images of phantoms, but this is much less common in clinical images.

As it stands, equation (1) implies a sum over all voxels for each new intensity value calculated. Since this is computationally very demanding, and

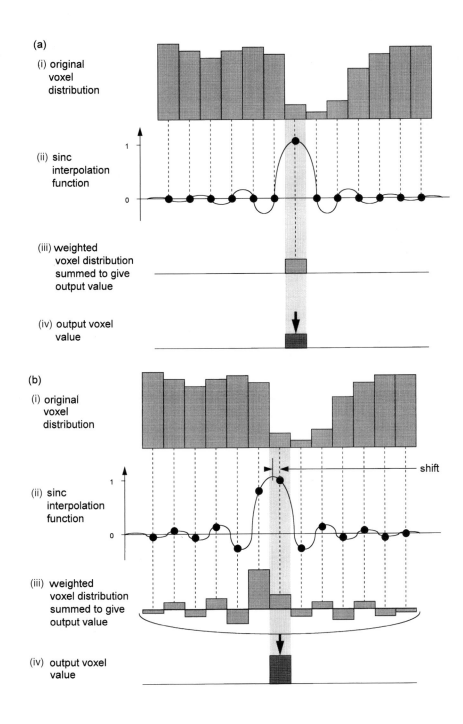

(a)

(i) original
voxel
distribution

(ii) sinc
interpolation
function

(iii) weighted
voxel distribution
summed to give
output value

(iv) output voxel
value

(b)

(i) original
voxel
distribution

(ii) sinc
interpolation
function

shift

(iii) weighted
voxel distribution
summed to give
output value

(iv) output voxel
value

Figure 10.4

Sinc interpolation for the case of a zero shift (a) and for a subvoxel shift (b). When the signal intensity distribution of an image (a(i), b(i)) is shifted relative to the fixed grid of voxels, new voxel intensity values must be synthesized. This is done by adding contributions from all voxels in a neighborhood, with each weighted by the value of a sinc function (a(ii), b(ii)). For the zero shift (no change, a(ii)), this just picks out the original voxel value (a(iv)), since all others are weighted by zero (a(ii), a(iii)). For the nonzero shift (b(ii)), many voxels contribute, some with a negative weighting (b(ii), b(iii)). The sum of all these contributions is the final interpolated voxel value (b(iv)). This procedure must be repeated in three directions to generate the new signal intensity value for each voxel in the image set.

distant voxels (for which the sinc weighting function is small) only contribute weakly, it is convenient in practical situations to truncate the interpolation. We do this by limiting the calculation to a cubic volume containing $(2R + 2)^3$ voxels centered on the target point for which an intensity is to be calculated, where R specifies the range of the interpolation. When R is set to zero, only the nearest neighbors are included. Because of the oscillating nature of the sinc function,

unacceptable truncation errors may result from this procedure. We therefore multiply each sinc function in equation (1) by an appodizing Hanning window function of the form

$$H(\alpha; R) = \frac{1}{2}\left(1 + \cos\frac{\pi\alpha}{R + 1}\right), \qquad (3)$$

where α is replaced by $x–X$, $y–Y$ or $z–Z$ as appropriate.

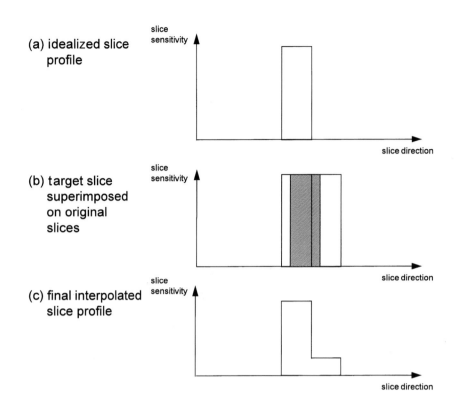

(a) idealized slice profile

(b) target slice superimposed on original slices

(c) final interpolated slice profile

Figure 10.5

Interpolation of multislice data. In order to shift the idealized slice profile (a) to a new position (shaded area in (b)) using linear interpolation, contributions from two neighboring slices are added in proportion to their proximity to the target slice position. This results in a modification of the slice profile (c) rather than the intended shift.

Image matching; chi-squared test

In addition to the capacity to accurately reproduce an image displaced by any angle of rotation or distance, we require a strategy for determining what the displacement needs to be in order to match one image with another. Techniques such as surface or landmark matching are not generally suitable for aligning images to subvoxel accuracy, because the criteria used to specify objects in images with these techniques are frequently only defined to the nearest voxel. In contrast, gray-scale correlation methods utilize the full information content of the images and produce data that may be used to match images to small fractions of a voxel. With a technique of this type, Woods et al[3,4] employed the standard deviation of the ratio of voxel intensities as an optimization criterion for automatic image registration. This proved to be a successful approach for both inter- and intramodality image matching. For matching MR images to one another, we prefer to use a least squares method. This has the advantages of conceptual clarity, ease of interpretation and ready availability of appropriate optimization algorithms. It also provides a direct estimate of the statistical uncertainty of the positional match that is achieved.

Our program employs the Levenburg–Marquardt algorithm[5] to minimize a function χ^2 defined by

$$\chi^2 = \sum_{\text{voxels}} (\mathbf{I}_B - \mathbf{I}_A)^2 / N_{\text{voxels}}, \qquad [4]$$

where $\mathbf{I}_A$ and $\mathbf{I}_B$ are the intensities of corresponding voxels in the images A and B that are to be positionally matched, and N_{voxels} is the number of voxels used in the calculation. The value of χ^2 is reduced by calculating new values for $\mathbf{I}_B$ as image B is moved relative to the voxel grid using rigid-body rotations and translations. To avoid making unproductive calculations, only those voxels for which $\mathbf{I}_A$ is greater than a user-defined threshold and for which there is data in image B are included in the evaluation of χ^2. A similar approach was adopted by Woods et al, but in their case there was an added concern, since the ratio of image intensities becomes unstable when the intensity used for the denominator is small.

The optimization procedure requires subvoxel shifts, and thus image interpolation plays a central role in the registration procedure. Interpolation errors influence the value of the optimization cost function (χ^2), and can lead to errors in the registration procedure. We have employed sinc interpolation in our program, thus allowing χ^2 and its derivatives to be correctly calculated regardless of the positional shifts employed. In practice, the program becomes very slow if the range of interpolation is large, and therefore a compromise must be sought in which the fidelity of the interpolation is traded off against computation time.

Reformatting; production of positionally matched images

Once a minimum value of χ^2 has been found, the three translations and three rotations that were applied to align image B with image A are stored in a file. The registration coordinates are then used to reformat image B to match image A using sinc interpolation. The range of interpolation used for reformatting data need not be the same as that used for determining the registration coordinates. In general, we use a larger value of R for reformatting, since it may be important to minimize intensity errors in individual voxels in the final images.

The precision of the positional match achieved depends on two distinct factors: competition between structure and noise in the images and genuine differences that exist between the tissues and fluids depicted in the images. The minimum value of χ^2 that can be achieved for two images that differ only in their noise content is simply the sum of the variances of their noise, which we assume to be uncorrelated. Under these conditions, an unbiased estimation of the standard deviations of the registration coordinates can easily be calculated from the inverse of the Hessian matrix of second derivatives of χ^2.[5] This is done routinely by our program once an optimal value of χ^2 has been found. A minimal value of χ^2 that is greater than the sum of the noise variances of the images implies either that the program has failed to find the global minimum or that the images contain structural differences not associated with noise.

Image segmentation

Where genuine structural differences exist, the optimization procedure results in a positional match that balances these against differences induced by positional shifts. Where a localized change is anticipated, an appropriate course of action is to register the images twice. Those voxels that show residual signal differences after the first registration can be excluded from the calculations made during the second registration. This will then produce a positional match that is unaffected by the putative local changes. In practice, highly localized changes generally have a negligible effect on the registration coordinates, because their contribution to χ^2 is small and χ^2 rises rapidly with changes in registration coordinates owing to the vast majority of voxels that represent unchanged structures.

A common cause of structural changes in in vivo images is variable deformation of soft tissues in the head and neck outside of the skull. This may be due to the manner in which the scalp and facial tissues are positioned when the patient is inside the scanner or to other differences such as whether the patient's mouth is open or closed. Under these circumstances, the registration coordinates are altered in a manner that represents a global compromise, but which may lead to unsatisfactory local matches everywhere in the images. Restricting the registration calculation to those parts of the images that are relevant is a key step in the successful application of subvoxel registration. For brain applications, we always segment the images to remove the skull, scalp, facial and neck tissues so that only the brain and immediately adjacent tissues and fluids are used for registration. This is done by replicating the A image set and then editing it using an automated segmentation algorithm[6,7] to leave only the brain and its immediate surrounds with all other voxels set to zero. A nonzero threshold in the registration program then restricts the calculation to the relevant voxels.

Image subtraction

To test our methods, we use difference images produced by subtracting registered scans. For serially acquired images that contain unchanged anatomic features, precise positioned matching and accurate interpolation ensures that tissue signals are reduced to the background noise level after image subtraction. If this is achieved, residual signals that are then detected on the registered subtraction images can be ascribed to irreconcilable image differences due to real change in the subject over time.

Implementation

Pulse sequences

Images to be registered were acquired with true 3D radiofrequency (rf)-spoiled T_1-weighted pulse sequences on a 1.0 T Picker HPQ scanner (Picker International, Cleveland, OH). For whole head studies, a nonselective rf excitation pulse was employed ($TR = 21$ ms, $TE = 6$ ms, flip angle 35°), and images were acquired in the sagittal plane with the frequency-encoding direction head-to-foot to avoid aliasing. Data matrices of $152 \times 256 \times 114$ with two NEX or $192 \times 256 \times 140$ and one NEX were acquired in a volume of 25 cm $\times$ 25 cm $\times$ 18 cm with isotropic nominal phase-encoded resolution of 1.6 mm or 1.3 mm. For angiographic studies, a slab-selective sequence was also employed, with a flip angle of 20°. A transverse slab was acquired with a $192 \times 256 \times 40$ data matrix providing 0.9 mm $\times$ 0.8 mm $\times$ 0.8 mm resolution.

For comparison, T_1 and T_2-weighted spin echo (SE) scans (SE720/20, SE2500/20 and SE2500/80 [TR/TE] ms) 192×256 matrix of 3–6 mm slice thickness were obtained in each case. All images were zero-filled to 256×256 inplane prior to Fourier transformation.

Image registration

Registration proceeded in the order Segmentation, Translation, Rotation and Interpolation, Chi-squared TEst, and Reformatting (STRICTER). For each subject, one of the volume image data sets was designated as the base line image set. In adults, this was usually the first scan acquired; but in children with more than two scans and whose head had grown significantly, it was sometimes advantageous to choose an intermediate scan and match it to both the previous and later ones in order to minimize the difference between any two images. The images in the base line set were duplicated and then segmented to isolate the brain, with all other voxels set to zero, using a semi-automated algorithm.[7] Each follow-up 3D image set from the same subject was then positionally matched to the segmented baseline set of images and reformatted before being compared with the original unsegmented base line images. Typical matching accuracies of less than 0.01 mm in each axis and less than 0.01° in each rotation angle were achieved. Difference images were produced by subtracting the baseline images from registered follow-up images or by subtracting one registered follow-up image set from another. These cancelled constant features, and revealed areas that had changed between the two studies concerned.

Volunteers and patients

The images used for this chapter were selected from over 120 examinations of volunteers and patients. Consistent patient head positioning to within 5–10° in each direction was used to control for the effects of gravitation on brain position. Contrast enhancement with intravenous Gadodiamide 0.1–0.3 mmol/kg was used in selected patients.

Although virtually all 3D images were acquired in the sagittal plane, the registered source images and difference images were also presented in either the transverse or coronal planes for radiological assessment.

Validation

Validation was performed on phantoms and human volunteers. In addition, errors introduced by the use of two-dimensional images and linear interpolation are illustrated. The value of segmentation in avoiding errors in the positional match of the brain due to extraneous changes in soft tissues is also illustrated.

Phantom studies

To test the registration algorithm, single-slice and true 3D images of phantoms were acquired. Positional changes were achieved by alteration in scanning coordinates rather than movement of the object. This was done to ensure precise control of the displacement/rotation employed. Changes in the acquisition coordinates directly modified the raw (Fourier-domain) data acquired by the scanner. After Fourier transformation, this resulted in independent images in which the object was shifted with respect to the matrix of voxels that defined the image space. Subsequent image matching was performed purely in the image domain.

The sinc interpolation algorithm was tested and compared with linear interpolation as follows: a T_1-weighted spin echo image of a phantom (Fig. 10.6a)

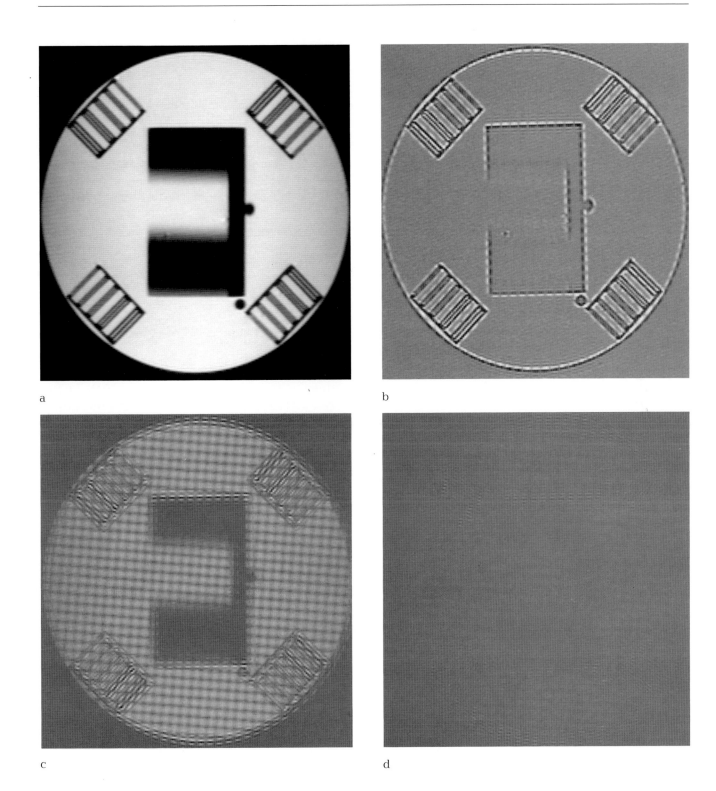

a

b

c

d

Figure 10.6

Rotation of a standard spin echo image of a phantom ($TR = 300$ ms, $TE = 20$ ms, 25 cm FOV, 256×256 resolution, 5 mm slice) by $+10°$, followed by rotation of the resulting image by $-10°$ and subtraction from the original image. Positive phantom image (a), errors introduced by the two rotations using linear interpolation (b), errors introduced by the rotations using sinc interpolation with range $R = 2$ voxels (c) and errors introduced with sinc interpolation using $R = 6$ voxels (d). The error is less with sinc interpolation than with linear interpolation, and least with $R = 6$ voxels.

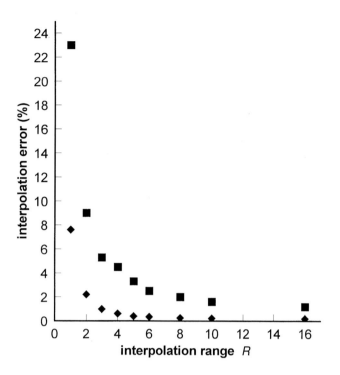

Figure 10.7

Interpolation range: graph of root mean square (RMS) and peak interpolation errors introduced by successive positive and negative 10° rotations of the phantom in Fig. 10.6(a) using sinc interpolation. Error magnitude as a percentage of the maximum phantom signal is plotted against interpolation range R in voxels. Peak errors are indicated by squares and RMS errors by diamonds. The errors decrease as R is increased, and the RMS error is less than 1% for $R > 2$.

was rotated by +10° using the interpolation method under test to generate new voxel values; this new image was then rotated by –10° using the same interpolation scheme, and finally subtracted from the original image. Figures 10.6(b), (c) and (d) show difference images for linear interpolation, sinc interpolation ($R = 2$ voxels range) and sinc interpolation ($R = 6$ voxels range) respectively. Linear interpolation resulted in errors of up to 23% of the peak signal, whereas sinc interpolation reduced this to less than 9% for a range of two voxels and to 2.5% for a range of six voxels. The residual check patterns in Figs 10.6(c,d) are due to truncation errors in the apodized sinc interpolation. The root mean square (RMS) and peak errors as a function of the range R of the sinc interpolation are shown in Fig. 10.7.

The patterns of errors obtained with the two interpolation methods are very different. With linear interpolation, the errors reflect the structure of the object, whereas with sinc interpolation, there is a nonlocalized low-level truncation error, with larger errors occurring only at isolated voxels.

Registration of phantom images is illustrated in Fig. 10.8. The phantom (Fig. 10.8a) was scanned twice with a 2½ voxel offset between the images obtained. This results in clear difference signals when the two images are subtracted (Fig. 10.8a); however, after image registration and reslicing using sinc interpolation, these differences are reduced to the noise level (Fig. 10.8b).

Normal volunteers

An example of registration of serial scans in a normal volunteer is shown in Fig. 10.9. In this case an adult male volunteer was scanned twice on the same day using true 3D rf-spoiled T_1-weighted acquisitions. Figure 10.9(a) shows a sagittal slice from the base image set, and Fig. 10.9(b) shows the corresponding slice from the second set of images. A raw difference image, 10.9(b) minus 10.9(a), prior to registration is shown in Fig. 10.9(c). Figure 10.9(d) shows a registered difference image in which only the brain was used for the registration calculations. Almost all structures within the brain have been reduced to below the noise level in this image, but the scalp and facial soft tissues show clear residual signals. The straight sinus can just be seen (arrow), probably indicating a change in size between scans. The statistical uncertainty of the registration was less than ±0.003 voxels and ±0.003° for all three translational and all three rotational coordinates.

Registration of multislice images with linear interpolation in the slice direction

For comparison with the T_1-weighted 3D acquisitions used in the rest of this chapter, a normal adult male subject was scanned twice with a conventional T_1-weighted multislice SE sequence. Figures 10.10(a,b) show approximately matched levels from the two multislice data sets. A change

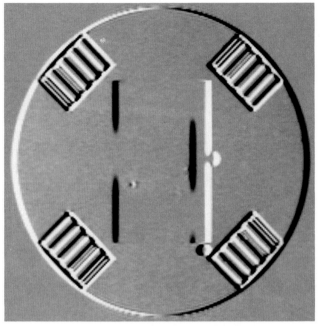

a

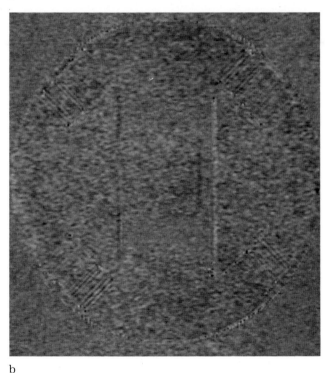

b

Figure 10.8

Registration of phantom images. The phantom in Fig. 10.7(a) was imaged twice with an inplane differential offset of 2½ voxels (approximately 2.5 mm). Subtraction of the unregistered images shows substantial difference signals (a), which are reduced to the noise level if the images are registered and resliced using sinc interpolation prior to subtraction (b).

in angulation of the slice is apparent as an anatomic mismatch. Figure 10.10(c) shows subtraction of 10.10(a) from 10.10(b). After registration and reslicing the image in Fig. 10.10(b) to match Fig. 10.10(a) using sinc interpolation in plane, but linear interpolation through plane, the image shown in Fig. 10.10(b) was transformed into that in Fig. 10.10(d), in which major anatomic landmarks matched those in Fig. 10.10(a). However, subtraction of Fig. 10.10(a) from Fig. 10.10(d) revealed persistent signal differences in Fig. 10.10(e) that were only a limited improvement on the unregistered difference image (Fig. 10.10c). This is because the linear interpolation function was not appropriate for reslicing the images in the through-slice direction without error (see Fig. 10.5). The same is true of a sinc function for 2D acquisitions.

Registration with and without segmentation

The importance of segmentation to separate the brain from extraneous soft tissues is demonstrated in Fig. 10.11 in the case of a 44-year-old man who had suffered minor head trauma. He was hit on the head with a mobile telephone, and developed a superficial hematoma. There was no loss of consciousness. The parasagittal image in Fig. 10.11(a) was acquired 1½ h after this event, and a follow-up examination (Fig. 10.11b) was performed three days later. By this time, the hematoma had substantially resolved. The brain anatomy is approximately matched in the two scans, but clear differences can be seen. Figure 10.11(c) is the image obtained by subtracting Fig. 10.11(a) from Fig. 10.11(b). Figure 10.11(d) is the difference image produced after the two volume sets were registered using all tissue signals that exceeded the background noise level. Differences are still seen in both the brain and extracranial tissues. Figure 10.11(e) shows a segmented version of Figure 10.11(a) in which all voxels that did not correspond to brain or CSF around the brain were set to zero. When only the segmented region (brain, adjacent CSF etc) was used to determine the registration coordinates required for reformatting the follow-up image (Fig. 10.11b), the difference image in Fig. 10.11(f) was produced. In this image virtually all structure in the brain has been reduced to the noise level, indicating that no detectable change had occurred

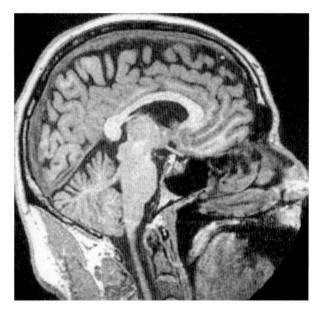

a

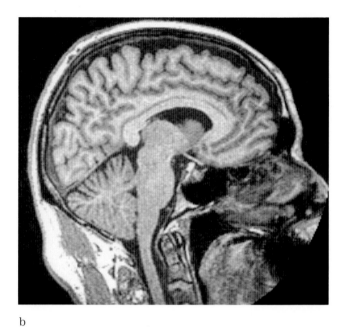

b

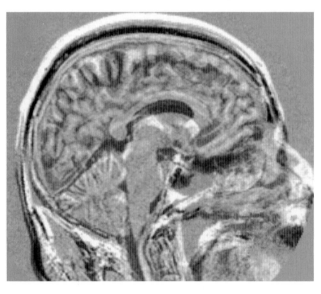

c

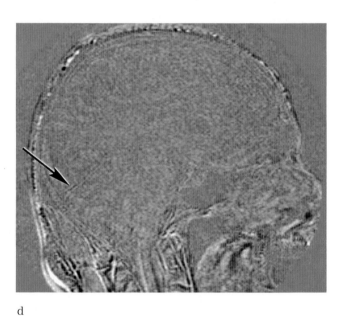

d

Figure 10.9

Normal male: registration of 3D rf-spoiled T_1-weighted images (TR = 21 ms, TE = 6 ms 35° flip angle, 25 cm FOV, 192 × 256 × 140 matrix with 1.3 mm slice thickness) of a normal volunteer who was scanned twice on the same day. Midline sagittal image from the first (a) and second (b) sets of images, unregistered difference image between these two images (c), and difference between the two scans after registration using sinc interpolation (d). The differences seen in (c) were almost reduced to the noise level in (d), except for the superficial tissues, which were excluded from the registration procedure by segmentation and which normally undergo small changes during and between examinations. Some residual signal is just seen in the straight sinus (d, arrow) probably because of a small decrease in its size.

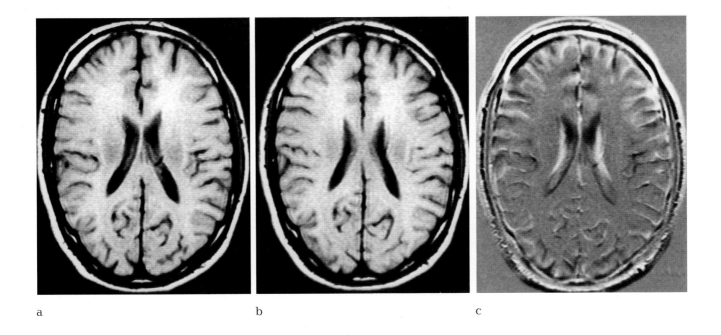

a   b   c

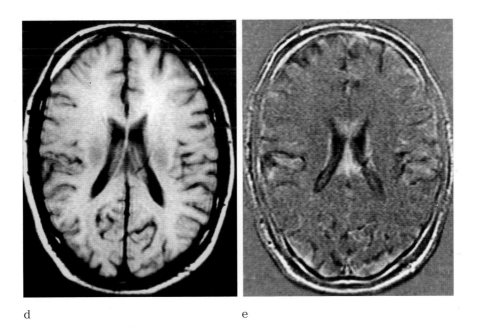

d   e

Figure 10.10

Registration of multislice images. (a,b) Approximately matched slices from two sets of T_1-weighted 2D multislice images (TR = 500 ms, TE = 20 ms, 192 × 256 resolution, 5 mm slice) acquired from a normal male volunteer. (c) Slight anatomical differences are seen on the unregistered difference image. Registration of scan (b) to match it with (a) using sinc interpolation in plane but linear interpolation through plane results in image (d), which is in good qualitative agreement with (a). However, subtraction of (a) from the registered image (d) reveals difference signals in (e) that are only a limited improvement over the original unregistered subtraction of (a) from (b) shown in (c). This unsatisfactory result arose because the voxel intensity values were corrupted by the linear interpolation in the through-plane direction.

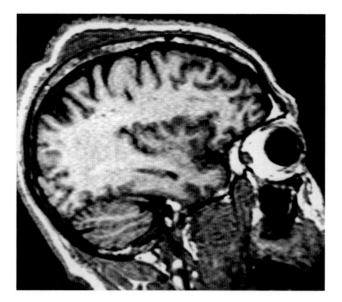

a

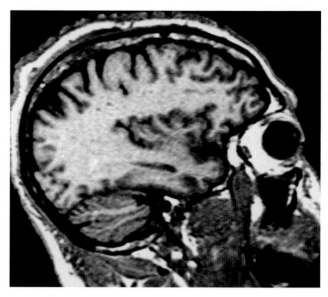

b

Figure 10.11

Sagittal slices from true 3D T_1-weighted images of a 44-year-old patient who suffered minor head trauma. (a) One and a half hours after the event, a superficial hematoma was seen. (b) This had largely resolved after three days. The brain anatomy in (a) and (b) is approximately matched, but overall misregistration is obvious on the subtraction image (c). (d) After registration using the full anatomic content of the images (without segmentation and removal of the scalp and skull from the match) and 3D sinc interpolation, the differences are reduced. However, the large changes in the superficial tissues have influenced the optimal position of the match, leaving residual differences in the brain region. (e) By segmenting the baseline image to isolate the brain, the superficial changes can be excluded from the registration procedure for determining the translations and rotations required to match (b) to (a). Reformatting (b) and subtracting (a) then results in the difference image (f). Almost all of the brain has been reduced to the background noise level, indicating that the brain itself was not changed by the trauma. The bright line at the top of the brain and dark line at its base (arrows) reveal that the brain has shifted superiorly within the cranial cavity between the first and second examinations. The position shown on the second scan was maintained on a third examination one week later, suggesting that the brain had been displaced inferiorly at the time of the initial trauma.

within the brain itself. However, the brain as a whole appeared displaced with respect to the surrounding skull (or vice versa), as manifested by the uniform white line superiorly and the dark line inferiorly in Fig. 10.11(f) (arrows). This was confirmed on a repeat examination one week later, suggesting that the brain had been displaced inferiorly at the time of the injury and had subsequently returned to its original position.

The smooth contour on the difference image reflects the fact that the brain as a whole has been centered between the two images, and the meninges and skull appear to have encroached on the CSF within the subarachnoid space above the brain, giving a high signal intensity there. The meninges and skull had moved away from the subarachnoid space below the brain, giving a low signal there.

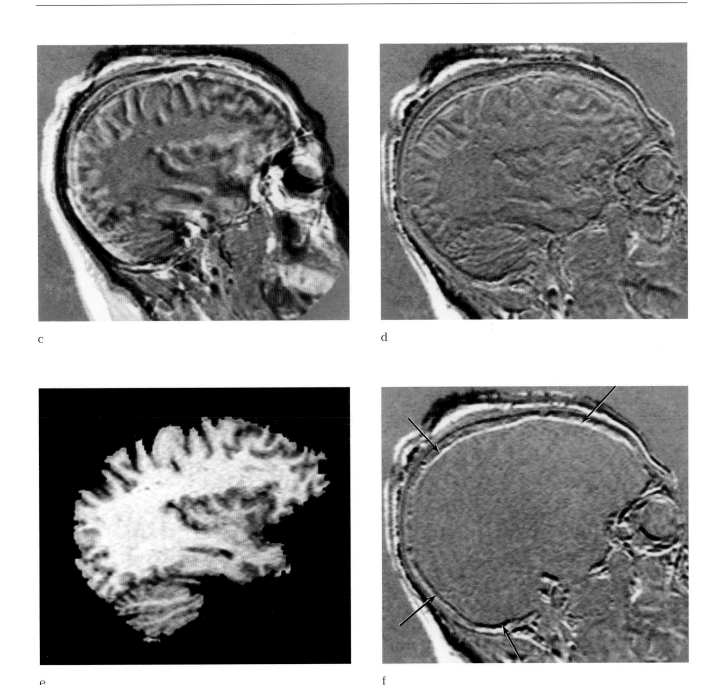

c

d

e

f

Figure 10.11 *continued*

Choice of pulse sequence

With the techniques described in this chapter, 3D data is essential to permit precise interpolation in the through-slice direction. While an unselective rf pulse was used in most of this study, a slab-selective pulse can be employed where it is useful to limit spatial coverage. In addition, the 3D scan needs to be isotropic to avoid errors being introduced by rotation, which might result in lower resolution data being obliqued to overlay higher-resolution signals.

The pulse sequence employed needs to produce high lesion contrast so that the signals from the lesion are well differentiated from those of surrounding normal brain (or other tissue or fluid). For this purpose, highly T_1- or T_2-weighted sequences are usually most effective, although in particular instances different sensitivities may be more effective. Examples include susceptibility-sensitive sequences for detecting acute hemorrhage and diffusion-weighted sequences for detecting acute ischemia.

To detect changes in site, shape or size of the brain, high contrast is required in the region of its boundaries. High brain-to-CSF contrast can be achieved with both heavily T_1-weighted (brain signal greater than CSF) and heavily T_2-weighted sequences (CSF signal greater than brain). Both approaches also show gray–white matter contrast, which is of value for demonstrating internal boundary regions.

Since many of the important changes occur at or close to the internal and external surfaces of the brain, sufficient spatial resolution to discriminate between white matter, gray matter, blood vessels, choroid plexuses, CSF and meninges is also important.

Flow effects need to be considered. While relatively solid tissue like brain is stable, differences of flow in CSF and blood may produce differences in signal intensity. Unselective rf pulses applied over the whole head, as in most of this study, are relatively insensitive to flow, and are an advantage in many situations. Conversely, 3D angiographic sequences are useful for detecting differences in blood flow, and may help in detecting changes in blood vessel site, shape or size.

Use of registration for demonstrating contrast enhancement requires either a T_1-weighted sequence for longitudinal relaxation time effects or a T_2^*-sensitive sequence for susceptibility effects. The former is easily accomplished with conventional T_1-weighted volume sequences.

Tolerance of the sequence to artifacts, including those from susceptibility effects at interfaces, is another important consideration, with short-*TE* gradient echoes being better than long-*TE* gradient echoes. Machine stability is also a potential concern, and technically undemanding approaches may have an advantage in this regard.

The T_1-weighted, short-*TE* rf-spoiled gradient sequence used in this study was sensitive to proton density and T_1 differences as well as contrast enhancement, but insensitive to T_2, susceptibility, flow, chemical shift and diffusion effects. Other sequences such as 3D MP-RAGE[8] may show higher lesion contrast and offer a range of magnetization preparation options.

Limitations

The least squares minimization routine is essentially noise- (and artifact-) limited in that once the differences between the two image sets reaches the noise level, no further improvement is possible. However, in our experience typical alignments in linear dimensions of less than 0.01 mm were reached, and residual signals due to misregistration were reduced to the noise floor. The segmentation process used to prepare the baseline images need not be highly accurate, since its purpose is to isolate areas of the brain that are unchanged. Inadvertent exclusion of small regions from the match is unlikely to affect overall accuracy, since the program typically uses 5×10^4–5×10^6 voxels.

With large changes, the constant regions available for matching become smaller and the matching process becomes more problematic. Where there has been a large global change it may be useful to restrict the matching process to a limited area so that much smaller changes are compared and a more precise match can be obtained. Large changes can be easily recognized without registration, but there may still be merit in aligning portions of images in which there have been large changes as accurately as possible to improve measurement.

The requirement for an isotropic volume scan is a limitation for rapid serial studies. Even a low-resolution slab acquisition with 10–12 partitions typically takes 20–30 s. This imposes a limit on the time resolution, as well as on the extent of the region which can be covered.

Computing time is currently about 3 h per match. It is likely that improvements in the various algorithms and use of parallel processing or other hardware improvements will produce a substantial reduction in this.

Machine stability can also be an issue. Some sequences are inherently more robust (e.g. spin echo versus gradient echo), and issues such as maintenance of gradient strength stability are important. Changes in machine configuration (such as after an upgrade) may be of critical importance in longer-term studies. Use of standard phantoms should allow these factors to be kept under control.

New developments

Placing all images in a single spatiotemporal coordinate system may provide a basis for unifying all MR images from the same patient over his or her illness (or lifetime).

A variety of different pulse sequences may be used for this work, provided that they produce isotropic 3D images. These include variants of the 3D MP-RAGE sequence with T_1, T_2, T_2^* and diffusion weighting, as well as T_2-weighted volume scans.

The registration technique can be used for combining images acquired with different scanning parameters. Combinations of images with different T_1, T_2, diffusion, magnetization transfer and susceptibility weighting may be used to produce accurate single parameter maps. The technique may also be of considerable value in spectroscopy. Images acquired with surface coils can be registered with phantom data, which can then be used to correct for signal intensity inhomogeneity due to the coil sensitivity profile.

Not only can measurement of signal intensity on MR images be improved by ensuring that comparable areas are measured, but also shifts can be assessed. Such measurements may be of value in calculating rates of growth and atrophy.

Non-rigid-body transformations are likely to be required for study of soft tissues changes outside of the skull, spine and rigid skeleton. This will require the use of satisfactory models for change in tissue geometry combined with appropriate validation techniques that allow incidental deviations from the model to be recognized and distinguished from the changes that are being sought.

References

1. Hajnal JV, Saeed N, Soar EJ et al, A registration and interpolation procedure for subvoxel matching of serially acquired magnetic resonance images. *J Comput Assist Tomogr* 1995; **19**: 289–96.

2. Jain AK, *Fundamentals of digital image processing*. Prentice-Hall, Englewood Cliffs, NJ, 1989.

3. Woods RP, Mazziotta JC, Cherry SR, MRI-PET registration with automated algorithm. *J Comput Assist Tomogr* 1993; **17**: 536–46.

4. Woods RP, Cherry SR, Mazziotta JC, Rapid automated algorithm for aligning and reslicing PET images. *J Comput Assist Tomogr* 1992; **16**: 620–33.

5. Press WH, Teukolsky SA, Vetterling WT, Flannery BP, *Numerical recipes in C*, 2nd edn. Cambridge University Press, Cambridge, 1992.

6. Marshall S, Saeed N, Young H et al, System for automatic patient realignment of the head in magnetic resonance imaging. *IEE Proc Pt* 1990; **137**: 319–30.

7. Saeed N. Application of digital image processing in magnetic resonance scanning. PhD thesis, Signal Processing Division, University of Strathclyde, 1990.

8. Mugler JP, Brookeman JR, Three-dimensional T_1-weighted MR imaging with the MP-RAGE sequence. *J Magn Reson Imaging* 1991; **1**: 561–8.

11

Registration and subtraction of serial magnetic resonance images Part 2: Image interpretation

Graeme M Bydder and Joseph V Hajnal

Introduction

In Chapter 10 we described how it was possible to obtain accurately aligned serial MR images of the brain using three-dimensional (3D) acquisitions, image segmentation, rigid-body translation and rotation with sinc interpolation and a least squares optimization procedure.[1,2] The process of comparing precisely registered images acquired at different times is greatly facilitated by forming subtraction images from the positionally registered scans. On these images, signals from unchanged structures cancel to reveal changes against a neutral background, allowing differences to be identified more clearly. These images require a different approach to interpretation than conventional images. This chapter describes a method for analyzing them.

Methods

Images to be registered were acquired with true 3D radiofrequency (rf)-spoiled T_1-weighted pulse sequences on a 1.0 T Picker HPQ scanner (Picker International, Cleveland, OH). For whole head studies, a nonselective rf excitation pulse was employed (TR = 21 ms, TE = 6 ms, flip angle 35°), and images were acquired in the sagittal plane with the frequency-encoding direction head to foot to avoid aliasing. Data matrices of 152 × 256 × 114 with two NEX or 192 × 256 × 140 and one NEX were acquired in a volume of 25 cm × 25 cm × 18 cm, with isotropic nominal phase-encoded resolution of 1.6 mm or 1.3 mm.

Registration proceeded in the order Segmentation, Translation, Rotation and Interpolation, Chisquared TEst, and Reformatting (STRICTER) (see Chapter 10). The stages are illustrated in Fig. 11.1.

The procedure produces an optimal global match for brain tissues. Typical matching accuracies of less than 0.01 mm in each axis and less than 0.01° in each rotation angle were achieved. Difference images were produced by subtracting the baseline images from registered follow-up images or by subtracting the earlier registered follow-up image set from the later one. Registered images and difference images acquired in the sagittal planes were routinely reformatted into the transverse and/or coronal planes.

An example of two T_1-weighted images acquired a month apart and the subtraction image derived from them is shown in Fig. 11.2.

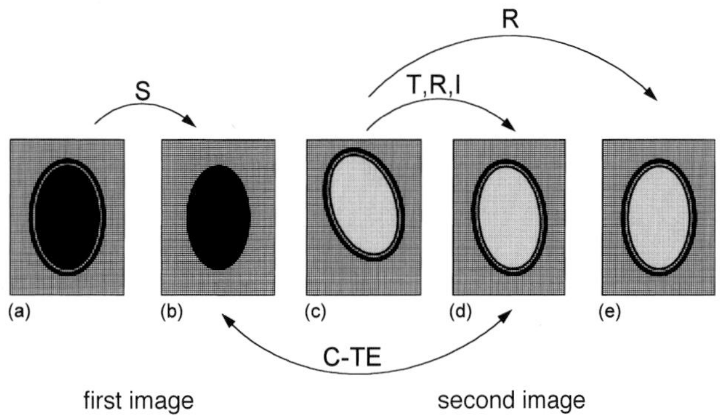

Figure 11.1

Implementation of registration (STRICTER). The first image obtained is shown on the left and is shaded black (a). The second image (shaded gray) is obtained at a different position in the same coordinate system (c). Segmentation (S) removes the skull and scalp from the first image (a) to give (b). Translation (T), Rotation (R) and sinc Interpolation (I) of voxel values are used to produce image (d), which is matched with the segmented version of the first images (b). A Chi-squared (C) TEst (*TE*) is used to assess the accuracy of this match. Following this first attempt at a match, more accurate values for the translation and rotation are chosen in order to reduce the value of χ^2, and the process is repeated. When the optimal match has been found in this way, the second image is Reformatted (R) into the same position as the first image. The original, unsegmented first image (a) can now be compared with the reformatted second image (e), which is precisely aligned.

Image interpretation

The information provided by subvoxel registration may be utilized at three different levels. Firstly, accurate alignment of images alone make detection of differences easier, since change in precisely corresponding areas can be properly attributed to genuine differences in the tissues or fluids under study. Secondly, it is possible to use the precisely registered images to produce subtraction images. Thirdly, precise registration provides a basis for accurate serial measurements, either directly from the images or through the use of computerized algorithms.

The overall approach has been to examine baseline, registered follow-up and subtraction images simultaneously. Collateral information may be obtained from regions apart from those of immediate interest, including from tissues other than brain. This provids a means of recognizing artifacts and checking the fidelity of the registration. On each image, validation of the registration process is assessed by examining regions where there are boundaries between tissues that produce steep changes in signal intensity and checking that these are reduced to the noise level of the difference image. The large amount of data acquired in the volume images and availability of slices in different planes ensures that this can be performed at many different locations.

Interpretation of accurately aligned baseline and follow-up images

This follows established principles. In this study, the sequence that was most often used was sensitive to tissue mobile proton density and T_1 changes. Disease processes that increase mobile proton density and T_1 include inflammation, demyelination, edema and most tumors. Diseases that decrease proton density and T_1 include late scar formation, calcification and subacute hemorrhage. The effect that these changes produce on image signal intensity can be determined using simple models.[3–5]

Interpretation of precisely registered difference images involves additional considerations. Once residual changes due to artifacts and misregistration of deformed or displaced extracerebral tissues have been discounted, changes in signal intensity on difference images are due to (i) change in signal intensity of one or more tissues or fluids; (ii) change in site, shape or size of one or more tissues or fluids; or (iii) a combination of (i) and (ii). These changes can generate either positive or negative signals on difference images (e.g. Fig. 11.2c).

Interpretation of changes in signal intensity on difference images

A pure change in signal intensity is illustrated in Fig. 11.3.

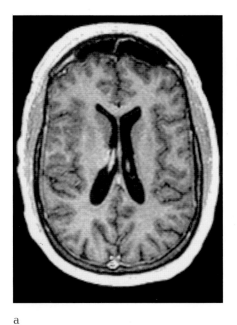
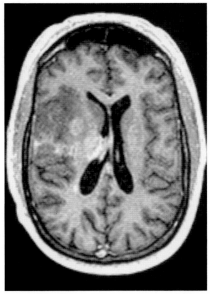
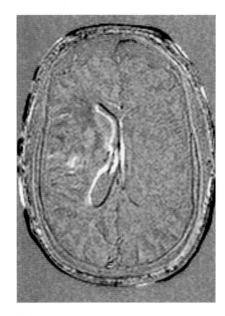

a   b   c

Figure 11.2

Astrocytoma grade III: registered contrast-enhanced T_1-weighted rf-spoiled images before (a) and four weeks after treatment with Temozolamide (b). The difference image, (b) – (a), is shown in (c). The white line around the right lateral ventricle is largely due to an interplateau shift (c). There are also increases in signal intensity in (c) due to increased contrast enhancement. Border zone shifts are seen in the right hemisphere (c).

Detection of signal intensity changes is usually simpler on difference images than on source images, because signals from unchanged tissues and fluids are reduced to a common background level. This can be particularly useful in regions where the anatomy is complex and where there are variable partial volume effects (such as in boundary regions). Difference images are also useful for recognizing signal changes in tissues with intensities at the extremities of the image intensity range. Whereas on the source images these are at the top or bottom of the gray scale, on the difference images they are referred to the neutral (zero-change) level. Global changes in signal intensity may only become obvious on difference images where the brain has a nonzero signal in relation to the noise on the image outside of the scalp.

Image registration can be useful in ensuring that pre- and post-contrast images are precisely matched. In most circumstances it is unlikely that any structure in the brain will significantly change in site, shape or size in the time between the pre

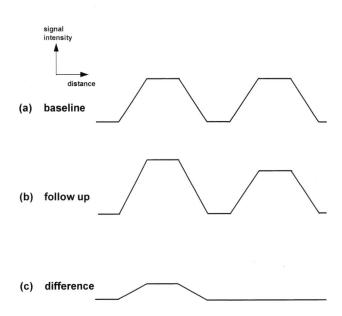

Figure 11.3

Profiles of tissue and/or fluid signal intensities with distance showing the effect of a local change in signal intensity on the difference image. The follow-up scan (b) shows a small change in one region. The difference in this region is more clearly shown by subtracting (a) from (b) to give (c). This shows the local increase in signal intensity.

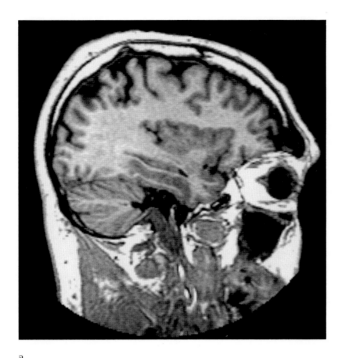

a

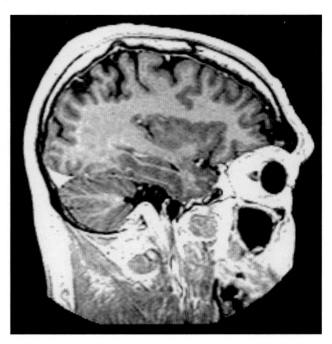

b

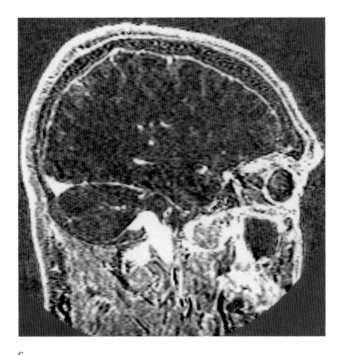

c

Figure 11.4

Contrast enhancement: normal volunteer aged 63 years. Registered T_1-weighted rf-spoiled images before (a) and after (b) intravenous gadolinium DTPA, with difference image, (b) – (a), shown in (c). Enhancement is seen in the gray matter, meninges, vascular layer of the scalp, skin, veins, sinuses and nasal mucosa in (c).

and post scans, so that differences on registered images are almost always due to pure changes in signal intensity (Fig. 11.4).

Normal enhancement occurs in tissues such as the meninges or cortical veins. These areas are subject to considerable partial volume effects from adjacent tissues, such as brain and CSF, producing variable baseline intensity values. By performing accurate registration, it is possible to provide the same set of partial volume effects. As a result, more uniform enhancement of meninges, cortical veins and the ependyma is seen on difference images than on conventional images. It is possible to perform double subtractions (i.e. the difference between the contrast enhancement differences) to show changes in contrast enhancement with time from one examination to the next.

The facts that on T_1-weighted images the contrast agent normally only gives positive enhancement and that there should be no change in brain site, shape or size provide an additional check on the fidelity of the registration procedure. Under these circumstances, immediate post minus pre difference images should only show positive changes whereas misregistration artifacts typically show both positive and negative effects. In some cases we have found that the image differences introduced by the contrast agent appear to be partially offset by a very slight positional mismatch when χ^2 is minimized. This results in weak negative signals that tend to follow high-contrast boundaries. It can be avoided by modifying the definition of χ^2 to include only those voxels for which the post-contrast scan has lower intensity than the pre-contrast scan. This ensures that the pattern of enhancement does not influence the spatial match.

Interpretation of changes in site, shape or size on difference images

Changes in site, shape or size are manifest as a local shift in position of at least some part of the brain and its surrounding tissues or fluids. The size and distribution of these local shifts provide information about the nature of the overall change (i.e. whether it has been one of site, shape, size or a combination of these).

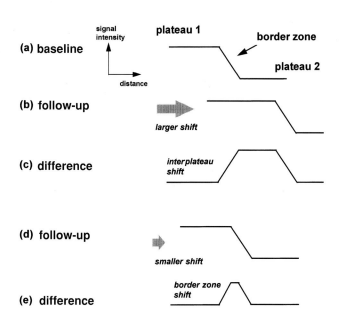

Figure 11.5

Plateaus and border zones, showing interplateau and border zone shifts. A tissue or fluid with a higher signal intensity is shown in plateau 1 and one with a lower signal intensity is shown in plateau 2 (a). This is appropriate for central white matter (plateau 1) and CSF (plateau 2) using a T_1-weighted pulse sequence. There is a border zone (region of partial volume effects) between them, in which signal intensity changes with distance. A larger, interplateau shift of the image is shown in (b), and subtraction of (a) from (b) is shown in the difference profile (c). This has a central full-scale change (plateau 1 minus plateau 2), with two intermediate zones on either side. A smaller border zone shift, which is less than the border zone in width, is shown in (d). This results in a difference profile (e) that is smaller than (c) in both amplitude and width.

Model for analyzing shifts

The effects of shifts can be analyzed using a simple model of two tissues (and/or fluids): one with a higher plateau of signal intensity, the other with a lower plateau, and a border zone (region of partial volume effects) between them (Fig. 11.5a). (Although Fig. 11.5(a) is shown in one spatial dimension, the model is used in three dimensions.) At the ventricular margin with a typical T_1-weighted pulse sequence, white matter or central gray matter forms the higher plateau and CSF the lower one. Likewise, within the brain, white matter forms the higher plateau and gray matter the lower one. (With a heavily T_2-weighted pulse sequence, the central white matter of plateau 1 would have a low signal intensity and the CSF would have a high signal intensity.) It is sometimes useful to regard the cortex as part of a composite (or double) border zone between central white

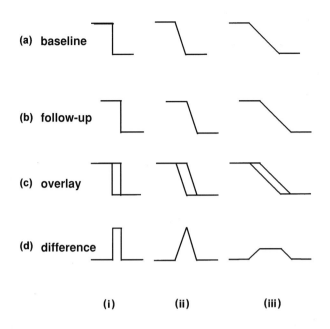

(a) baseline

(b) follow-up

(c) overlay

(d) difference

(i)   (ii)   (iii)

Figure 11.6

Profiles of two plateaus and a border zone, showing the effect of change in signal intensity gradient size for a constant border zone shift. Initial image profiles (a), shifted image profiles (b), overlays (c) of (b) on (a), and subtraction (d) of (a) from (b) are shown for vertical signal change (infinite slope) (i) and decreasing slopes (ii), (iii) and (iv). As the slope is decreased, the width of the difference profile is increased, and the height decreases after image (ii). This makes the change less easy to detect against background noise (not shown). The area under the curves (d) is the same in each case for the constant shift that is illustrated.

matter and CSF. Shifts can be thought of as larger, in which one plateau crosses the border zone so that it overlays the other plateau, and smaller, in which the displacement is less than the width of the border zone.

Larger (interplateau) shifts produce a high and constant (full-scale) central signal change on difference images (Figs 11.5b,c). The full-scale signal change on the difference image is locally monophasic. It is positive when the high-signal plateau has shifted into the region of the low-signal plateau (e.g. Fig. 11.2, lateral margin of right lateral ventricle), and vice versa. There are also intermediate regions on either side of the full-scale change corresponding to the two border zones on the source images. The origin of interplateau shifts is usually clear from the source images. The size of the shift in the direction of the maximum signal

intensity gradient is equal to the width of the full-scale region plus a fraction of the width of the border-zone region (see below).

Smaller shifts (where higher and lower plateaus do not overlap) primarily involve border zones. On difference images, they produce smaller changes in signal intensity than the full-scale changes seen with interplateau shifts (Figs 11.5(d,e) and Fig. 11.2, right hemisphere). The precise effect depends on the size and direction of both the local signal intensity gradient and the shift.

Effect of signal intensity gradient size

In the limit of a vertical slope (idealized maximum signal intensity gradient), there is a step function change in signal intensity on the difference image over the width of the shift (it is really an interplateau shift) (Fig. 11.6). With smaller signal intensity gradients (less than vertical slopes), the same shift results in a rise that is more gradual and to a lower height but over a wider area. The area under the difference curve is the same in each case (i.e. the area of a parallelogram, base × height). The steep gradient produces the highest contrast-to-noise ratio; eventually, as the slope decreases, the change on the difference image becomes so slight that it merges into the noise of the image, and so is not detectable.

Effect of signal intensity gradient direction

At the junction between the higher signal tissue plateau (e.g. white matter) and the border zone, it is possible to draw a contour (which is a line of constant signal intensity and hence zero signal intensity gradient). The local direction of maximum signal intensity gradient is perpendicular to this (Fig. 11.7). The same applies to the junction between the border zone and the lower-signal-intensity plateau. The size of the gradient generally decreases as the width of the border zone increases, since the two plateaus have a constant signal intensity difference. A contour divides the image into voxels of higher signal intensity on one side and voxels of lower signal intensity on the other. It is convenient to indicate the signal intensity gradient direction with an

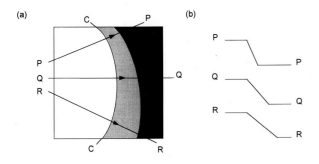

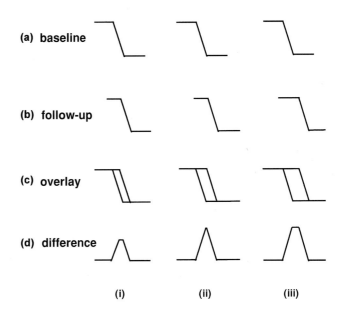

(a) baseline

(b) follow-up

(c) overlay

(d) difference

(i)   (ii)   (iii)

Figure 11.7

Plan (a) and profiles (b) of two plateaus and a border zone, showing signal intensity gradients in different directions. The profiles (PP, QQ and RR) show the signal intensity changes in passing from one plateau across the border zone to the other plateau. The contour (CC) marks the edge of the high-signal plateau. At each point on CC the maximum signal intensity gradient is perpendicular to the contour. The direction of the gradient defined as being from higher to lower signal intensity is indicated by the arrows. An estimate of the slope of the signal intensity gradient through PP, QQ and RR can be obtained by noting that the slope is inversely related to the distance between the two plateaus.

Figure 11.8

Effect of shift size. Baseline image profiles (a), successively displaced image profiles (b), overlays (c) of (b) on (a), and differences (d) are shown for increasing shifts (i)–(iv). As the shift is increased, the height of the difference increases to a maximum, and the width of this maximum then increases. The area under the difference curve is directly proportional to the shift distance.

arrow showing the direction of *decreasing* signal intensity across a contour because then, if the shift has a component parallel to the direction shown, there will be an *increase* in signal on the difference image. If the shift has a parallel component, but in the opposite direction, there will be a decrease in signal on the difference image. A high signal intensity gradient in plane generally corresponds to a low signal intensity gradient through plane, and vice versa.

of the magnitude of the signal intensity gradient. Using the plateau model, the size of the component of a shift that is parallel to the local gradient direction will be the width shown on the difference image multiplied by the mean difference signal as a fraction of the full-scale signal intensity.

Effect of size of a shift

As shown in Fig. 11.8, the initial effect of a shift is to show a small change on the difference image (i.e. a border zone shift). If the shift is increased, this reaches a peak when one plateau just crosses the boundary zone to reach the other plateau. This peak is maintained in intensity, and widens as the shift is increased further (i.e. an interplateau shift). The area under the curve on the difference image increases in direct proportion to the size of the shift (i.e. area of a parallelogram), and is independent

Effect of shift direction

Shifts are usually both in-plane and through-plane but may be thought of as predominantly one or the other. With in-plane shifts, it is possible to visualize on the same image the tissue or fluid that has shifted (or will shift) (e.g. Fig. 11.2) whereas with through-plane shifts, the tissue or fluid moving into the slice comes from adjacent slices. In order to visualize plateaus and border zones in three dimensions, it is therefore necessary to consider adjacent slices (which are one voxel apart with 3D acquisitions).

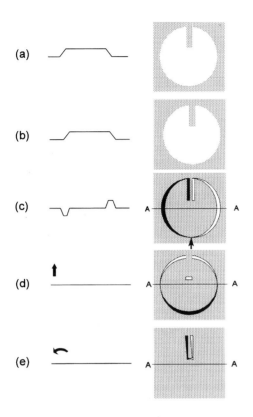

Figure 11.9

Effect of the shift direction (in-plane). Profiles (left) and plans (right) of an object are shown in the initial position (a), with shift to the right (b) and on the corresponding difference image (c). Difference image profiles along the lines AA and plans are shown for an upward in-plane displacement (d) and counterclockwise rotation (e). The changes in signal on the difference images can be directly related to the signal intensity gradients and shifts. A shift that is perpendicular to the local signal intensity gradient direction produces no change on the difference image (e.g. (c), arrow).

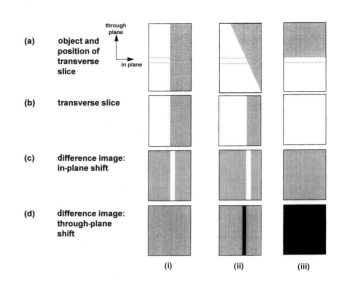

Figure 11.10

Effects of in-plane and through-plane shifts. Three objects with differently oriented boundaries between regions of high and low signal are shown in (a)(i–iii). The position of a transverse slice through each object is also shown (dotted lines). The corresponding images are shown in (b)(i–iii). For an in-plane shift to the right, the difference image shows a linear change in both (c)(i) and (c)(ii), but no change in (c)(iii). For a through-plane shift, a variety of patterns are seen. There is no change in (d)(i), change along a line in (d)(ii), and a change within the whole plane in (d)(iii). In the last case there is a steep gradient through plane, which is not apparent from the image (b)(iii). In-plane shifts produce predictable difference signals where there are in-plane edges (c)(i,ii). However, through-plane shifts, which reveal the presence of through-plane intensity gradients, can produce either linear or regional difference patterns (d)(i,ii). In this diagram white indicates positive signal, gray is zero and black is a negative signal.

The effect of in-plane shifts is shown in Fig. 11.9. There is an increase in signal intensity on the side to which the high-signal tissue or fluid has shifted on the difference image. The difference is maximal at the point of the maximum signal intensity gradient in the direction of the shift. When the displacement is perpendicular to the local intensity gradient, no signal intensity change is seen. This effect is seen in the right lateral ventricle in Fig. 11.2(c), where a positive change is seen at the lateral margin and a negative change is seen at the medial margin.

The effect of rotation is to produce differential shifts. These produce changes on the difference images where there is a radial edge, since this has a circumferential intensity gradient component

that is parallel to the local shift direction. The displacement increases with radial distance from the center of rotation.

The mechanism for signal change produced by through-plane shifts is the same as for in-plane shifts, i.e. changes are produced on difference images whenever the shift has a component parallel to the local signal intensity gradient. However, the visual appearance of difference signals produced by through-plane shifts is more heterogeneous than that produced by in-plane shifts (Fig. 11.10).

The practical effects of both in-plane and through-plane shifts for a transverse and a coronal slice taken from the same 3D data set are shown in Figs 11.11 and 11.12. The images were

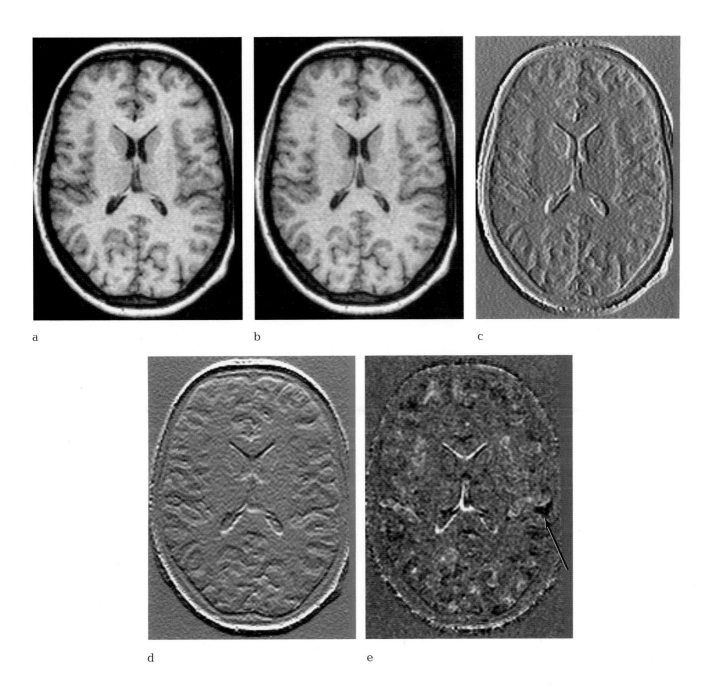

a   b   c

d   e

Figure 11.11

Simulated effects of in-plane and through-plane shifts on anatomic images: a volume data set with cubic voxels (0.97 mm on each side) was copied and displaced by one voxel in each of three orthogonal directions, and then the original data were subtracted from it. A transverse slice from the volume set (a), the adjacent slice (b), and difference images for left–right (c), postero–anterior (d) and head–foot (e) displacements are shown. Image (e) results from subtracting (a) from (b). The differences produced by in-plane shifts (c,d) show monophasic and multiphasic curvilinear changes that can easily be related to the anatomy in (a). Intense signals with a simple geometry can be seen around the skull and scalp (c,d). The pattern of through-plane changes (e) is less clearly related to the anatomy shown in (a). The ventricular system produces curvilinear features as expected from Figs 11.9(a–d)(ii). However, there are more widespread changes, which are patchy or mottled (arrow) rather than curvilinear. These arise from through-plane differences between (a) and (b) that have little or no in-plane component. Close inspection is necessary to relate the differences in (e) to the source images (a) and (b).

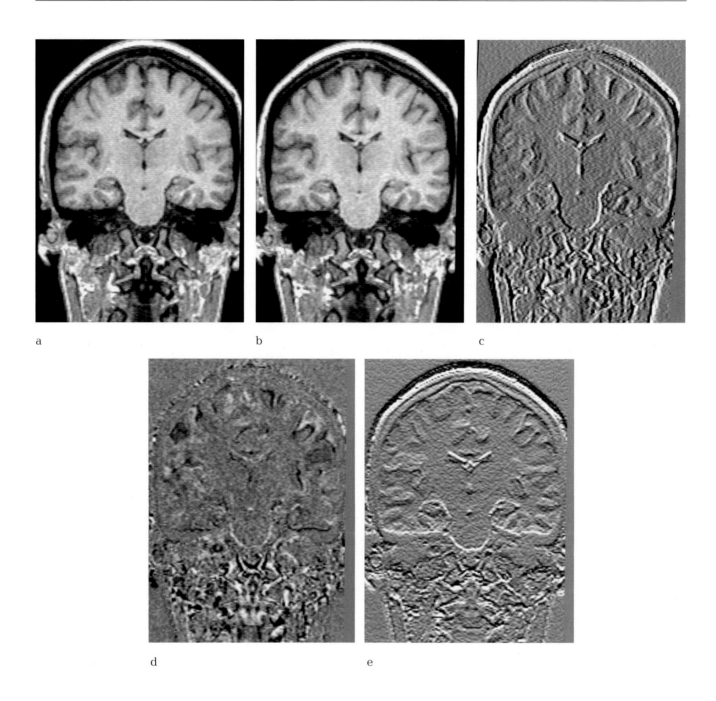

a   b   c

d   e

Figure 11.12

The same image data as in Fig. 11.11 is shown, but reformatted into the coronal plane. Anatomic image (a), adjacent slice (b), and differences produced by a one voxel shift in the left–right (c), postero–anterior (d) and head–foot (e) directions are displayed. Note that

the through-plane direction is now postero–anterior (d), and this image shows nonspecific changes in signal intensity as well as monophasic and multiphasic curvilinear changes.

produced by shifting the volume data by a single voxel (approximately 0.97 mm) in each of the principal matrix directions in turn and then subtracting the original images from the displaced images.

Figure 11.11(a) shows a transverse slice taken from the volume set, and Fig. 11.11(b) shows the adjacent slice. The difference images in Figs 11.11(c–e) show respectively the effect of left–right, postero–anterior and head–foot shifts of just one voxel. The in-plane shifts in Figs 11.11(c,d) produce predictable results in which edges (border zones) in Fig. 11.11(a) are accentuated as high or low signal according to the pattern of the local signal intensity gradients.

The result of the through-plane displacement (Fig. 11.11e) is more complex. The origin of individual regions of positive or negative signal difference can be determined by careful comparison of Figs 11.11(a,b), since Fig. 11.11(e) is simply 11.11(b) minus 11.11(a). However, while some regions contain curvilinear changes of the same type seen with in-plane shifts, in many areas the overall effect does not correspond overtly to the anatomic structures visible in Fig. 11.11(a) or (b). This is because the regions on the difference image where the largest signal intensity changes occur are those with the maximum *through-plane* signal intensity gradient. These are just the places that tend to have the smallest *in-plane* signal intensity gradients, because they arise where tissue boundaries are parallel or nearly parallel to the slice plane (cf. Figs 11.10(a–d)(iii)). Small in-plane gradients imply a relatively uniform appearance in the source image, with little hint of the through-plane differences.

A similar effect is seen in Fig. 11.12, but this time it is the postero–anterior shift (Fig. 11.12d) that produces through-plane differences from the slice in Fig. 11.12(a) to that in Fig. 11.12(b). Note that simply by reformatting to the coronal plane, the head–foot displacement that was difficult to interpret in Fig. 11.11(e) is transformed to the anatomically linked pattern in Fig. 11.12(e).

A through-plane shift in a case of cerebral atrophy is shown in Fig. 11.13. The movement of the upper surface of the corpus callosum upwards into the region of the pericallosal sulcus and gray matter produces an increase in signal on the transverse difference image (Fig. 11.13c).

Effects of change in shape (without change in signal intensity)

Change in shape involves change in site of some (at least) of the tissue or fluid, but it does not necessarily produce a change in size. A change in shape will in general be accompanied by corresponding shifts elsewhere in the image. Recognition of these may be straightforward for simple structures and larger changes, but difficult for complex structures and smaller changes. It requires an overview of the site and direction of the shifts at different locations in the brain.

Effect of change in size (without change in signal intensity)

This will also involve change in site and possibly shape. The associated shifts may be focal or general. The focal changes may be centered on a particular region, while general changes are centered on the structure itself. Change in size is typically not associated with compensatory (i.e. equal and opposite) changes in the corresponding regions. Recognition of change in size also requires an overall assessment of the site, size and direction of shifts.

Etiology

Changes in site (as well as shape and size) are typically due to mass effects. The latter term includes displacement of otherwise normal tissue by a disease process. Mass effects are typically associated with tumors, but may be seen with many other diseases, such as abscesses, hematomas, trauma, edema and demyelination.[3-5] The effects may be local or general. Reduction in size may take the form of localized or generalized atrophy. This occurs typically in degenerative conditions, but also in cerebral infarction, trauma etc.

Interpretation of changes in signal intensity as well as changes in site, shape or size on difference images

Changes in signal intensity and shifts frequently occur together (e.g. Fig. 11.2), since many pathologies that increase T_1 and T_2 also produce mass effects, and the region of greatest T_1 and T_2 may also be the region of greatest mass effect.

The increase or decrease in signal intensity may take it beyond the plateau levels in the model used to describe shifts. As a result, shifts may produce

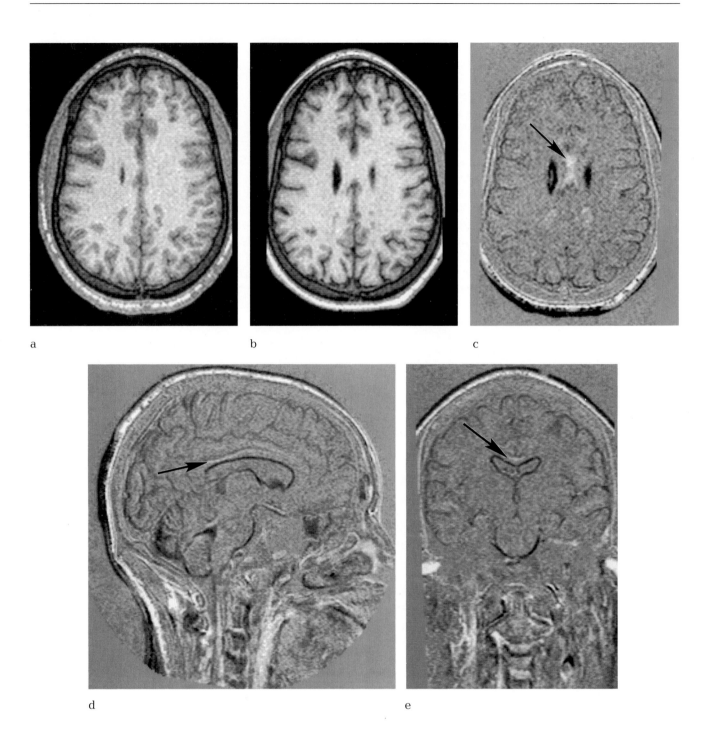

a   b   c

d   e

Figure 11.13

Through-plane shift: registered transverse T_1-weighted rf-spoiled images prior to bone marrow transplantation (a) and eight months later (b). The difference image is shown in (c). The corresponding registered difference images in the sagittal (d) and coronal (e) plane are also shown. With the cerebral atrophy, the corpus callosum has shifted superiorly and its superior surface encroaches on the region previously occupied by the pericallosal sulcus and gray matter giving the high signal in (c) (arrow). The small size of the shift is apparent in (d) and (e) (arrows). Cerebral atrophy has developed, and this produces low signal margins around the ventricular system and the external surface of the brain.

signal differences that are beyond the 'full-scale' of the model. Using the sequences described here, this occurred with very short T_1 lesions owing to either subacute hemorrhage or contrast enhancement. A lesion involving the higher plateau (e.g. white matter) that lengthens its T_1 decreases the size of the difference between the two plateaus, so the interplateau difference is less than full-scale.

When the changes in signal intensity and shifts are at different sites, they can be treated independently (as with displaced but otherwise normal tissue around a space-occupying lesion). When they occur together, some further consideration is necessary. The key concept is that a difference in signal intensity of a tissue or fluid in the boundary zone not only produces a change in its own right, but also changes the signal intensity gradient so that the effect of a shift may be increased or decreased. The detailed change depends on the pulse sequence being employed. For example, with the T_1-weighted sequence, a lesion that increased T_1 would decrease its signal intensity and also decrease the gradient at its interface with CSF. The decreased signal intensity would produce a negative signal on the difference image, and the effect of any shift in producing a change on the difference image would be reduced.

When a lesion is characterized only by an increase or decrease in its signal intensity relative to the surrounding normal tissue (and has no mass effect), it may be difficult or impossible to distinguish a change in its signal intensity from a change in its size. The change in signal intensity usually changes the signal intensity gradient in the border zone, and this determines the threshold for detecting the border of the lesion in relation to the image noise and artifact level. In this situation a decrease in signal intensity difference between the lesion and its surroundings usually appears to be accompanied by a decrease in size, but if the signal intensity gradient in the border zone is maintained then the lesion size may appear unchanged. A 'pure' change in signal intensity may thus be inextricably linked to a change in size of the lesion.

Regional and tissue specific appearances on difference images

In this section specific anatomic regions are considered in more detail and a wider range of tissues and fluids are discussed.

The ventricular system

The ventricles are smooth, continuous and regular, and their signal intensity gradients are predictable both in plane and over adjacent slices (Figs 11.12 and 11.13). The border zone for shifts in certain directions is quite narrow. In this situation full-scale changes due to relatively small interplateau shifts are readily seen when the shift is parallel to the maximum signal intensity gradient. Locally monophasic curvilinear changes are typically seen with smaller border zone shifts.

Changes within the ventricles may be complicated by the presence of the choroid plexus and other structures, which may produce multiphasic effects. Large shifts may lead to complete overlap of the ventricular system with the brain, and there may be changes in the shape of the ventricles as well as size.

There is also variation in ventricular size as a function of brain position due to gravitational effects, so that positioning needs to be accurate (see Chapter 12). Small changes have also been seen in different phases of the menstrual cycle.

The brainstem and cerebellum

The brainstem also presents continuous and predictable boundaries, although the cerebellar folia show a more complex, but still regular, pattern. The signal intensity gradients associated with the cerebellar folia sensitize them to shifts in the superior–inferior and postero–anterior directions.

The cerebral cortex

In contrast to the ventricular system and brainstem, the cerebral cortex is convoluted, and the signal intensity gradients are highly variable in both magnitude and direction. The sulci are generally wider in the frontal lobes than in the occipital lobes. The major fissures (central and lateral) are wider again. Because of the many different gradient directions the cortex is sensitive to shifts in many different directions. It can be divided into (i) a superficial part representing the external surface and including the tips of the gyri, and (ii) a deeper part consisting of infolded cortex below the external surface. The superficial gyri form part of the general external shape of the brain, and have a reasonable degree of regularity about their position. Their signal intensity gradients reflect this and it is possible to recognize shifts of the superficial cortex using the simple plateau model, although the plateaus are not so well defined as with the ventricular system.

The deeper infolded cortex is notable for the fact that there are frequently two border zones in close proximity with signal intensity gradients that are opposed ('reverse slopes') or obliqued. The cortex is subject to shifts that may move both of these border zones in the same direction producing biphasic changes (e.g. Fig. 11.2, right hemisphere). There are also other processes that move the sulcal border zones in opposite directions, either towards one another (as in generalized brain swelling) or apart (as in cortical atrophy, e.g. Fig. 11.13). Combinations of the different signal intensity gradients and different inplane shifts in both border zones within sulci (and fissures) of different widths result in a variety of appearances, some of which are illustrated in Fig. 11.14.

Adjacent to the cortex are blood vessels as well as meninges, and shifts involving these may result in more complex multiphasic changes.

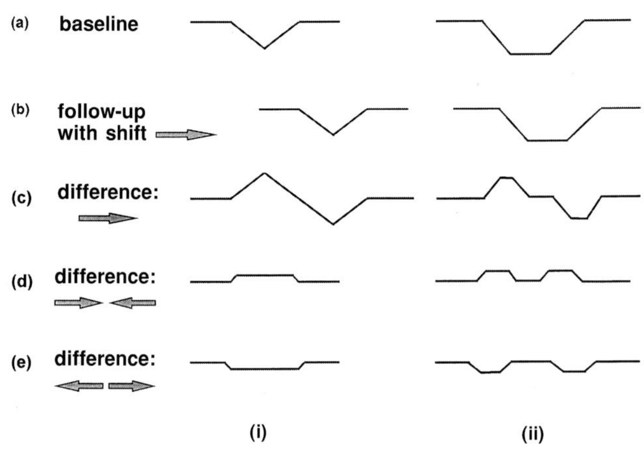

Figure 11.14

Intensity profiles showing effects of shifts on sulci and fissures. Wedge (i) and trough (ii) profiles are shown in (a). A displacement is shown in (b), and the corresponding differences in (c). Effects of sulci moving together (d) and apart (e) are also shown.

Global change in brain size

When there is a global change in brain size, the matching process effectively aligns the central portion of the two-volume images of the brain. As a result, the more peripheral regions are progressively displaced from their original positions. If slices are imaged perpendicular to a radius from the center out to the periphery, there will be a progressive through-plane shift that reaches a maximum at the outer surface. This effect will generally be greatest for transverse slices at the superior aspect of the brain and at the inferior aspect of the cerebellum. For parasagittal slices, the largest changes are at the lateral extremities of the hemisphere, since these are furthest from the center of the brain. The effect is reversed for generalized reduction in size. To obtain more accurate images of local changes, the matching process can be restricted to smaller volumes around the area of interest.

Blood vessels and venous sinuses

With the T_1-weighted sequence used in most of this study, only minimal inflow effects were seen in proximal arteries, but changes in signal intensity were more obvious with angiographic sequences. The signal intensity in many vessels reflected the T_1 of blood, which is intermediate between those of the brain and CSF. The blood vessels may be circular, elliptical or triangular in cross-section, and subtraction of these following an increase or decrease in size may produce different effects, which can be predicted from the plateau model (Fig. 11.15). There may also be shifts of blood vessels.

A change in the straight sinus is illustrated in Fig. 11.16.

Meninges

Because the images are matched to the brain, shift of the brain within the cranial cavity may appear as a shift of the dura and skull into the subarachnoid space surrounding the brain. This shift then shows up along the smooth outline of the dura and adjacent skull rather than the convolutions of the cortex.

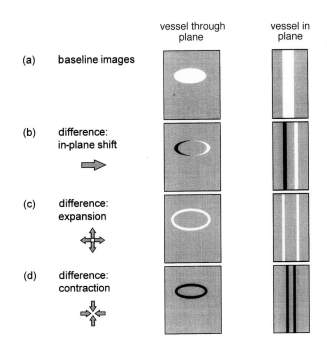

vessel through plane | vessel in plane

(a) baseline images

(b) difference: in-plane shift

(c) difference: expansion

(d) difference: contraction

Figure 11.15

Views of blood vessels (in-plane and through-plane) and surrounded by CSF for a T_1-weighted image are shown in (a). The difference for an in-plane shift is shown in (b), and the effects of expansion (c) and contraction (d) on difference images are also shown.

Other extracerebral tissues and fluids

The process of registering the brain also aligns tissues and fluids surrounding it, as long as these are in fixed relation to the brain. If they are not in fixed relation, differences will be seen on the subtraction images. Such tissues may undergo changes in their own right, and these need to be interpreted with reference to the brain. Susceptibility effects from air in the nasal sinuses may impact on brain signal with $T_2{}^*$-weighted sequences. The scalp shows changes in most subtraction images consistent with differences in the distribution of blood within it. Changes were seen in the neck consistent with changes in the relative position of the head and neck at the craniovertebral junction. Marked contrast enhancement is seen in blood vessels, the nasal mucosa, scalp and the skin.

Artifacts

Difference images are subject to all of the artifacts present on the source images, and subtraction usually makes these more obvious. Artifacts may be produced by global motion of the subject as well as more localized motion of structures such as the eyes and the pharynx. The use of phase encoding in two directions as required by the 3D acquisition increases the vulnerability of the sequence to motion artifacts in different directions. Susceptibility artifacts may be very largely replicated if the patient is in virtually the same position on both examinations. However, they are inherently anisotropic with respect to $\mathbf{B}_0$, and may not therefore be correctable by rigid-body translation and rotation. The problem is likely to be greater with $T_2{}^*$-weighted sequences than the T_1-weighted sequences mainly used in this study.

Failed registration

The difference images provide an inbuilt check of the fidelity of registration. If the program fails to obtain a satisfactory match, monophasic or multiphasic changes will be seen in border zones. Inter-plateau shifts may also be seen. The changes may be widespread and generally have the character of a whole brain shift superimposed on any underlying changes. Unregistered images provide a useful guide in this context. The differential diagnosis is widespread change of physiologic or pathologic origin, for example in growth during childhood. In the latter case there is usually a systematic pattern of change around the ventricles, cortex and other structures.

To date, in 120 cases, there have been three failures of registration. One occurred when an unenhanced image was badly matched to the post-enhancement image taken two months later in a patient with a cerebral tumor that had grown significantly over two months. The other images in the series (first examination, post-enhancement and second examination, pre-enhancement) were correctly aligned. The other two failures were associated with problems in signal intensity scaling that probably resulted from changes in coil loading. Systematic changes of this type are manifest by nonzero mean signal on the difference images. This can be easily recognized in relation to the surrounding noise, and is simple to correct.

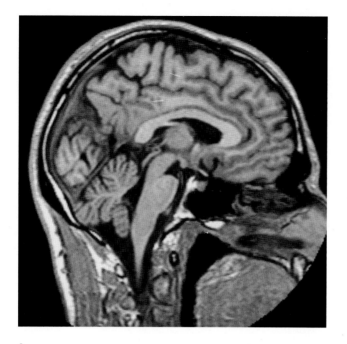

a

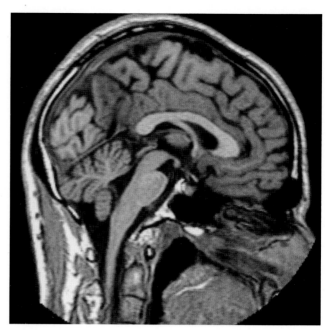

b

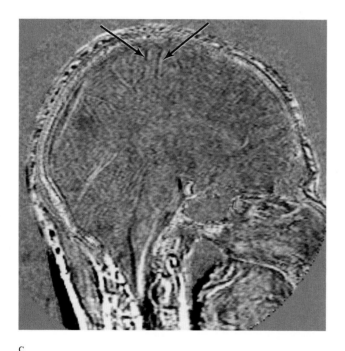

c

Figure 11.16

Change in the superior sagittal and straight sinuses with head flexion: sagittal T_1-weighted images in upright position (a) and with head flexion (b). The registered difference image, (b) – (a), is shown in (c). The signal from the inferior sagittal sinus has increased, probably as a result of an increase in size. The superior sagittal sinus shows a more complex change posteriorly (c). Border zone shifts are noted in the region of the superior cerebral sulci (c).

Approach to diagnosis of changes to the brain on difference images

It is necessary to relate the causes of changes on difference images (i.e. pure changes in signal intensity, through-plane and in-plane border zone shifts and interplateau shifts) to the appearances they produce, i.e. (i) nonspecific changes in signal intensity, (ii) monophasic curvilinear changes, (iii) multiphasic curvilinear changes and (iv) inter-plateau changes. Changes of different types may be present on the same image. Their relation to the underlying causes is summarized in Table 11.1.

A formal approach to image interpretation is described in Table 11.2.

Table 11.1 Typical appearances of changes on difference images

Cause	Pure change in signal intensity	Through-plane border zone shift	In-plane border zone shift	Interplateau shift
	→	↘ →	↗ ↘	→
Overall appearance	Nonspecific change in signal intensity	Monophasic curvilinear change	Multiphasic curvilinear change	Interplateau change
Signal intensity	Often monophasic (locally) variable	Monophasic (locally) less than full scale	Multiphasic (locally) less than full scale	Monophasic (locally) full scale
Site	Anatomic, physiologic, pathologic distribution	In-plane plateau but through-plane border zone. Ventricular margin, brainstem margin, etc	Cerebral cortex, cerebellar hemisphere, etc	Brain margins, i.e. around ventricles and subarachnoid space (for brain/CSF)
Shape	Variable	Curvilinear	Curvilinear	Follows brain margins (for brain/CSF)
Size	Variable	Local, size of border zone	Local, size of border zone	Often extensive, but may be local, with or without reversed phase
Segments	Mottled, patchy or circumscribed area	Narrower curvilinear directional dependence	Broader curvilinear etched, bas relief, directional shadowing	Uniform central region

Notes
(i)   Shifts are shown from smallest (pure change in signal intensity, zero shift) to largest (interplateau).
(ii) The specificity of appearances also increases from left to right across the page.
(iii) Interplateau shifts may be through plane and/or in plane, and are accompanied by smaller changes due to through-plane and in-plane border zone shifts.
(iv) Through-plane border zone shifts produce a heterogeneous range of appearances, i.e. nonspecific change in signal intensity as well as monophasic and multiphasic curvilinear changes.
(v)   In-plane border zone shifts produce monophasic and multiphasic curvilinear changes.
(vi) Monophasic curvilinear changes typically occur at ventricular margins, brainstem margins etc, where interplateau shifts first appear with larger shifts.
(vii) Reformatting into a perpendicular plane may convert a nonspecific through-plane shift to a more specific in-plane shift.

Table 11.2 Approach to image interpretation

(1) *Review source images:* Define any signal intensity changes and shifts.

(2) *Review difference images:* Define significant abnormalities (i.e. non-artifactual areas of increased or decreased signal intensity). These should fit into one or more of the four categories described in Table 11.1, i.e. nonspecific change in signal intensity, monophasic curvilinear change, multiphasic curvilinear change or interplateau change.

(3) *Assess inter-plateau shifts:* For interplateau changes, determine the shift direction (in plane or through plane) by direct reference to the source images, including different slices. The shift size is equal to the width of the full-scale region on the difference image plus a fraction of the width of the associated border zone region (see below).

(4) *Assess signal intensity gradients:* In the regions of other changes on the difference images use the source images to define the in-plane contours and signal intensity gradients (which are perpendicular to the contours), noting the direction of decreasing signal. Define the through-plane signal intensity gradients in the slice of interest (these tend to be reciprocally related to the in-plane gradients). Define the through-plane signal intensity gradients between slices by comparison of adjacent source images in the relevant areas.

(5) *Assess border zone shifts:* Determine shifts in the border zones by noting
 (a) signal on the difference image is produced by a shift with a component parallel to the maximum signal intensity gradient;
 (b) the difference image signal is positive when the shift is in the direction of decreasing gradient, and vice versa;
 (c) the size of the shift in the direction of the maximum gradient is equal to the width of the change on the difference image multiplied by the average fraction of the full-scale signal intensity;
 (d) local changes in signal intensity may exaggerate or minimize the signal difference produced by a shift;
 (e) profiles from source and difference may help to resolve shift direction and size.
 (f) reformatting the images into a perpendicular plane may transform a nonspecific change in signal intensity due to a through-plane shift to the curvilinear change of an in-plane shift.

(6) *Assess overall pattern of shifts:* Review the overall pattern of shifts for changes in brain site, shape or size on a focal or general basis.

(7) *Assess pure changes in signal intensity:* Note that with a pure change in signal intensity no shift is detectable. (A pure change in signal intensity may, however, be accompanied by an inseparable change in lesion size.)

Conclusions

The production of accurately registered images from serial examinations acquired over time allows comparisons to be made with a precision that has not been possible previously. A crucial aspect of this work is the use of subtraction images that demonstrate changes against a neutral background. The interpretation of these images involves considerations that are not part of routine radiological practice at present. An approach to interpreting images of this type has been presented in this chapter.

Acknowledgements

We wish to thank the Medical Research Council, the Wellcome Trust and Nycomed for their continued support.

References

1. Hajnal JV, Saeed N, Soar EJ et al, A registration and interpolation procedure for subvoxel matching of serially acquired magnetic resonance images. *J Comput Assist Tomogr* 1995; **19:** 289–96.

2. Bydder GM, Detection of small changes to the brain with serial magnetic resonance imaging. *Br J Radiol* 1995; **68:** 1271–95.

3. Stark DD, Bradley WG (eds), *Magnetic resonance imaging*, 2nd edn. Mosby-Year Book, St Louis, MO, 1992.

4. Atlas SW (ed), *Magnetic resonance imaging of the brain and spine*. Raven Press, New York, 1991.

5. Grossman RI, Yousem DM, *Neuroradiology*. Mosby-Year Book, St Louis, MO, 1994.

12

Registration and subtraction of serial magnetic resonance images Part 3: Applications

Graeme M Bydder and Joseph V Hajnal

Introduction

Chapters 10 and 11 have described a technique used for registration and subtraction of serial MR images and how these images can be interpreted. In this chapter some physiological and clinical applications of the technique are described.

There are many potential uses for this technique, and the applications we describe merely constitute a starting point that reflects local interest. Monitoring of physiological changes was necessary to establish a baseline for recognition of changes in patients. In fact, patient positioning appears to be of critical importance since small differences in the angle at which the head is studied can result in changes to the shape of the brain.

Bone marrow transplantation provided an unexpected model of cerebral atrophy where a controlled insult was applied to normal or nearly normal brain. Contrary to expectations, we found atrophy rather than edema, the cause of which is still not clear.

Children were of interest because of the additional effects of growth and development. These could be readily identified. Of particular interest was the increased growth found in the brain adjacent to the site of neonatal infarction. This raised questions about plasticity and regeneration of the brain in infancy.

Another unexpected finding was a reduction in brain size (atrophy rather than edema) during the third trimester in patients with pre-eclampsia. We have also observed both atrophic change and swelling in first episode schizophrenia over a 6–12 month period. Many other applications of this technique are possible, and results from these are awaited with considerable interest.

Physiological changes

Effect of head position

Flexing the neck by 13° in a normal male volunteer produced multiphasic curvilinear changes around the superior sulci consistent with a change in the shape of the brain (Fig. 12.1, arrows). When the subject was repositioned in the original head orientation, the sulcal signals were no longer detected. In all subjects tested, signal differences could be detected above the noise level when the head orientation was altered by more than 5° in any direction. Change due to slight alteration to head position are a major factor determining the threshold for minimal detectable changes in this work, and this puts a premium on accurate positioning of the head in serial studies. Changes

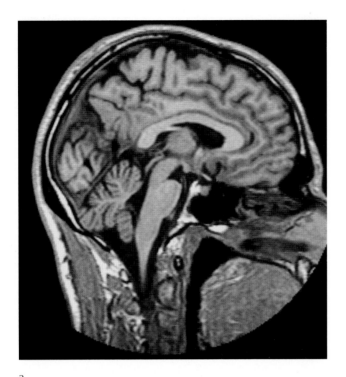

a

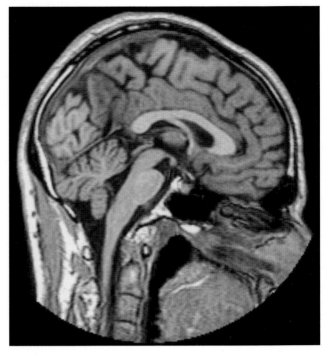

b

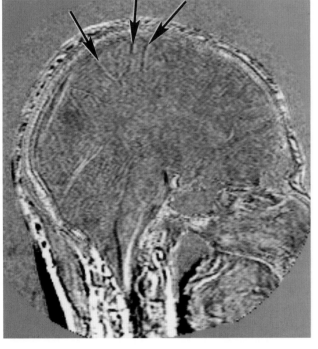

c

Figure 12.1

Positional changes in a normal volunteer: (a) Initial sagittal image; (b) second image with head flexed 13°; (c) registered difference image. Biphasic curvilinear changes are seen on the region of the superior sulci (arrows). Increased signal is also seen in the straight sinus (c). Widespread differences are seen in the neck, arising from its flexure during the change in position. These extrenuous effects were excluded from the registration process by image segmentation (see Chapter 10) and so did not affect the brain comparison.

may be seen both at the ventricular margins and in the cortical regions. Figure 12.1 emphasizes the role of image segmentation in limiting the region of the anatomy that is used in determining the positional match. The large changes in the neck in Fig. 12.1(a) reflects its flexion during this change in head position. These changes were excluded during the matching process, so ensuring that they did not influence the residual changes in the brain, which reflect a real local change in shape.

Figure 12.2 shows interplateau and border zone shifts (see Chapter 11) produced by changing head

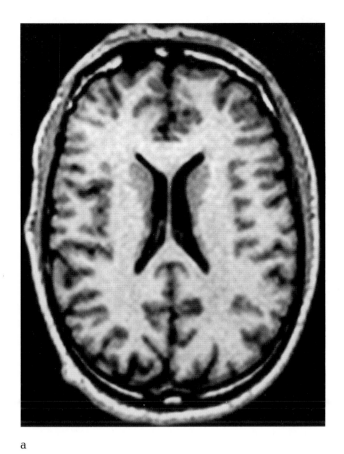

a

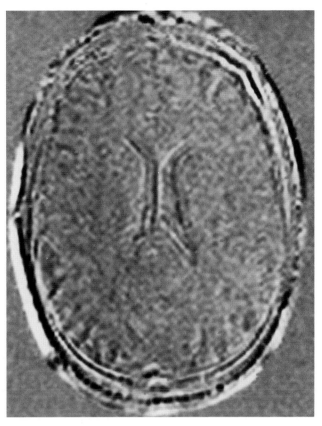

b

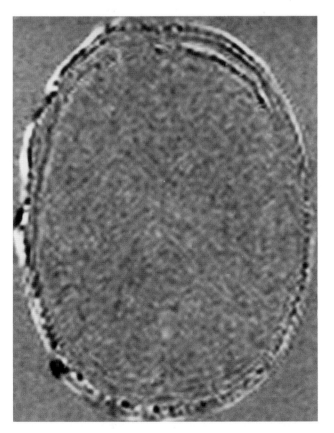

c

Figure 12.2

Gravitational effects on the brain: transverse slice
acquired from a normal adult male volunteer with his
head right-side down (a) and registered subtraction of
images acquired with the volunteer positioned with his
left-side down minus the right-side down (b). In (b)
the margins of the lateral ventricles show interplateau
and border zone shifts (black and white lines), while
the gyri show border zone shifts. (c) On returning to
the right-side-down position, the differences in the
brain are no longer apparent.

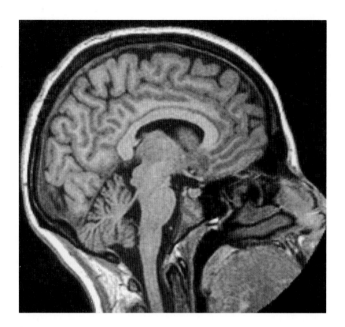

a

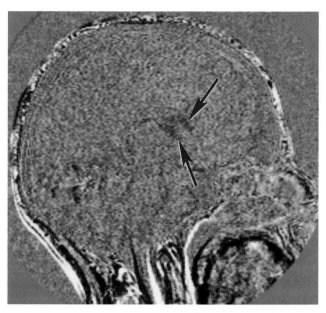

b

Figure 12.3

Menstrual cycle in a normal adult female: mid-cycle image (a) and registered difference image produced by subtracting the mid-cycle image from the corresponding late-cycle image (b). There are low- signal regions on (b) (arrows) consistent with a through-plane border zone shift. They are indicative of an increase in ventricular size.

orientation from right-side down to left-side down. The image shows shift of the ventricular system and changes in many gyri. These changes may provide a basis for measuring brain compliance in health and disease, including quantification of the elastic properties of the brain.

Menstrual cycle

In the four normal females studied, registration of repeated examinations showed very small changes. The most consistent finding on the differ- ence images was a border zone shift related to the lateral ventricles consistent with an increase in their size at the end of the second half of the menstrual cycle (Fig. 12.3b, arrows). This change is consistent in sign, but may be smaller in size than the previously reported finding of increase in CSF volume later in the menstrual cycle detected with a volume measurement technique.[1]

Contrast enhancement

Normal enhancement in the meninges, diploic veins, scalp, skin and other structures was more clearly demonstrated than with conventional unregistered images. In addition, abnormal enhancement was more clearly demonstrated in patients with meningeal disease and other condi- tions[2] (Fig. 12.4).

Registration and subtraction were of particular value in the following situations.

(a) *Recognition of small degrees of enhancement.* When the level of change was small, differ- ences may be much less than those produced by misregistration, particularly when the changes are at boundaries. Diffuse generalized enhancement may also be more readily recog- nized on subtraction images in relation to the noise level of the surrounding images. This type of change may be missed with conven- tional display strategies.

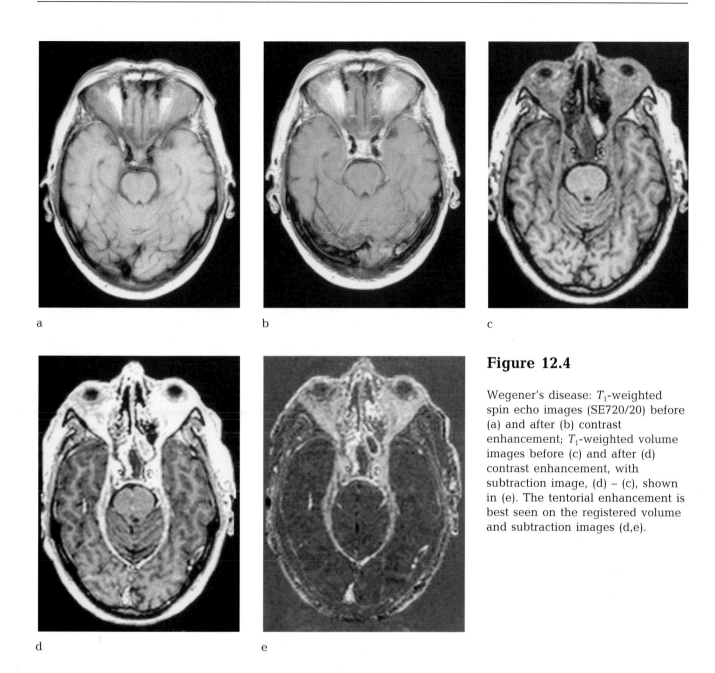

a b c

d e

Figure 12.4

Wegener's disease: T_1-weighted spin echo images (SE720/20) before (a) and after (b) contrast enhancement; T_1-weighted volume images before (c) and after (d) contrast enhancement, with subtraction image, (d) – (c), shown in (e). The tentorial enhancement is best seen on the registered volume and subtraction images (d,e).

(b) *Enhancement in tissues or fluids with very high or very low baseline signals.* The usual window level and width settings may place the changes due to enhancement off the top or the bottom of the display gray scale, and so render changes difficult to recognize. Subtraction reduces all tissues and fluids to a common baseline, and makes changes of this type easier to visualize.

(c) *Enhancement at interfaces, boundaries and other regions of complex anatomy.* In these situations there are frequently partial volume effects, and even a small displacement of the brain between pre- and post-contrast images produces a difference in these effects, resulting in spurious changes in signal intensity. Precise registration provides the same partial volume effects on the before and after images, so that enhancement can be readily recognized.

(d) *Assessment of enhancement when thin slices are used.* While use of thin slices reduces partial volume effects, it may increase problems due to overt misregistration. The

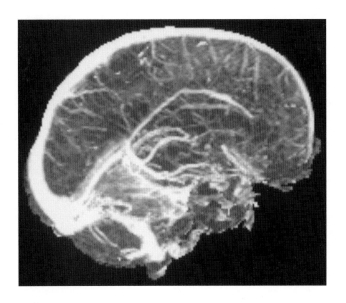

Figure 12.5

Angiography: maximum intensity projection (MIP) of subtracted registered T_1-weighted volume images taken before and after intravenous Gadodiamide shows detail of both arteries and veins. For clarity, superficial tissues were segmented off prior to performing the MIP.

same absolute displacement may appear as only a slight difference in position of a thick slice, and so permit valid image interpretation, but when a narrow slice thickness is used, the same displacement may take the region of interest into a completely different slice and create uncertainty in interpretation. Precise registration enables the patient position to be maintained, and allows the advantage of thin slices to be utilized.

(e) *Follow-up studies.* Assessing changes in the degree of enhancement between examinations may be rendered difficult by misregistration between examinations. This problem can be overcome by accurate alignment of images on serial examinations.

The technique may also be used to provide angiography (Fig. 12.5).

In a number of conditions, such as detection of metastases and demonstration of enhancement in multiple sclerosis (MS) plaques, scans delayed by one to two hours may be more useful than immediate post-injection scans. Misregistration problems are usually increased in this situation, since the patient is taken out of the scanner and positioned back again later. Results from this technique may be improved by registration. It may also be possible to reduce the dosage of contrast enhancement if subtraction is used routinely. The need for triple-dose enhancement may also be reduced.

A limitation is the need for an isotropic volume scan. Even slab imaging takes 20–30 s. As a result, the technique is not particularly suited to the timescale of dynamic studies.

Bone marrow transplantation

Bone marrow transplantation (BMT) has revolutionized the management of chronic myeloid leukemia (CML), and provides the only possibility of cure for this disease. Conditioning regimens are essential to the success of transplantation. A typical regimen consists of a cytotoxic drug (e.g. cyclophosphamide 60 mg/kg per day for two days), followed by total body irradiation (TBI) of 1320–1440 cGy given in several fractions over 2–3 days.

Neurological complications are unusual, but damage to white matter is well recognized. The role of chemotherapeutic agents and radiation, either individually or in combination, in causing brain damage may be difficult to determine. Cytotoxic and immunosuppressive agents such as methotrexate, cytarabine and cyclosporin A can each cause brain damage. Radiation can also cause damage, but the dose to the brain for conditioning (e.g. 1320–1440 cGy) is less than that used either in prophylactic cranial irradiation in acute leukemia (e.g. 2000–4000 cGy) or treatment of cerebral tumors (e.g. 4000–6000 cGy).

In order to determine the nature and frequency of changes to the brain in patients undergoing chemoradiotherapy and BMT, we performed registered serial MRI studies in 15 patients with CML (13 allografts and two autografts).

Repeated studies performed 4–339 days after transplantation showed ventricular enlargement and cortical atrophy in all 13 patients who had allografts.[3] The changes were evident at 4–6 days, and became more obvious in later follow-up cases (Fig. 12.6). Similar changes were seen in one patient with an autograft, but no significant change was seen in the other autografted patient or in the normal controls.

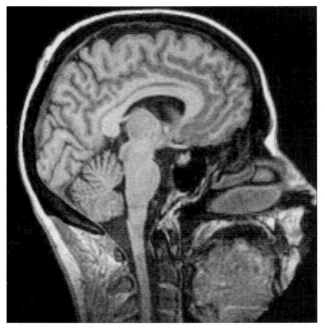

a

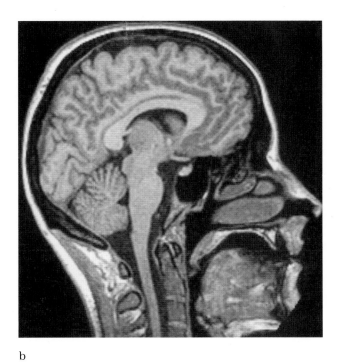

b

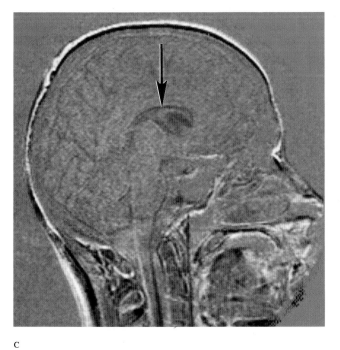

c

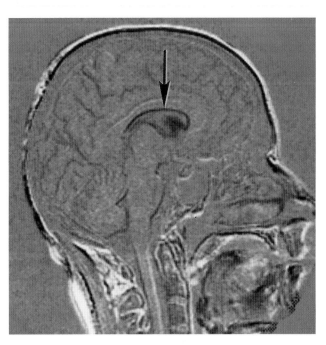

d

Figure 12.6

A female patient aged 43 years imaged before (a) and six days after (b) whole body conditioning radiotherapy and bone marrow transplantation, and again three months later. The registered subtraction of the first scan (a) from the initial follow-up scan shows a small change at the margins of the ventricles (c)

(arrow). After a further three months, the registered difference image (second follow-up minus pre-treatment scan) revealed additional ventricular enlargement (d, arrow) as well as more extensive interplateau and boundary shifts consistent with a further decrease in brain size.

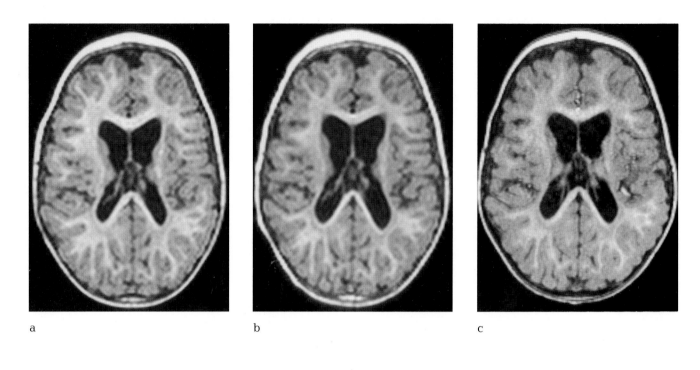

a   b   c

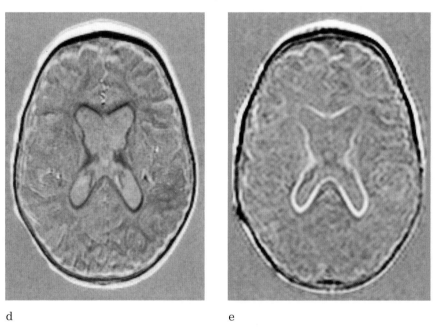

d   e

Figure 12.7

Growth and development in a child aged 10 months (a), 14 months (b) and 17 months (c) on registered T_1-weighted images and subtraction images (d) (= (b) − (a)) and (e) (= (c) − (b)). The white line around the gyral tips of the brain in (d) (interplateau shift) indicates growth of the brain, while the dark line (interplateau shift) is due to enlargement of the lateral ventricles, which has been symmetrical during the period from 10 to 14 months. In (e) there are white interplateau and monophasic border zone shifts around the external surface of the brain, indicating further growth, but there is now a white line around much of the ventricular system, which reveals that the brain in this region is expanding into the ventricular system to overly what was CSF at the age of 14 months.

Cerebral atrophy has been described following the long-term administration of steroids, and reversibility of the findings may follow decrease or cessation of steroid use. The appearances are typically described with long-term use (6 months to 5 years) and cumulative doses of 4000–58 000 mg of prednisone. Assessing the potential effect of steroids is complex. All 15 patients in this study had steroids at some stage in their illness. The total dosage for allograft patients varied from the equivalent of 100–20 250 mg of prednisolone. There was no evidence of reversibility of ventricular size in any patients. This might have been expected in patients having a reduction in their dosage or stopping treatment with steroids. The onset of brain changes occurred at the same time as treatment with steroids, cyclophosphamide and TBI, but there did not appear to be a particular association with steroids given in the previous 48 h.

Reversible cerebral atrophy has been described in patients with anorexia nervosa. Some of the patients had suffered substantial weight loss. At the last follow-up, 11 had lost weight, one had retained the same weight and two had increased weight. Changes in the brain did not reverse in these latter three patients. Of the two patients who had autografts, the patient who lost 11 kg showed brain changes, while the patient who lost only 2 kg showed no change.

The toxicity associated with cyclosporin A is specific, and involves hypertension, severe visual disturbances and occipital lobe changes. These complications were not seen in this study. It is possible that some other drug besides steroids and cyclosporin A may have caused the MRI changes. High-dose methotrexate has been associated with cerebral atrophy in late follow-up scans when it was used for treatment of osteosarcoma. However, the dosage was much higher than in the cases described here. Neuronal loss may be a cause of atrophy in this context, but the changes appeared relatively early for this complication.

folding, myelination and decrease in brain proton density, T_1 and T_2. The surrounding tissues and fluids may also change. Growth of the skull means that much larger changes are generally seen in children than in adults, where the skull generally imposes rigid limits on changes in brain size. Because of the large changes in children, it is often useful to match examinations in successive pairs so that the difference between any two image sets is minimized. The small subarachnoid space over the cortex also makes segmentation more difficult than in adults.

Changes in children may be quite complex, with, for example, the ventricular system showing changes due to expansion and contraction at different phases of growth (Fig. 12.7).

In the late phase of neonatal infarction (one to nine months) increased growth can be seen at the margins of the lesion (Fig 12.8). This was also seen after hypoxic ischaemic encephalopathy (Fig 12.9).

The rapidly proliferating tissue seen in the late phase of infarction did not have the features of gliosis (long T_1 and T_2), and followed the configuration of the brain. It may provide an anatomical substrate for neurological plasticity. In studies following prenatal surgical removal of the frontal association cortex in rhesus monkeys, Goldman and Galkin[4] observed the formation of new sulci and gyri at the borders of the lesion. The surgical lesions were created at about 100–110 days of gestation, when the rhesus monkey brain is relatively lissencephalic. Because of the difference in species, stage of gestation, nature of the primary lesion and other factors, it is difficult to extrapolate from these results to our patients, but the phenomenon we observed also appears very similar to that observed in the newborn cat.[5]

The technique was of value in separating out the different components of basal ganglia haemorrhage (Fig. 12.10).

The effect of acetazolamide in treating hydrocephalus could also be monitored (Fig. 12.11).

Paediatrics

In children, physiological, pathological and therapeutic changes of the type described above may be present. These may be complicated by growth and development, which may be normal or abnormal. Growth and development includes not only increase in size of the brain, but also cortical

Multiple sclerosis

There is considerable interest in monitoring the progress of multiple sclerosis (MS) with and without treatment, and some cohorts have now been studied for many years. The expected annual change in lesion burden is about 5–10%. This is of

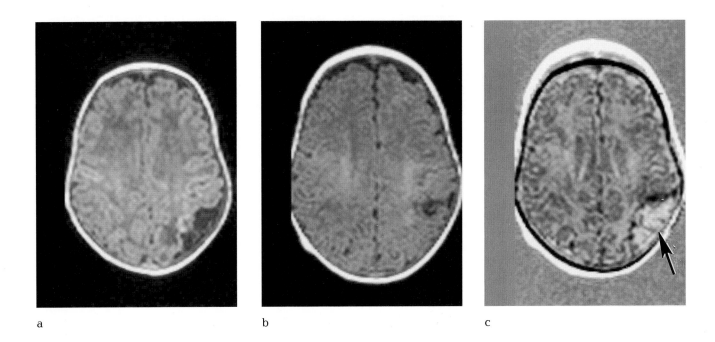

a   b   c

Figure 12.8

Neonatal infarction: T_1-weighted scan at four weeks (a) and at 14 weeks (b), with registered difference image (c). The highlighted area in (c) arrow shows that growth in the brain adjacent to the infarction has been more rapid than elsewhere.

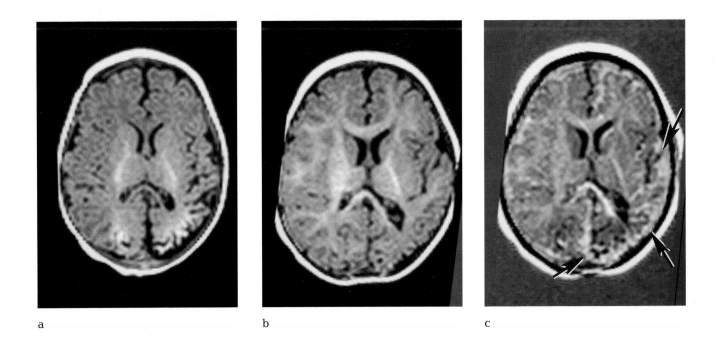

a   b   c

Figure 12.9

HIE grade II: registered T_1-weighted 3D scans at two months (a) and six months (b), with difference image (c) (= (b) – (a)). There is evidence of increased growth in the left hemisphere (c) (arrows).

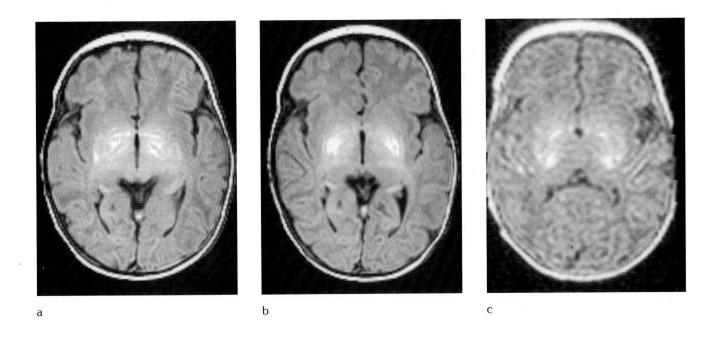

a   b   c

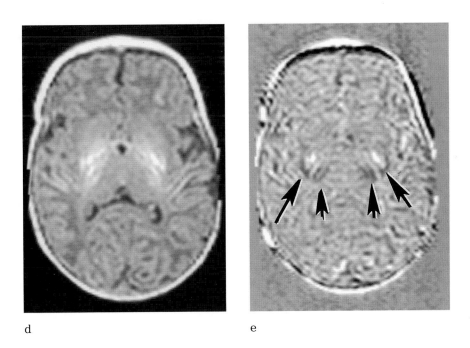

d   e

Figure 12.10

Basal ganglia hemorrhage: T_1-weighted spin echo (SE 820/20) (a) and five days later (b); T_1-weighted image from a 3D set at the corresponding level (c) and five-day follow-up (d), with registered difference image (e). The loss of signal in the thalamus (arrow heads) and lateral lentiform nuclei (arrows) are best seen on (e), together with the increase in signal in the medial lentiform nucleus.

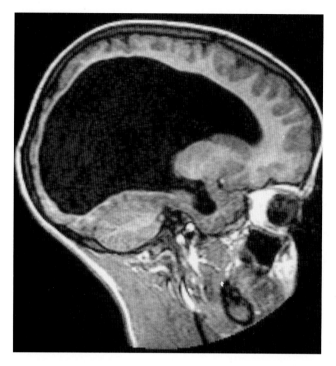

a

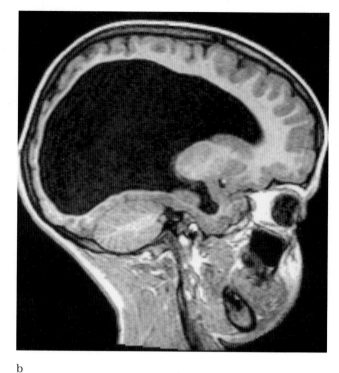

b

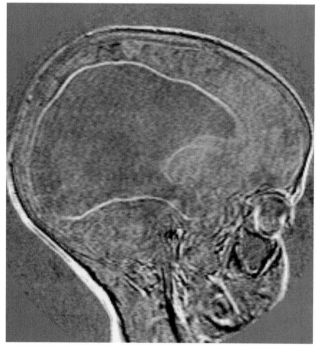

c

Figure 12.11

Treatment of hydrocephalus with acetazolamide: parasagittal T_1-weighted image before treatment (a), after three months treatment (b) and difference image (c). The highlighted margin in (c) shows that the lateral ventricle has decreased in size.

the same order as misregistration errors inherent with conventional techniques, so assessing the effectiveness of new therapies such as interferon may be difficult in short-term studies.

We have now studied 12 patients on two or more occasions. Registration not only allowed changes to be identified within lesions, but also differences in contrast enhancement could be separated from other changes using 'difference of difference' images (i.e. difference of post minus pre contrast enhancement scans at two different times). Changes in unenhanced lesion T_1 were much more

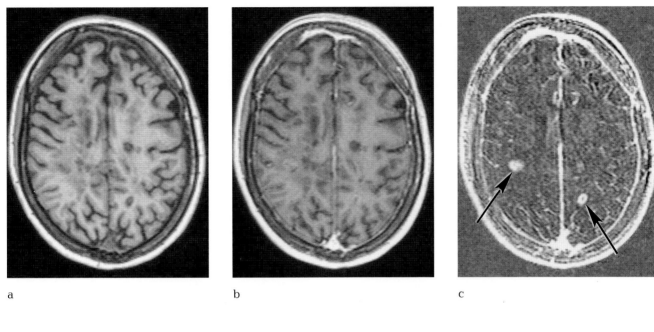

a   b   c

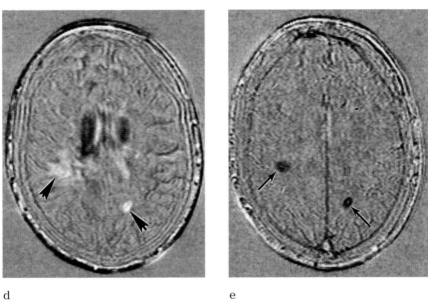

d   e

Figure 12.12

A 31-year-old female with MS: initial unenhanced (a), enhanced (b) and registered subtraction (c) images. A repeat pre- and post-enhancement scan was performed six months later. The difference image of the unenhanced scans six months apart is shown in (d), and the difference between the earlier 'post minus pre' scans and the later 'post minus pre' scans is shown in (e). The enhancing lesions are seen better in (c) (black and white arrows). The ventricular system has increased in size, giving a through-plane shift in (d), and there is evidence of decreased brain size. Some lesions appear bright because they have shortened their T_1 time (d, arrowheads). Lesions that were enhancing in (b) now appear dark on (e) (they no longer enhance) (black and white arrows). Some lesions without obvious mass effects have changed signal intensity in (d), and it is not possible to be certain whether they have also changed in size (although this is likely).

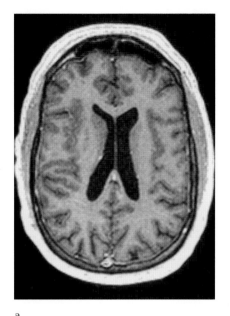 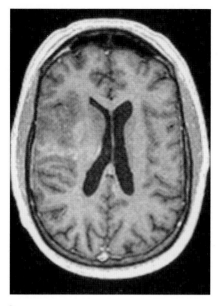 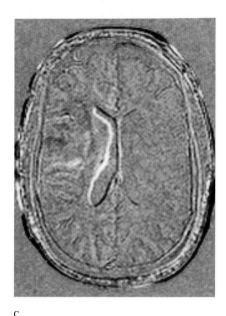

a   b   c

Figure 12.13

Astrocytoma grade III in a 42-year-old male examined
with IV Gadodiamide (a) and again one month later
(b), with subtraction of (a) from (b) shown in image (c).
The increase in tumor size can be seen on the aligned
source images, but the extent of the mass effect is
better seen in (c). Positive and negative interplateau

shifts are seen around the right lateral ventricle.
Border zone shifts are seen on the right hemisphere.
Smaller negative interplateau shifts are seen at the
ventricular margins on the left, as well as more subtle
border zone shifts anteriorly and posteriorly within the
left hemisphere.

readily recognized with the subtraction images,
including effects due to both increased and
decreased T_1. Obvious changes were seen in the
T_1 of areas where no enhancement was observed.
Decrease in brain size was observed in patients
who had treatment with steroids and others who
did not have this treatment.

Subvoxel registration revealed that many lesions
are more complicated than they appear at first
sight, with some undergoing remission and others
in very close proximity undergoing exacerbation
with both parallel and discordant contrast
enhancement. We also observed shortening of T_1
(as well as lengthening) in the acute phase.

For example, a 31-year-old woman with MS
was examined with and without contrast
enhancement on two occasions six months apart.
Many contrast-enhancing lesions were either
much better seen or only seen on the registered
images. There were changes in lesion signal

intensity and the degree of enhancement, as well
as evidence of decreased brain size on the follow-
up scans (Fig. 12.12). This may have been due to
brain swelling at the time of the initial examination that had partly or completely resolved when
the follow-up study was performed. It may also be
due to progressive atrophy. The patient did not
receive steroids.

Tumors

On the registered difference images, increased
tumor size was manifest as encroachment on the
ventricular system and subarachnoid space. Figure
12.13(a) shows an astrocytoma grade III before

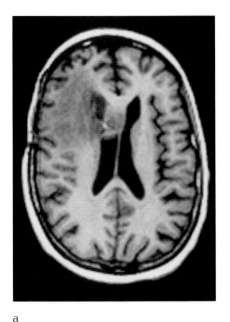 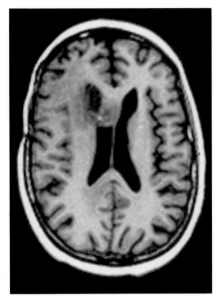 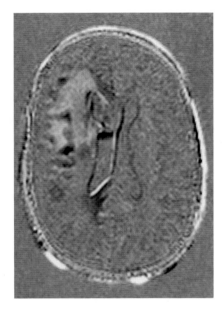

a   b   c

Figure 12.14

Astrocytoma: T_1-weighted scans before (a) and six weeks after (b) treatment with temozolamide; (c) difference image. Most of the tumor has decreased in size and shortened its T_1 following treatment. Many of the features are the reverse of those seen in Fig. 12.11.

treatment. After one month, the registered difference image (Fig. 12.13b) shows tumor expansion in spite of treatment. Differences in contrast enhancement were also demonstrated by comparison of the subtracted (post minus pre contrast) images on each examination.

Tumor growth was demonstrated in one astrocytoma, no changes in another and regression in the third case. The changes were more apparent on the registered images than on the unregistered scans. In each of these cases the pattern on contrast enhancement paralleled the tumor response to treatment.

In tumor regression following treatment, T_1 may be decreased. This produces an increased signal on the difference image. Decreased mass effect can also be demonstrated (Fig. 12.14).

Registration may allow earlier recognition of tumor growth and response to therapy than conventional techniques. We are studying a cohort of inoperable and partially resected meningiomas to assess their rate of growth (Fig. 12.15).

Pre-eclampsia

There are many reports in the CT and MR imaging literature describing cerebral edema during pre-eclampsia (see e.g. Digre et al[6]). Using image registration to compare appearances of the brain in the third trimester and those six weeks after delivery in women with pre-eclampsia, the brain was found to be atrophic rather than edematous prior to delivery in all four subjects studied (Fig. 12.16).

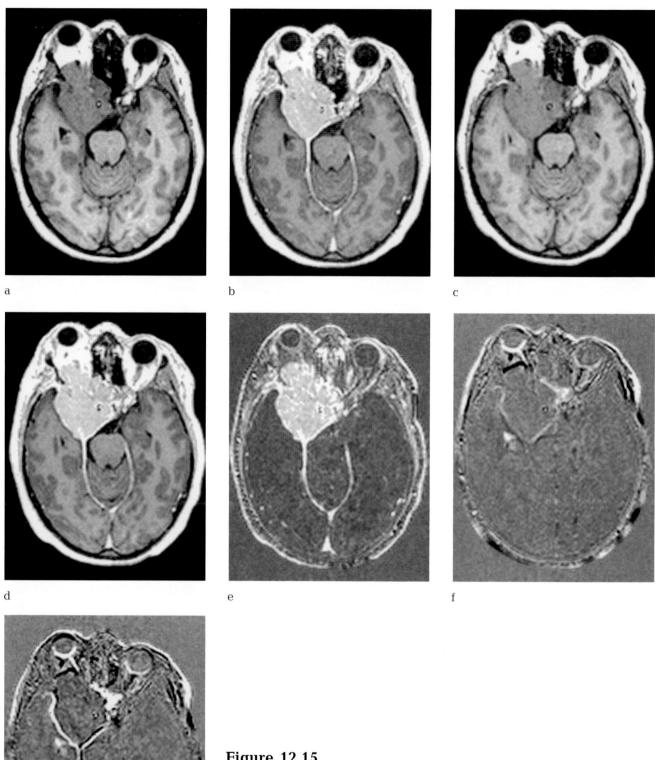

Figure 12.15

Meningioma: T_1-weighted images from volume acquisitions before (a) and after (b) contrast enhancement; registered images at the same level before (c) and after (d) contrast enhancement 13 months later. Subtraction of (c) from (d) show the pattern of enhancement on the second examination in (e). Subtraction of (a) from (c) in image (f) shows that the tumor has grown over the 13 months between the scans. The same changes are seen with the addition of the effect of contrast enhancement in (g), which is (d) – (b).

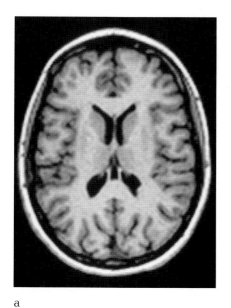
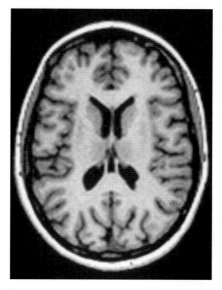
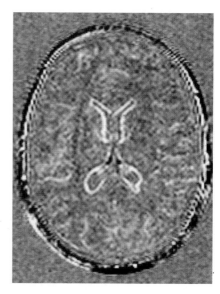

a   b   c

Figure 12.16

Pre-eclampsia: T_1-weighted images during the third trimester (a) and six weeks following delivery (b). The subtraction image (c) shows that the brain has expanded between the two examinations. This indicates that the brain has undergone (reversible) atrophy during the phase of pre-eclampsia.

There have been two previous reports in which the finding of edema in pre-eclampsia or eclampsia has been questioned. One of these was based on pathological studies in which the brain was not increased in weight.[7] The other was a CT study of 44 patients in which nine patients showed atrophy on CT.[8] Patients with pre-eclampsia may receive treatment with fluid restriction and/or diuretics. It is possible that this treatment may not be of benefit to the brain.

antipsychotics.[11] Using registration, atrophic changes were demonstrated in the five first-episode schizophrenics who were studied six months apart (Fig. 12.17). Another three patients showed evidence of brain swelling, two studies were equivocal and one was negative. These changes may reflect different phases of the first episode of the illness.

Schizophrenia

The first study with CT showing ventricular enlargement in schizophrenia was published 20 years ago.[9] It was a cross-sectional study. Longitudinal studies without registration have shown no change in the brain with CT[10] and increase in size of the caudate nucleus in patients treated with

Post-operative changes

Although three published serial studies of the brain following coronary artery bypass surgery (CABS) have been negative except in patients who had clinical evidence of strokes,[12-14] registration of serial scans has shown abnormalities in each of the five patients studied to date (Fig. 12.18).

A 63-year-old man had studies before, within one hour after and seven days after a left carotid

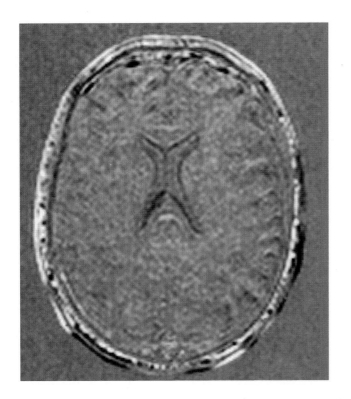

Figure 12.17

Schizophrenia: registered subtraction image, showing differences that developed over six months after first admission. The ventricles have increased in size, and abnormalities (biphasic changes) are seen in the left temporal lobe.

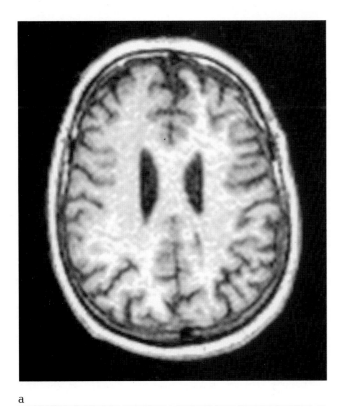

a

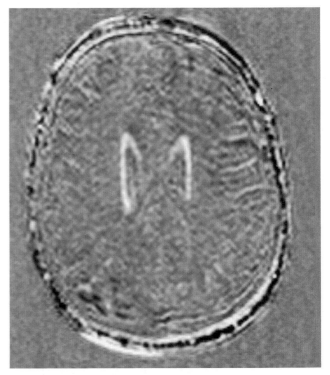

b

Figure 12.18

Study before and eight days after coronary artery bypass surgery: T_1-weighted scan (a) and difference image (b). The brain has increased in size.

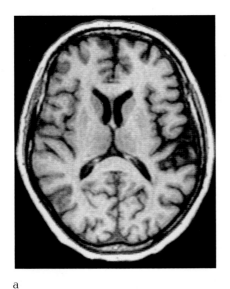 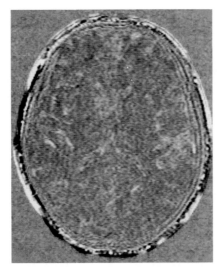 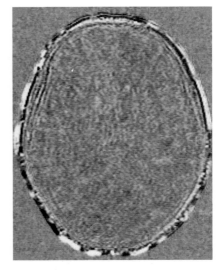

a b c

Figure 12.19

Carotid endarterectomy: pre-operative transverse image (a), difference image derived from immediate post-operative image minus the pre-operative image (b) and difference image from seven day post-operative image minus pre-operative image (c). There is an increase in signal intensity related to sulci and the ventricular system, which could be due to brain swelling, shortening of T_1 of CSF by molecular oxygen or both (b). The appearances have largely returned to the pre-operative state after seven days, as shown by (c).

endarterectomy. There were changes to the brain and/or its surroundings on the immediate postoperative scan, which resolved seven days later (Fig. 12.19). These may have been due to the inhalation of 40% oxygen shortening the T_1 of CSF or to swelling of the brain.

In monitoring the effect of treatment, effects of drugs on brain size need to be recognized. In particular, steroids and ACTH may produce a change in brain size that is due to treatment not to the primary pathologic process. Likewise, alcohol and states of hydration may affect brain size.

technique may also be of value in distinguishing infarction from low-grade glioma.

Alzheimer's disease

Fox, Freeborough and Rosser[15] have used essentially the same technique to demonstrate atrophic change in Alzheimer's disease. They found marked changes in eight patients compared with controls. There were also some presymptomatic patients with intermediate changes.

Infarction

Registration can be used to show atrophic changes associated with adult infarction (Fig. 12.20). The

Conclusions

Use of image registration allows changes to be detected on serial examination in many diseases

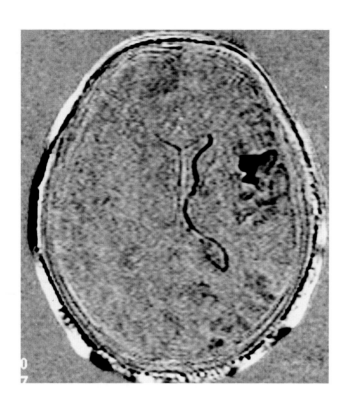

Figure 12.20

Cerebral infarction: registered difference image from two T_1-weighted scans obtained 10 months apart after the infarction. The scan shows the infarct as low signal as well as associated atrophic changes, which are mainly in the left (ipsilateral) hemisphere.

when conventional approaches produce equivocal or negative results. This is likely to increase the sensitivity of MRI for many neuroradiological applications. Effects due to treatment may also be monitored with this technique. Paediatrics is notable for the fact that there are also changes due to growth and development, and these may be affected by disease and treatment. The technique appears likely to have a very wide application.

Acknowledgements

We wish to thank the Medical Research Council, the Wellcome Trust and Nycomed for their continued support.

References

1. Grant R, Condon B, Lawrence A et al, Is cranial CSF volume under hormonal influence? An MR Study. *J Comput Assist Tomogr* 1988; **12**: 36–9.

2. Curati WL, Williams EJ, Oatridge A et al, Use of subvoxel registration and subtraction to improve the demonstration of contrast enhancement in magnetic resonance imaging of the brain. *Neuroradiology* (in press).

3. Jager HR, Williams EJ, Savage DG et al, Assessment of the brain before and after conditioning and bone marrow transplantation for chronic myeloid leukemia using subvoxel registration and subtraction of serial magnetic resonance images. *AJNR* (in press).

4. Goldman PS, Galkin TW, Prenatal removal of frontal association cortex in the fetal rhesus monkey: anatomical and functional consequences in postnatal life. *Brain Res.* 1978; **152**: 451–85.

5. Isaacson RL, Nonneman AJ, Schumaltz LW, Behavioural and anatomical sequelae of damage to the infant central nervous system. In: *The neuropsychology of development* (ed RL Isaacson), 41–78. Wiley, New York, 1968.

6. Digre KB, Varner MW, Osborn AG, Crawford S, Cranial magnetic resonance imaging in severe pre-eclampsia and eclampsia. *Arch Neurol* 1993; **50**: 399–406.

7. Sheehan HL, Lynch JB, *Pathology of toxaemia of pregnancy*, 524–553, Churchill Livingstone, Edinburgh, 1973.

8. Milliez J, Dohoun A, Boudraa M, Computed tomography of the brain in eclampsia. *Obstet Gynecol* 1990; **75**: 975–80.

9. Johnstone EC, Crow TJ, Frith CD et al, Cerebral ventricular size and cognitive impairment in chronic schizophrenia. *Lancet* 1976; **ii**: 924–6.

10. Jaskiw GE, Julaino DM, Goldberg TE et al, Cerebral ventricular enlargement in schizophreniform disorder does not progress. A seven year follow-up study. *Schizophrenia Res* 1994; **14**: 23–8.

11. Chakos MH, Lieberman JA, Bibler RM et al, Increase in caudate nuclei volumes of first-episode schizophrenic patients taking antipsychotic drugs. *Am J Psychiat* 1994; **151**: 1430–6.

12. Vik A, Brubakk AO, Rinck PA et al, MRI: a method to detect minor brain damage following coronary bypass surgery? *Neuroradiology* 1991; **33**: 396–8.

13. Sellman M, Hindmarsh T, Ivert I, Semp BK, Magnetic resonance imaging of the brain before and after open heart operations. *Ann Thorac Surg* 1992; **53**: 807–12.

14. Schmidt R, Fazekas F, Offenbacher H et al, Results of pre- and postoperative MRI in coronary artery bypass surgery (CABS). *Neurology* 1993; **43**: 775–8.

15. Fox NC, Freeborough PA, Rosser MN, Visualising and quantifying rates of atrophy in Alzheimer's disease from registered 3D MRI of the brain. *Abstracts 4th Ann Mtg Int Soc Magn Reson Med, New York, 1996 ISMRM*: 234.

13

A dedicated MR system in a neonatal intensive therapy unit

Alasdair S Hall, Ian R Young, Frank J Davies and Surya N Mohapatra

Introduction

There is growing interest in the use of magnetic resonance (MR) for the clinical evaluation of premature and critically ill neonates. This has principally involved the study of cerebral ischemia and infarction with both MRI and MRS. The first MR studies of the neonatal brain were performed in 1983 and used ^{31}P MRS.[1] More recently, proton spectroscopy has been used to provide very early prognosis in hypoxic ischemic injury.[2] See Fig. 13.1.

Diffusion-weighted MRI is also being used to make an early assessment of brain damage.[3] With the increasing interest in the use of neuroprotective therapy for treatment of hypoxic ischemic brain damage,[4,5] it is becoming more important to be able to study the neonate within the first six hours of birth. See Fig. 13.2.

In many institutions, including Hammersmith Hospital, the neonatal intensive therapy unit (ITU) is remote from the MR systems, and the journey between the two can involve relatively long distances and the use of elevators. Staff supervising very premature and critically ill neonates are generally loathe to take them outside the ITU and into situations in which full support and resuscitation facilities might not be easily available at short notice. These concerns apply to single examinations. They apply even more strongly to serial studies. In order to overcome these problems, we

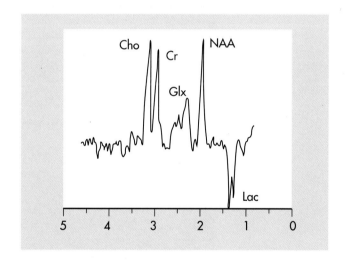

Figure 13.1

Proton MR spectrum (chemical shift imaging, *TE* = 135 ms) in a term infant with HIII grade III, eight hours after the insult, from a 4.5 cm³ volume within the basal ganglia. The lactate (Lac) peak is markedly increased. The Glx (glutamate/gluatmine) peak is also increased.

have developed a highly specialized MR system, which has been installed in our neonatal ITU.

This chapter discusses the specification and concept of the machine, describes its engineering and installation, and concludes with some early results.

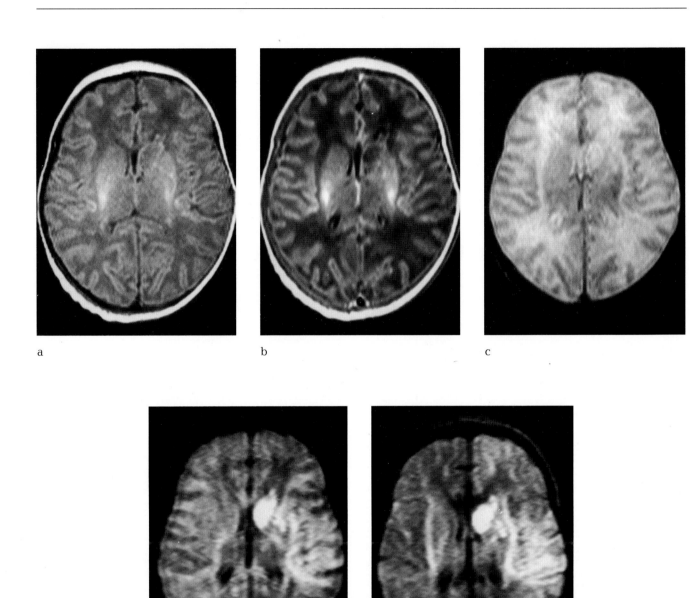

a   b   c

d   e

Figure 13.2

MR imaging in HIE grade II spin echo (SE 120/20) (a),
IR 3000/30/900 (b) 8E 2500/120 (c), antero-posterior
sensitized diffusion-weighted image (d) and left–right
sensitized diffusion-weighted image (e). The
conventional images (a)–(c) show the abnormality in the
head of the left caudate nucleus. There is also
extensive change in the left fronto-temporal region,
which is only shown on the diffusion-weighted images.

System specification

Two requirements have already been mentioned, namely that the system be capable of spectroscopy and that it should perform diffusion-weighted imaging. The former factor suggested that the minimum field suitable would be 1.0 T. At the time of the system's specification, proton spectroscopy had not been demonstrated at 0.5 T. This has since happened,[6] and might have influenced the choice of field strength, particularly if useful phosphorus MRS could also be demonstrated at 0.5 T.

Another important design consideration was that the neonates should be as accessible as possible to clinicians during scanning. This meant that it was desirable that the region of good field should be as close to the magnet face as possible. It was also important that the magnet should be actively shielded, since it was to be installed in the ITU (and immediately above an adult cardiac ITU) with sophisticated electronic equipment close to it.

The region of interest that was specified was discus-shaped, with a diameter of 160 mm and central thickness of 70 mm. It was planned that the imaging strategy would evolve to be similar to that used in spiral-scan computed tomography (CT), with the patient being moved through the field in order to cover more extensive regions of the body. The target field specification (after shimming) for the region of interest was ±10 ppm over the full volume; improving to ±3 ppm over a central volume of diameter 120 mm and thickness 50 mm, with ±1 ppm over a volume of 60 mm diameter by 25 mm thickness. Details of the magnet as it finally evolved are given below.

The requirement for diffusion-weighted imaging led to the gradient strength being specified at greater than 30 mT/m. The wish to make the MR examinations short, so as to minimize the time the patients were away from their cots, put a premium on fast imaging techniques (such as echo planar imaging, EPI).[7] Gradient rise times of less than 200 µs were therefore specified.

It was felt important that the babies should be disturbed as little as possible during the examination, and the primary radiofrequency (rf) system was therefore chosen to be a transmit/receive birdcage.[8] These coils were large enough to allow a baby in a nonmetallic incubator to be slid through them. As a result, the filling factor of the coils was low. Provision was therefore made for surface and other coil systems, including receiver arrays, to be used as well.

Considerable thought was given to the arrangements for patient handling, including provision for the analog of CT spiral imaging mentioned previously. Another key issue was the life support systems and monitoring equipment. These were specified to be as comprehensive as would be available for the baby in his or her ITU cot.

Implementation

Magnet

The magnet was designed and built by Oxford Magnet Technology Ltd (Eynsham, Oxford, UK). It has a homogeneous field of 1.0 T and a warm bore of 500 mm. The bore length is 380 mm, which is uniquely short. This was achieved with a combination of iron at liquid helium temperature and a powerful main winding. The magnet tapers outwards to its maximum thickness of 500 mm at a face diameter of 1000 mm. The overall magnet diameter required to accommodate the outermost shielding winding is 2 m. The magnet is cooled only by liquid helium, and, with its refrigerator, has a specified hold time of six months between helium refills.

As mentioned previously, the volume of homogenous field is discus-shaped. Its center is 190 mm from the faces of the magnet at the outer diameter of the bore. In practice, as will be discussed later, the gradients determine the openness of access to the patient rather than the magnet configuration.

The magnet's 5 G footprint is 3 m radially and 4 m axially distant. To achieve this, the shielding windings have to be very powerful, leading inevitably to a requirement for great strength from the main-field generating windings. This combination means that the field at the surface of the magnet at around 1000 mm diameter (at the colored ring shown in Fig. 13.3) is in the region of 2 T. This places even greater importance than usual on ensuring that ferromagnetic objects are not brought too close to the magnet, though it does have the (minor) compensating effect that iron objects tend to be attracted away from the magnet bore and towards the ring, so providing some protection for the patient (if not for a clinician or nurse standing next to the magnet).

A photograph of the magnet during installation is shown in Fig. 13.3. It weighs 3.6 tonnes, and is

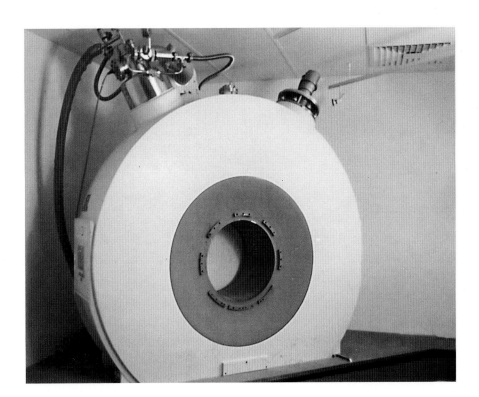

Figure 13.3

View of the magnet during installation. The magnet is supported by a pair of stainless steel beams straddling the corner of the room.

supported by a pair of stainless steel beams, which in turn are supported at their ends by the walls of the building (the system is located on the fourth floor of an old building). Homogeneity targets were exceeded with ±7.5 ppm over the larger volume of 160 mm diameter by 70 mm thickness; ±2.9 ppm over the volume specified at ±3 ppm, and ±0.7 ppm over that specified at ±1 ppm.

field includes a substantial radial component. This gives rise to unbalanced axial forces on the coils, which have to be transferred to the magnet cryostat. As a result, the coils had to be fixed with considerable care. While the ends of the gradient coils are more or less flush with the front of the magnet, the coil structure extends externally at the rear by around 50 mm. This is to allow for connections, including those necessary for the cooling water.

Gradients

The gradients presented a number of design problems. In order to avoid obscuring the patient access, they had to be very short, with very substantially truncated windings. They had to be actively shielded because of the proximity of cold metal structures. Because of the requirements for EPI and diffusion-weighted imaging and the use of substantial duty cycles, they were water-cooled. At 200 A, all three axes generate between 40 and 45 mT/m, with a rise time of less than 100 µs. They comfortably exceed the target specifications.

An unusual problem, because of the shortness of the magnet, is that a significant fraction of the gradient windings lies in regions where the main

Radiofrequency (rf) coils and system

As mentioned previously, the prime coil system is a transmit/receive quadrature birdcage. Provision is also made for a transmit-only birdcage, with facilities for surface or array coils (four digital receive channels are available, with the capability for an increase in that number if this is thought necessary). The rf transmitter amplifier has a power of 2 kW, and the transmitter coil produces a peak rf field of greater than 125 µT. A square rf pulse can thus invert the magnetization in less than 95 µs.

Table 13.1   Sites and transfers of baby from neonatal nursing station to magnet room

Site of baby	Neonatal ITU nursing station	Cot carrier	Magnet room
Monitoring	HP Merlin behind Ohio station	Nellcor pulse oximeter on shelf	HP Merlin in rf enclosures (Fig. 2.5)
Ventilation	SLE2000 breathing system on stand-by station	Non-magnetic cylinders under cot shelf	SLE2000 in rf enclosures (6 m run length for tubes and cables)
Infusions	Infusion pumps on stand-by station	Syringes and coiled lines on shelf under cot (lines lengthened by 2 m)	Wall-mounted infusion pumps (outside 100 G)

Transfer: station to cot carrier	Transfer: cot carrier to magnet
Metal check baby Modify life support/monitoring Clamp lines to cot	Attach magnet room life support/monitoring

Computer and electronics system

The electronics system of the machine is essentially that of a Picker Vista 1.0 T scanner (Picker International Inc, Cleveland, OH). This is equipped to handle all the scanning modes envisaged, including proton spectroscopy and EPI.

Patient handling system

This is unique to the machine. Table 13.1 shows the various locations of the life support and monitoring facilities and transfers involved in taking the baby to the MR system. It demonstrates the role of the cot carrier unit in transporting the baby to the machine bore. Figure 13.4 shows a diagram of the system.

The baby is placed in one of two Perspex carriers. The one for larger babies is a fixed semicircular channel with closed ends, while the one for smaller babies opens to lie flat. The smaller carrier allows the baby to be picked up and put down without the operator's hands being obstructed by the walls of a fixed container.

The patient holder is transported using a belt drive, which can be operated during scanning so that, if necessary, the patient can be moved through the region of high-quality field. Using this arrangement the whole head and body of the patient can be scanned.

Installation

The general layout of the system is shown in plan view in Fig. 13.5.

The magnet is set on a pair of stainless steel girders across the corner of the machine room. This allows its weight to be taken directly on the walls of the building. The rf shielding does not include the space near the door inside the room (rf enclosures in Fig. 13.5). This is used to house the magnet power supply and the patient monitoring equipment. The cables for this are fed through a boom so that the various connections hang over the area where they are wanted. The faces of the instruments can be seen through the rf window.

The control area is separated from the machine room by a further rf window. This provides an excellent view of the equipment for the operator.

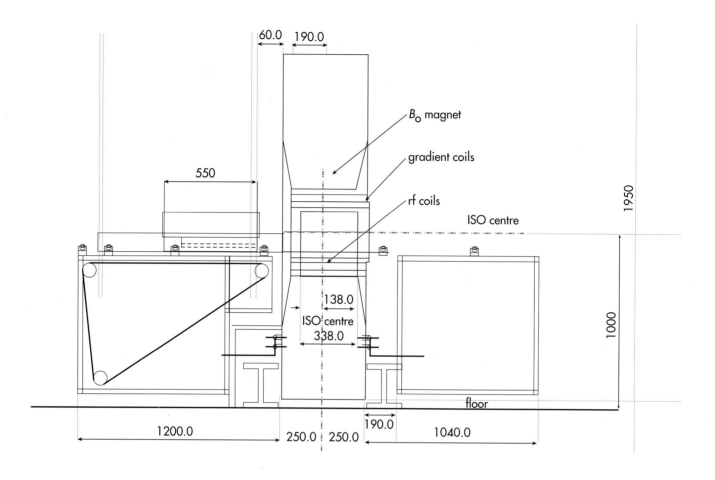

Figure 13.4

Sectional drawing showing the general arrangement of the system and its patient handling (dimensions in mm). The patient holder is belt-driven through the region of interest.

Including the equipment and control rooms, the total area occupied by the system is 6.7 m by 5.6 m (or about 34 m²).

The proximity of the relevant part of the ITU created the security and safety issues that had to be addressed. A corridor leading to a fire escape passes the door, while the ITU cots are on its far side. With the large team of nurses needed for such work, and with parents of babies moving round the ITU, even the near location of the nursing station is no guarantee that people will not enter the magnet room unless physically prevented from doing so. The door is on a magnetic latch controlled from the console, and the room is kept locked at all times when the scanner is not actually being used for patient studies.

Scanning requires two people at any one time, one operating the machine from the console and the other monitoring the patient using direct observation and the equipment in the area external to the rf screened room.

Patient monitoring

The patient monitoring equipment comprises the set of Hewlett Packard Merlin units used in the ITU itself. These include ECG, pulse oximeter and CO_2 gas monitoring. As mentioned above, the enclosures are housed external to the screened room in the cubicle marked 'rf enclosure' in Fig. 13.5. Gases for the patient are provided via inlets on the wall just behind and to the left of the magnet.

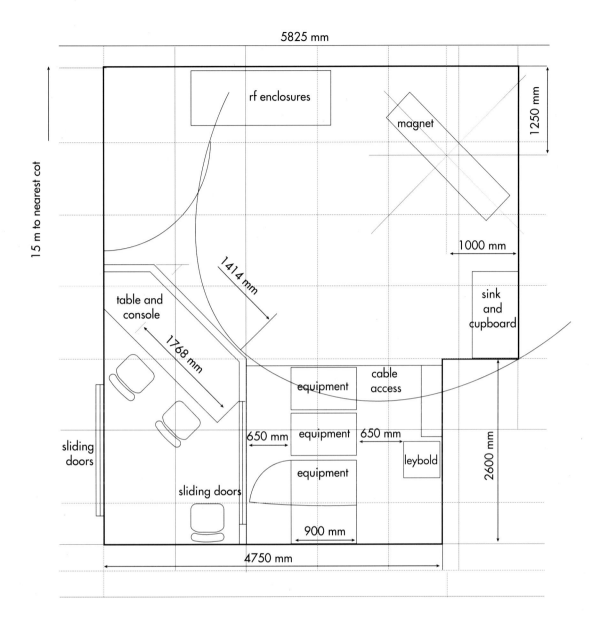

Figure 13.5

Layout of the neonatal machine in the ITU, together
with its immediate surroundings.

Facilities

The machine is configured for all likely clinical
protocols, including EPI and spectroscopy. The
capability to scan as the bed is moved does not
depend on the choice of a specific scanning protocol. It is unlikely that the bed will be shifted during
a spectroscopy study because of the extent of
averaging needed.

Preliminary results

Technical aspects

The very short lengths of the main and gradient
fields introduce some additional difficulties with
the imaging. The net result of the rapid change in
static field with distance is that regions outside the

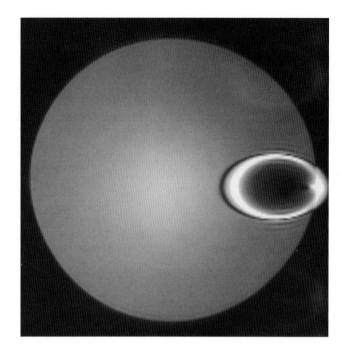

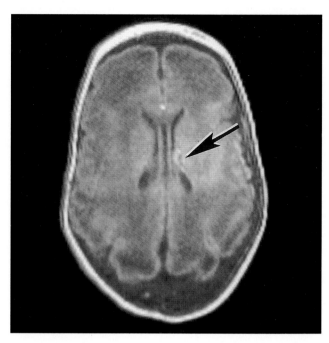

a

Figure 13.6

Image of a phantom taken using a non-optimum sequence to illustrate data being aliased back from outside the region of good field.

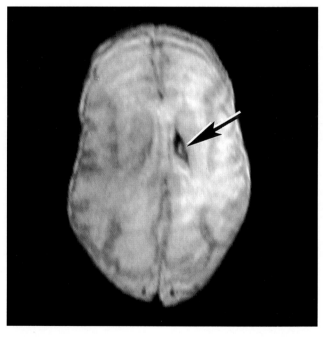

b

desired central imaging volume in which both B_1 transmitter and receiver are sensitive are excited, and the signals from them are mixed with those from the center. This aliasing is illustrated in Fig. 13.6, which is an image of a simple cylindrical phantom.

There are a variety of solutions to this problem, many of which are readily implemented. Typical methods are to reduce the sensitive volume of the transmitter or receiver coils, either by forms of active rf shielding[9] or by the use of surface coils rather than the whole body detectors. Other methods include increasing the gradient amplitudes, particularly at the time of excitation. For any given selective volume, this also implies reducing the width of the rf pulses (which requires an increase in the pulse amplitude). The effect of the increased gradient amplitude is to push the places at which the conjunction of gradients and main fields can result in unwanted excitation further away from the machine center, and so into regions that are less sensitive from an rf point of view.

Figure 13.7

First case examined: intraventricular and parenchymal hemorrhage in an infant of 34 weeks. (a) SE 824/20 and (b) SE 2700/120 with the parenchymal abnormality (arrows) seen on both scans.

Clinical studies

The machine is at an early stage of its work at the time of writing, so that only preliminary imaging and spectroscopy results are available. Figure 13.7 shows results from the first case examined with this system. These results should not be taken as typical of what will ultimately be achievable by the system or the final repertoire of operations that will be performed.

Conclusions

This machine represents a first attempt to install an MR system in a neonatal ITU. The scanning volume is a mere 15 m from the nearest neonate cot in which one of the patients is being cared for, following the path that the patient transport has to follow. It will be a matter of great interest to see if this system can realize the potential that those involved with the project hoped for. We expect it to provide considerable benefit to the patients scanned as well as results of considerable interest in the scientific study of very premature and critically ill infants.

Acknowledgements

Oxford Magnet Technology Ltd, Eynsham, Oxford, UK supplied the magnet. They also provide service and support the magnet, and have funded the salary of a physicist to work on the machine. Tesla Engineering Ltd, Storrington, Sussex, UK built and contributed part of the gradient coils. Picker International Inc, Cleveland, OH, USA supplied the back-end of the system, and designed and contributed part of the gradient coils.

References

1. Cady EB, Dawson JM, Hope PL et al, Non-invasive investigation of cerebral metabolism in newborn infants by phosphorus nuclear magnetic resonance spectroscopy. *Lancet* 1983; **i**: 1059–62.

2. Hanrahan JD, Sargentoni J, Azzdpardi D et al, Cerebral metabolism within 18 hours of birth asphyxia: a proton magnetic resonance spectroscopy study. *Pediatric Research* 1996; **39**: 584–90.

3. Cowan FM, Pennock JM, Hanrahan JD et al, Early detection of cerebral infarction and hypoxic encephalopathy in neonates using diffusion weighted magnetic resonance imaging. *Neuropediatrics* 1994; **25**: 172–5.

4. Edwards AD, Protection against hypoxic–ischaemic cerebral injury in the developing brain. *Perfusion* 1993; **8**: 97–100.

5. Gluckman PD, Williams CE, When and why do brain cells die? *Dev Med Child Neurol* 1992; **34**: 1010–14.

6. Prost RW, Mueller W, Yetkin Z et al, 0.5 T 1H spectroscopy as an adjunct to diagnosis in indeterminate CNS lesions: results from 40 patients. *Proc 3rd Ann Mtg Soc Magn Reson*, 1995, 1711.

7. Mansfield P, Multi-planar image formation using NMR spin echoes. *J Phys C (Solid State Phys)*, 1977; **10**: L55–9.

8. Hayes CE, Edelstein WA, Schenck JF et al, An efficient, highly homogeneous radiofrequency for whole body NMR imaging at 1.5 T. *J Magn Reson* 1985; **63**: 622–9.

9. Burl M, Young I, Surface receiver coils with asymmetric sensitivity on either side for MR imaging and spectroscopy. *Proc 2nd Ann Mtg Soc Magn Reson, San Francisco*, 1994, 1128.

14

Interventional MRI

George J So, Gasser Hathout, Keyvan Farahani,
Antonio deSalles, Shantanu Sinha, Dan Castro,
Keith Black and Robert B Lufkin

Introduction

Despite its relatively short history, magnetic
resonance (MR) imaging has become a major
diagnostic tool in almost all clinical specialties. The
multiplanar capabilities, increasingly high spatial
resolution, excellent soft tissue contrast, and the
absence of ionizing radiation and beam hardening
from bony structure all have contributed to MRI's
development as a powerful tool to guide interventional procedures.

New designs of MR open scanners allow
improved patient access for MR-guided interventional procedures.[1] MR-compatible needles and
catheters, developed for interventional purposes
and composed of high-nickel-content stainless
steel and other MR-compatible materials, reduce
the torque from the static magnetic field and
minimize susceptibility artifacts.

Studies of interventional MR applications
currently underway include aspiration cytology,
stereotactic depth electrode placement for
electroencephalography, chemoablation, cryoablation, and thermal ablation using lasers, focused
ultrasound and radiofrequency.[2-4] Because of its
high spatial resolution and soft tissue contrast, MR-
guided aspiration and biopsy is becoming more
popular. Lesions are easily localized without expos-
ing either patient or physician to ionizing radiation.
Once a needle has been positioned to reach a
lesion for diagnosis in the MR suite, subsequent
treatment of the lesion can be performed via
thermal ablation, freezing (cryosurgery) or
chemoablation (ethanol injection) through the same
access. MRI allows not only precise localization but
also sensitive monitoring of tissue changes during
therapy. In vital organs, such as the brain, where
destruction of a small area may result in significant
neurological deficits, MRI potentially provides critical information on the degree and extent of tissue
destruction during interventional procedures.

This chapter will briefly discuss the various
facets of interventional MRI, including dedicated
instrumentation, interventional techniques and
emerging clinical applications.

Instrumentation

MR-compatible instruments

MRI is notoriously sensitive to local magnetic field
variation. Any material of magnetic susceptibility
significantly different from the diamagnetic soft
tissues of the body can lead to geometric image
distortion. In addition, some of these materials also
experience significant torque and accelerate into
the magnetic field, creating a potential hazard
(Fig. 14.1).

Several artifacts that may affect interventional
MRI procedures have been described. The most
common artifacts are those due to local magnetic
field variations (susceptibility) induced by needles
or canulas used in IMRI procedures. There is also
a possibility of electronic interference from interventional equipment, such as radiofrequency (rf)
generators.

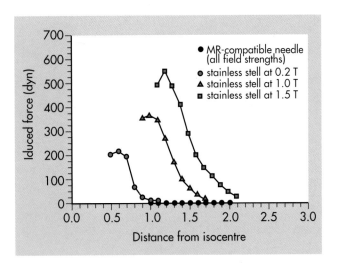

Figure 14.1

Graph of torque experienced by MR-compatible and noncompatible needles at various field strengths.

Susceptibility artifacts also depend on the pulse sequence applied. For instance, spin echo sequences are less sensitive to time-independent local magnetic field variations, while gradient echo sequences are sensitive to both time-dependent and time-independent local field changes. The degree of image distortion is also dependent on the magnitude of the main magnetic field, and increases with higher field strengths.

By optimizing pulse sequences, such as by using a shorter echo time, thinner slices, smaller field of view (FOV) and higher readout gradients, and by replacing standard medical-grade stainless steel with high-nickel-content stainless steel or other nonferrous alloys, induced forces on interventional equipment and their associated artifacts can be minimized (Fig. 14.1). MR-compatible needles, forceps, scissors and canulas (Cook Inc, USA; EFMT, Bochum, Germany; EZ-EM Westbury, NY; Micromed Inc, Bochum; Radionics, Inc, Burlington, MA) are available from many sources (Fig. 14.2). Similar modifications have been made with other support instrumentation such as anesthesia monitoring equipment, lasers and radiofrequency generators, as well as tracking systems.

Open MR systems and MR sequences

Current designs of interventional MRI scanners have focused on allowing the maximum direct access to the patient so that therapy, monitoring

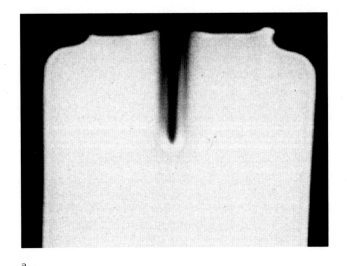

a

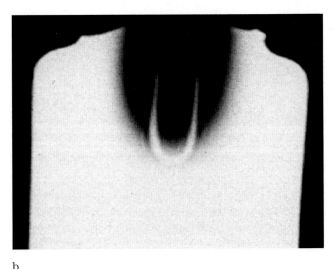

b

Figure 14.2

Comparison of magnetic susceptibility artifacts from (a) MR-compatible and (b) noncompatible (stainless steel) needles. Images obtained at 1.5 T. The standard needle produces a large artifact.

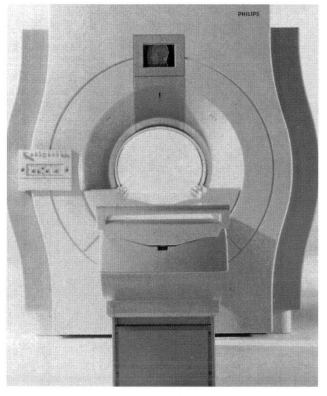

a

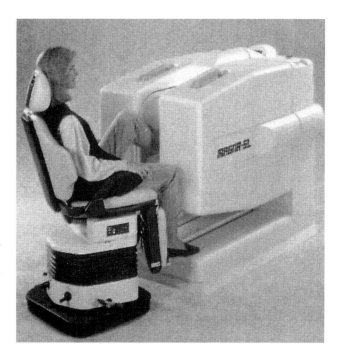

c

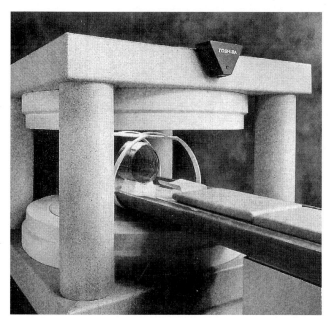

b

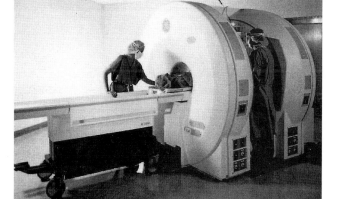

d

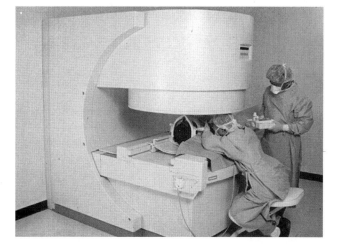

e

Figure 14.3

(a) 1.5 T system based on a modified superconducting MR system (Philips). (b) Double-donut design with horizontal orientation (Toshiba). (c) Double donut design with vertical orientation (GE). (d) Vertical C-shaped design magnet at 0.3 T (Magna-vu). (e) Horizontal 0.2 T C-shaped design system by Siemens.

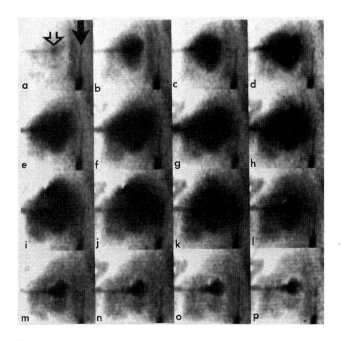

a

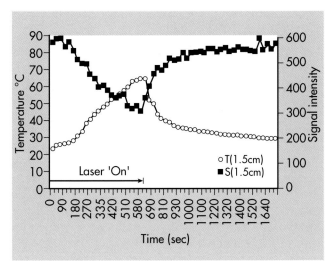

b

Figure 14.4

(a) Tissue phantom images obtained using gradient echo sequences over time. There is one image every 20 s. The reversible signal loss reflects T_1 changes due to tissue heating. (b) Graph of temperature and MR image signal intensity versus time. Note that the MR signal change closely parallels the temperature. (Images courtesy of Dr Keyvan Farahani.)

and anesthesia can be achieved. Several designs are now available. Of the so-called 'open' systems that have been announced or are in development, that with the highest field strength (and the least open design) is the 1.5 T Gyroscan (Philips Medical Systems, Eindhoven, Netherlands) (Fig. 14.3a).

Two manufacturers have built systems using a 'double-doughnut' configuration. The 0.64 T ACCESS (Toshiba, San Francisco, CA) has a horizontal orientation, and a 0.5 T model from General Electric has a vertical orientation (Figs 14.3b,c).

The C-arm configuration is also popular, with this design being used in machines from at least two manufacturers: the 0.3 T Magna-SL and the 0.2 T Siemens Open (Figs 14.3d,e). Finally, there is at least one company (Interventional MRI International, San Francisco, CA) that is involved with leasing and packaging interventional MRI equipment.

Interventional MRI pulse sequences

MRI temperature monitoring and related sequences

MR-guided thermal ablation therapy, using rf, high-intensity focused ultrasound (HIFU) or lasers, would be greatly aided by the development of accurate MR thermal monitoring. Although tissue heating may be monitored by implanted transducers such as thermocouples or thermistors, this is invasive, hazardous and can yield temperature measurements at only a few points limited by the number of the probes.

Because several MR parameters, such as T_1 relaxation,[5–9] the diffusion coefficient[10] D and the chemical shift of the water peak,[11,12] are temperature-dependent, MRI has long been proposed as a non-invasive technique to map in vivo temperature distribution.

Of the various parameters, changes in T_1 relaxation with thermal changes were first studied, and did seem to be relatively straightforward and provide a linear scale. The studies suggested a slight rise in T_1 with heating, and a signal decrease in T_1-weighted images over a limited range (28–43°C) (Fig. 14.4). However in vivo temperature measurement based on T_1 changes showed that these changes can be influenced by tissue perfusion, and proton density variations.[13,14] There is a significant hysteresis existing between signal intensity and temperature.[13,15] Another concern is that at high energy depositions during thermal ablation, the induced T_1 changes may be irreversible.[15,16] Moreover, a recent ex vivo study using brain and muscle demonstrated that the slope of the relaxation time was positive for muscle but negative for brain, so that the signal level may increase or decrease, depending on tissue differences.[13] Hence it is generally thought at present that T_1 temperature monitoring cannot yield unambiguous results.

The other parameter for MR temperature mapping is the diffusion coefficient of water, D. It was reported that in the physiological temperature range, the sensitivity of diffusion to temperature is about 2.4%, which is about twice as high as that of the T_1 relaxation time.[10] The drawback of the measurement of the diffusion coefficient in vivo is that, since diffusion imaging is very sensitive to bulk motion and tissue anisotropy, it also requires ultrafast acquisition schemes, such as echo planar schemes, to avoid motion artifacts, high signal-to-noise ratio and strong gradients.

MR thermometry using water proton chemical shift imaging[11,12] is also of growing interest. The temperature dependence of water proton chemical shift may be measured using the phase difference of a dynamic multiplanar rf-spoiled fast field echo sequence.[12] Chemical shift imaging seems to be a potentially robust technique. The ultimate accuracy and efficacy of water proton chemical shift imaging for in vivo MR thermometry needs to be proven in further investigations.

Fast scanning and MR fluoroscopy

The development of ultrafast pulse sequences for rapid acquisition and reconstruction represents another challenge. In order to approximate real-time imaging (fluoroscopic mode), both image acquisition and image reconstruction have to be of very high speed (Fig. 14.5). Spatial and temporal

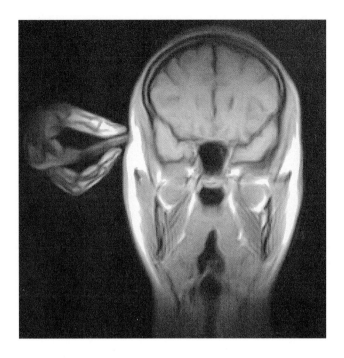

Figure 14.5

The ability to rapidly scan and localize during a procedure makes hand-held approaches for some procedures appealing.

resolution trade off against each other. Currently, submillimeter spatial resolution can be achieved in a 0.2 T system in 5 min with standard spin echo sequences. Although a gradient echo image (28 cm FOV, 128 × 256 matrix) can be obtained in 9 s, there is a decrease in signal-to-noise ratio and a greater sensitivity to magnetic susceptibility artifacts.

Many recent studies have focused on sequences with very short repetition time (*TR*) and a hybrid of echo planar and spin echo methods (SE–EPI). Echo planar sequences provide the shortest scan times, but have a low signal-to-noise ratio and are very sensitive to local field changes. Another rapid imaging strategy involves selective filling of *k*-space. Such 'restricted field-of-view' imaging limits updating of *k*-space to the lower-frequency domains, leaving the higher-frequency space untouched. 'Keyhole' imaging or LOLO (local look) techniques use subsampling methods to significantly shorten the imaging time.[17] LOLO utilizes single-shot Turbo spin echo sequences and can

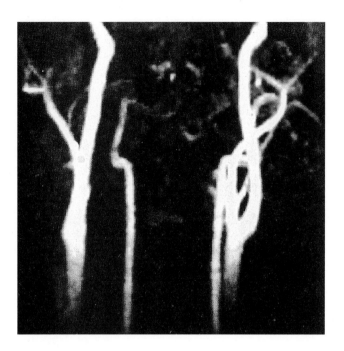

Figure 14.6

Simulation of real-time position tracking of a catheter using an MRA roadmap and rf tracking.

acquire a 'real-time' 128 × 128 image matrix in 50–150 ms. The particular choice of sequence will depend on available software and hardware, as well as the perceived need for real-time imaging.

Finally, high-speed tracking systems using optical or specialized rf tracking coils may allow rapid updating of positional information when combined with high-spatial-resolution data obtained from standard imaging or MRA sequences (Fig. 14.6).

Interventional approaches

Aspiration cytology/biopsy

Head and neck

MR-guided aspiration cytology for deep-sited head and neck lesions has been performed for nearly a decade, and has become a standard procedure at our institution.[3,18–24] Because of the complicated

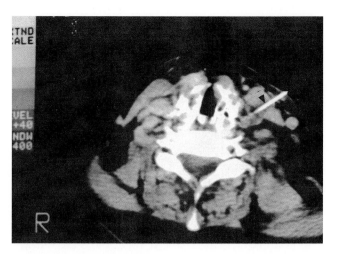

a

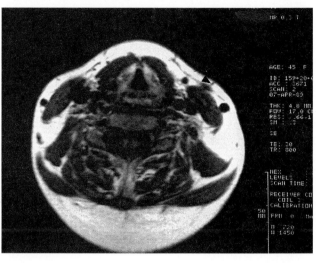

b

Figure 14.7

Comparison in CT and MR in guiding biopsy approaches to the low neck. (a) The CT image has considerable beam hardening artifact and poor soft tissue resolution. Note the needle for CT-guided biopsy of suspected mass. (b) The subsequent improved-quality MR image of the same patient reveals that there is no mass and that no biopsy is necessary.

anatomy and closely spaced structures, blind needle aspiration of the nonpalpable deep structures that lie close to the great vessels and the nervous system is not only technically difficult but

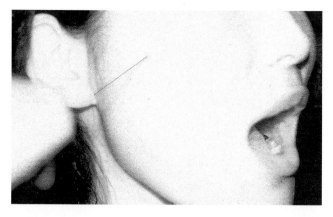

a

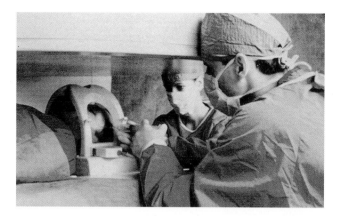

a

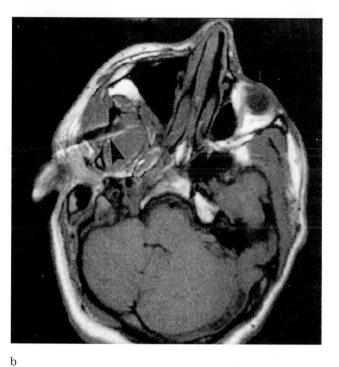

b

b

Figure 14.8

Subzygomatic approach to the skull base and intratemporal fossa. (a) The needle is directed below the zygoma and between the coronoid process and condyle of the mandible. (b) Axial MR image showing the path of the needle in a patient with suspected residual juvenile angiofibroma. The biopsy showed only granulation tissue.

Figure 14.9

Retromandibular approach to the poststyloid compartment. (a) Mock-up of approach to the patient in the scanner. (b) The needle is visible as a signal void (arrowhead). The aspiration revealed metastatic carcinoma.

also dangerous. MRI permits visualization of structures near the skull base, where beam-hardening artifacts greatly reduce the effectiveness of CT (Fig. 14.7). The multiplanar capability of MR also

allows localization along the course of the needle similar to that of ultrasound.

By using 26-gauge MR-compatible needles of variable lengths and curvatures, lesions in this

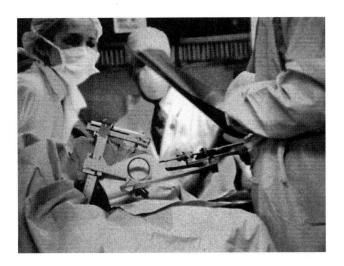

Figure 14.10

Frame-based stereotaxis in a patient undergoing MR-guided biopsy and rf ablation of a brain tumor. This approach is being replaced by frameless approaches at many centers.

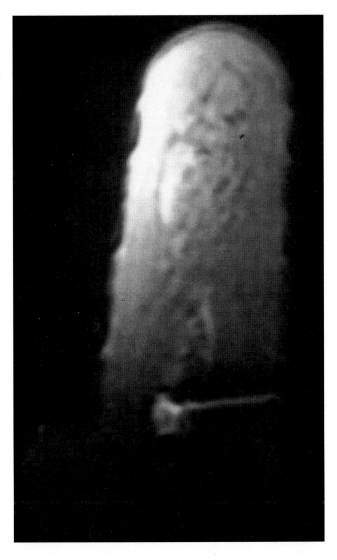

Figure 14.11

Image of MR-guided breast biopsy using a new breast biopsy coil. The needle is represented as a signal void. (Image courtesy of Dr David Gorczyka.)

small and closely spaced anatomy can be approached via different approaches.

The subzygomatic/infratemporal approach can be performed to access lesions in the parapharyngeal space, skull base and infratemporal fossa. The patient's mouth is held open during the insertion. The triangle outlined by the zygoma, coronoid process and the manibular condyle forms the landmark for needle insertion (Fig. 14.8).

The retromandibular approach is useful in accessing the paraoropharyngeal, parotid and lower masticator spaces. The needle is placed just posterior to the angle of the mandible and more than 1 cm below the tragus to avoid damaging the facial nerve (Fig. 14.9).

The submastoid approach can be used to access lesions in the skull base. The needle is inserted 1 cm inferior to the mastoid tip along the anterior aspect of the sternocleidomastoid muscle.

Stereotactic brain biopsy

With development of the MR-compatible stereotactic frame, stereotactic brain biopsy is now performed based on prebiopsy MR imaging in many institutions (Fig. 14.10). Stereotactic coordinates and optimum angle of probe insertion are calculated

with high accuracy based on MR imaging.[25] Dedicated interventional MR magnets now allow frameless stereotactic brain biopsy and treatment.

Breast

It has been reported that, with the use of dynamic contrast enhancement, MR can detect breast carcinomas that are not visible with standard mammographic techniques. Using a similar set-up to the mammographic system, the breast can be compressed and stabilized while the patient is in a prone position. Although experience is limited to date, successful biopsy under MR guidance has been performed on lesions that are not detectable or easily localized by other modalities.[26] Many experts feel that the single largest area of potential application for interventional MRI is in the detection and treatment of breast disease (Fig. 14.11).

Interstitial laser therapy

Despite its relatively long history, the potential for treatment of neoplasms with lasers has been limited by the poor deep tissue penetration achieved with surface illumination. Interstitial laser thermotherapy (ILT) is a new therapeutic technique that offers the advantages of transmitting energy directly into deep tumors through a fiber-optic probe. ILT causes thermal tissue injury through to laser energy deposition, resulting in coagulative necrosis (Fig. 14.12). Whereas in traditional *hyperthermia*, tissue is heated to 43–45°C for greater than 10 min, typically to augment other therapies, in *thermal ablation* using lasers or rf, the temperature is over 65°C to produce protein denaturation. This effect seems to be nonspecific for neoplasms unless a tissue-specific photosensitizer is used. ILT will create coagulative necrosis wherever sufficient energy is delivered through the fiber optics. Therefore accurate localization of fiber optics within a target tumor and careful monitoring with MR are essential for successful treatment.

ILT is one of the most promising recent thermal ablation techniques.[27–30] Nd : YAG is one of the most commonly used lasers for interstitial application. The major advantages of ILT as a thermal ablation technique are

- a powerful heat source that potentially destroys a large volume of tissue;
- few artifacts by laser on MR;
- the small caliber of the laser fiber does not require large-bore needle insertion;
- it is independent of radiation sensitivity (nonspecific thermal injury);
- minimal tissue damage to adjacent normal structures.

MR has the potential to allow the detection of the tumor, localization of the instrument within the

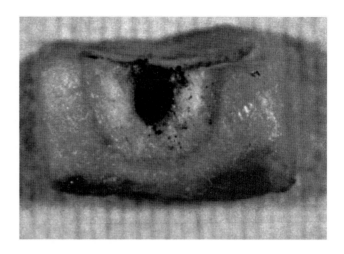

Figure 14.12

Gross pathology of laser-induced heat lesion in the rabbit model. Note the concentric rings of tissue change, indicating (from the center outward) carbonization, coagulation necrosis and edema.

target tumor, temperature monitoring during ILT, and demonstration of accurate thermal tissue injury. 2D FLASH sequences show increased signal within brain tumors as temperature increases during ILT.[29] T_2-weighted images of acute ILT lesions show low-signal coagulative necrosis with or without a central cavity, surrounded by high-signal edema on T_2-weighted images (Fig. 14.13).[31] Histopathological correlation in the chronic animal model showed that the lesion size increases up to one week following laser treatment, and then gradually decreases owing to infiltration of phagocytotic cells from adjacent vital tissue.[32] Granulation tissues will then form around the lesion, which then eventually progresses to a residual fibrotic scar.

Although high-power ILT can produce a larger lesion size than low-power ILT for a given total energy delivered, high-power ILT has a very steep thermal gradient. This means that the temperature around the laser fiber is extremely high, so that tissue vaporization (gas formation) or charring may occur inside the tumor. High-power ILT is not recommended for treatment of lesions in a closed space, such as the brain, where the development of a mass effect due to rapid gas formation may occur. Low-power ILT may require a longer treatment time, but provide a more gradual and

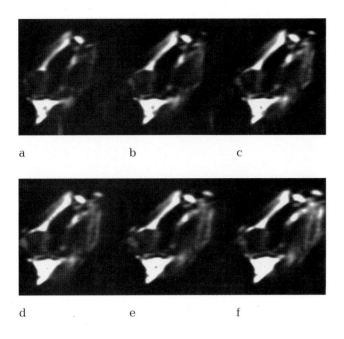

a   b   c

d   e   f

Figure 14.13

Sequential (a–f) T_2-weighted images obtained in the animal model (20 s apart) as the laser is fired into the tissue. Note the appearance of the evolving burn lesion.

homogenous heating effect. In most clinical ILT studies for brain tumors, the low-power (<4 W) setting has been used.

Radiofrequency ablation

Radiofrequency (rf) thermal ablation is a technique of tissue destruction by resistive heating using an rf (approximately 500 kHz) alternating current. A probe system with an active and a dispersive electrode is connected to the patient to complete an electrical circuit. The uninsulated tip of the active electrode or rf probe is placed at the center of the target tissue, from which the alternating current is conducted to the probe. Because of the impedance (resistance) of the tissue surrounding the probe, ionic agitation results in frictional heating,[33] which results in tissue damage secondary to coagulation necrosis. The size of the rf lesion produced is a function of the length and

diameter of the exposed electrode tip, as well as the energy delivered.

Prior to the development of MRI, rf ablation had been used extensively in many neurosurgical applications, including thalamotomy, pallidotomy and leucotomy for intractable pain and movement disorders.[34-36] Radiofrequency ablation for these functional disorders is controlled by simply observing the patient's unique symptoms, such as tremor, dyskinesia and pain. Imaging studies have not played a major role in rf ablation of functional disorders, other than localization of the rf probe. When rf ablation is applied to brain tumors, however, MR imaging is essential for controlling rf energy delivery and evaluation of the treatment.[37]

Radiofrequency has been used in the neurosurgical field for over three decades, and has proved to be a safe thermal ablation technique. The central temperature adjacent to the rf probe can be set to 80°C to cause coagulative necrosis, so that overheating of tissue (vaporization or charring) can be easily avoided.

The MR appearance of rf lesions is similar to those of lasers, i.e. a well-defined ellipsoidal coagulative necrosis surrounded by edema. MR is sensitive enough to detect acute thermal injury that can be missed by other imaging modalities.

MR studies indicate that the lesions are well delineated from surrounding normal tissue.[1,34] With the currently available accurate stereotactic technique,[25] and the recent development of an MR-compatible rf unit,[38] the use of dynamic MR to monitor the ablation of deep lesions in the body has become a practical and useful application of IMRI (Fig. 14.14).

Focused ultrasound ablation

By using high-intensity focused ultrasound (HIFU), focal hyperthermia can be induced and can cause destruction of lesions in soft tissue. This technique provides a nonincisional, transcutaneous ablation method using ultrasound energy to create thermal energy to cause direct thermal coagulation, necrosis and cavitation.

High-intensity ultrasound (frequency 0.5–10 MHz) beams are generated by piezoceramics. The beam is then focused by a combination of lenses and reflecting surfaces. The emitted beam converges to the focal zone, where the lesion is created, and then diverges. The relative ultrasound power deposition is highest in the focal

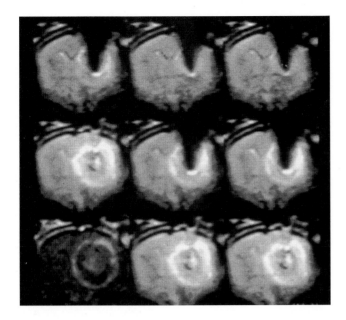

Figure 14.14

Sequential MR of rf energy applied to rapid brain, showing evolution of concentric rings of thermal injury. The linear region of signal void is the rf electrode.

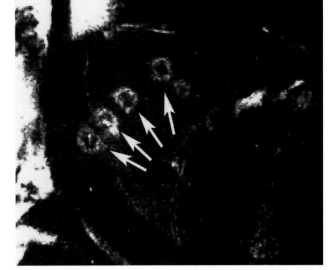

Figure 14.15

MR image of rabbit model following percutaneous high-energy focused ultrasound (HIFU) application. The concentric rings (arrowed) represent the tissue damage. (Image courtesy of Dr Hynonen.)

zone, and decreases significantly in the near and far fields. With sufficient intensity, very sharp temperature profiles can be produced, so that an intense rise of temperature can be attained within a few seconds in the focal zone, causing tissue destruction. Furthermore, unlike other energy delivery systems such as rf and lasers, the location of ablation can be moved easily and the focus of destruction can be made very small.

Destruction of tissues is achieved by two major mechanisms: (1) rapid increase of temperature locally, causing coagulation and denaturation of the cellular protein, and (2) generation of microbubbles similar to those of boiling water, which disrupt the cellular structure mechanically. Histological studies of HIFU ablation of the brain, liver and kidneys have shown that it is possible to produce a well-localized and well-demarcated necrotic lesion.[39,40]

Numerous studies and phase I clinical trials have been performed under ultrasound guidance, including the treatment of breast, liver and prostate tumors.[41-43] Some of the problems in ultra-sound-guided focused ultrasound ablation stem from acoustic coupling. The sonic path must be clear of air or bone to avoid reflection of sonic distortion. This precludes application in regions such as lungs, skeleton and bowel. Another drawback of HIFU ablation is the small lesion size obtained in single treatment. A recent study showed that it requires 50 min to treat a 1 cm³ lesion volume.[44] The profile of tissue destruction depends on the applied power, duration of sonication, tissue type and vascularity,[45,46] and must be closely monitored. Because MR imaging can provide excellent soft tissue contrast, and possibly temperature monitoring, MRI may be able to guide clinical applications of ultrasound ablation (Fig. 14.15).

Ultrasound-induced lesions are not only visible in MRI; in addition, the dimensions of the destroyed lesion correlate well with T_2-weighted images.[47] In addition, since T_1 and T_2 relaxation times and some other MR-measurable parameters such as diffusion coefficients are temperature-dependent, appropriate images may be used for monitoring.[48] Direct near real time imaging or destruction of tissue is possible by this method.

Cryoablation

Cryosurgery is a therapeutic method that involves freezing ablation of tissue by direct contact with a cryoprobe.[49] A cryogen, typically liquid nitrogen, is circulated through the probe, which is thermally insulated except at its tip. Thermal exchange occurs between the probe and the tissue, and a frozen region gradually extends outward from the probe tip. In experiments involving the rabbit brain, 8–10 min of freezing were required to create a lesion 5 mm in depth; thawing of frozen tissue also required approximately 8 min.[49]

With recent advances in imaging, there is promise that cryoablation may play a role in the treatment of tumors. Recently, intraoperative ultrasound has been used to guide cryosurgery in the prostate[50,51] and the liver.[52,53] Advances in MR imaging, and the field of interventional MRI, now make MR one of the more promising tools for the direction of cryoablation of deep tumors. Previous animal experiments have demonstrated the ability of MR to monitor the extent of the frozen region during surgery.[54] MR-compatible cryoprobes have recently been developed,[55,56] and a thorough investigation of MR-guided cryosurgery has been conducted on the rabbit brain model.[49]

The frozen region is apparent on all MR pulse sequences as a well-defined area of signal void, with a sharp interface to nonfrozen tissue, which can be tracked in time during the freezing process. The signal void of the frozen area is presumably due to a significant increase in the spin–spin relaxation rates as liquid water transitions to ice, rendering water protons invisible to MRI.[49,57]

T_1-weighted images, while less accurate for dynamic monitoring, display the interesting feature of a bright band at the boundary of the freeze front, which represents nonfrozen cooled tissue adjacent to the front.[49,58] Early results indicate that after freezing, there is Gd enhancement at the margin of the frozen region, which correlates with vascular damage and ischemic necrosis at the center of the lesion.[48,58–60]

MR images provide adequate spatial and temporal resolution of the expanding frozen lesion, as well as delineation of brain edema and blood–brain barrier breakdown post-thaw.

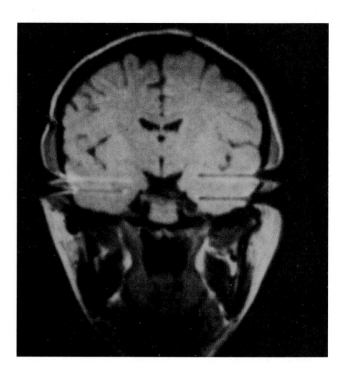

Figure 14.16

MR-compatible EEG electrodes are visible as a signal void in this patient with intractable partial complex seizures being studied for possible temporal lobectomy. In the future the seizure focus may be treated through the electrodes without open surgery.

Stereotactic depth electrode placement for electroencephalography

Intracerebral electroencephalography is sometimes used to monitor medically intractable epilepsy in order to define the site and extent of the epileptic focus. Until recently, the most widely used method has been stereoscopic angiography and a double-grid system to place the electrodes. Stereoscopic angiography with digital subtraction provides a safe trajectory for the electrode and avoids intracranial vessels such as the sylvian vessels and the vein of Labbe during temporal lobe electrode placement. This method, however, limits the working space available for implantation. Given the ability of MRI to provide detailed anatomy and angiographic information, interventional MRI may also provide feedback during insertion, assessment of positional accuracy and also freedom to choose both the target and the entry points (Fig. 14.16).

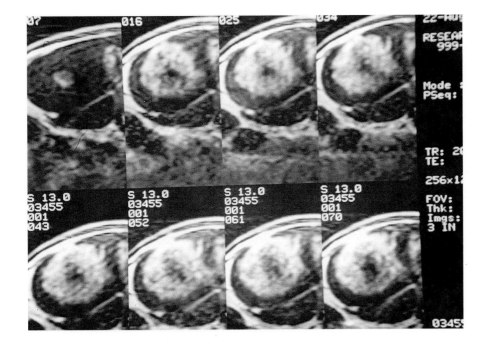

Figure 14.17

Sequential T_2-weighted MR images of application of ethanol to deep tissue in the animal model. The lesion of dehydration necrosis is clearly visible.

In the future, once an epileptic focus has been determined, possible treatment of the focus can be performed in an interventional MR suite using thermal, or cryoablation, instead of large partial temporal lobectomy.

signal is selectively suppressed using a fast inversion recovery sequence with water suppression.[62] Follow-up studies have demonstrated that tumors treated with ethanol show decreased signal on T_2-weighted images, possibly secondary to protein denaturation, and a resultant shortening of T_2.[63,64]

Chemoablation

Percutaneous ethanol injection (PEI) is an example of chemoablation, using a high concentration of ethanol to cause local dehydration necrosis. This technique has been used for treatment of liver tumors or parathyroid adenomas.[61–64] A more predictable ablation can be attained in encapsulated lesions, because ethanol infusion tends to follow anatomic tissue planes. The hydrophilic nature of ethanol makes it difficult to produce well-controlled uniform lesions of reproducible size and shape.[62] MR is used to guide the placement of needles and cannulas for the instillation of chemotherapeutics (Fig. 14.17). In ethanol ablation, it has been shown that MR can be useful in directly imaging ethanol in the interstitium to assess proper delivery. This is done by utilizing the minimal chemical shift of ethanol from water. The water

Clinical applications

Brain

Trials are currently ongoing to assess the use of MR-guided thermal ablation of brain tumors, using either Nd : YAG lasers or rf.[29,37] The advantages of this approach are

- it is less invasive than an open craniotomy for tumor resection (performed under local anesthesia with a 3 mm burr hole);
- it is focal therapy, with minimal adjacent vital tissue damage, and may be repeated as often as necessary;
- it can be performed following whole brain radiation or surgery;

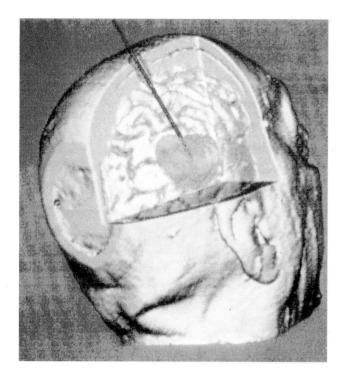

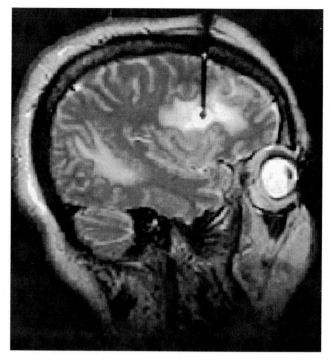

Figure 14.18

Rendered 3D MR image of patient showing electrode
track for MR-guided rf ablation of brain tumour.

Figure 14.19

Sagittal MR image of rf ablation electrode in place in
a patient with metastatic adenocarcinoma to the brain.
The red region indicates the intended region for heat
deposition.

- it is significantly less costly than open
  craniotomy.

The technique employed at the UCLA Center for
Interventional MRI is as follows (Fig. 14.18):[37]

(1) MR stereotaxis for localization of brain tumor;
(2) place biopsy needle if necessary or rf probe
    (Radionics, Burlington, MA) into the tumor
    through a 3 mm twist-drill hole;
(3) apply rf power to achieve an intratumoral
    temperature of 80°C for 1 min, under MR
    visualization;
(4) repeat treatment until the entire tumor volume
    is destroyed, under MR.

The brain lesion is detected as a central focus of
high signal on a noncontrast T_1-weighted image,
which presumably represents heat-induced methemoglobin, surrounded by a low-signal ring. A post-
gadolinium T_1-weighted image demonstrates a rim
of enhancement peripheral to the low-signal ring
seen on the noncontrast T_1-weighted image, which

represents the acute thermal lesion (Fig. 14.19). As
the lesion matures (3–7 days), a peripheral low-
signal area of hemosiderin is also noted on the T_2-
weighted image. The heat lesion and adjacent
edema increase in size up to 1 week post-therapy,
and gradually then decrease unless local recurrence occurs (Fig. 14.20).

Hence MRI-guided thermal ablation so far
appears to be a safe, minimally invasive treatment
of brain tumors. Unlike radiation, it is not
contraindicated by accumulative toxicity, and it
may serve as a palliative alternative for end-stage
patients not wishing to undergo open craniotomy.

Head and neck

Head, neck and skull base lesions have close
proximity to many cranial nerves and major
vessels. Wide local resection of those lesions may
result in functional and cosmetic deformities. Head
and neck tumors are usually treated by surgery

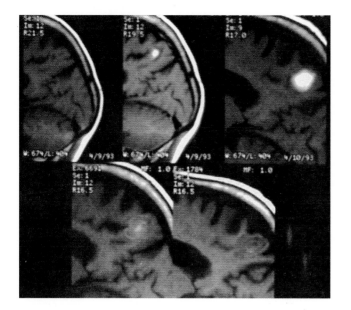

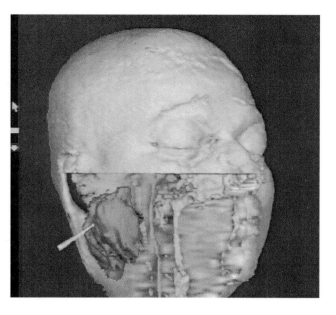

Figure 14.20

Sequential sagital T_1-weighted MR images showing the appearance of a metastatic tumor following rf treatment over time. The images were obtained immediately pre, post, and days, weeks and months following treatment.

Figure 14.21

Rendered 3D image showing an approach for MR-guided laser ablation of a patient with metastatic breast carcinoma in the parotid region.

and/or radiation therapy. MR-guided minimally invasive thermal ablation can be another alternative, if thermal energy delivery can be accurately controlled by MR (Fig. 14.21).

Preliminary clinical trials of interstitial laser therapy in this area have been reported.[27,65,66] Although the efficacy of this technique needs to be further proven in large series with long follow-up, results are promising. This technique may offer another treatment option to patients with recurrent head and neck cancer or a lesion in the skull base that requires a radical craniofacial resection.

Breast

Breast carcinoma is a leading cause of death for women in the United States. Because of high soft tissue contrast, MR has been reported to be able to detect breast carcinomas that are not visible with the usual mammographic technique. With the recent development of breast biopsy surface coils, the breast can be compressed and stabilized while the patient is in a prone position. Although experience is limited to date, successful biopsy under MR guidance has been performed on lesions that are not detectable or easily localized by other modalities.[26]

A preliminary clinical trial of interstitial laser therapy for human breast cancer followed by surgery was recently presented that showed excellent correlation of MR thermal lesion appearance and pathology.[67] The study suggests that MR-guided ILT for breast cancer is potentially a useful tool. Another study of MR-guided HIFU therapy for breast fibroadenomas has also been presented.[68] Although experience is limited, further studies are again necessary and warranted.

Spine

MR-guided percutaneous injections of long-acting anesthesia (Bupivacain) and steroid (Triamcinolon) to the facet joints and the sacroiliac joints have been performed to relieve pseudoradicular pain. Preliminary results have shown an over 90% response rate of relief of pain.[69] Percutaneous laser diskectomy in the lumbar spine is also under investigation as an alternative to spinal surgery.

Conclusions

Technological advances in health care, such as diagnostic MRI, are under increasing criticism for their high cost. However, because of its minimally invasive nature compared with other open surgical approaches, interventional MRI (IMRI) may actually emerge as a means of lowering the cost of medical care.

Interventional MRI is clearly in its early stages of development. The future of MR-guided therapy remains to be proven with large clinical studies to define its ultimate effectiveness. With the new dedicated interventional MR units that are available, this work should be forthcoming. Now, as we look on to the millennium, it is possible to imagine dedicated interventional MR units for combined radiological and surgical approaches in what may be the archetype for operating rooms of the 21st century.

References

1. Anzai Y, DeSalles A, Black K et al, Interventional MR imaging update. Scientific Exhibition in RSNA, 1993.

2. Mueller P, Stark D, Simeone J et al, MR-guided aspiration biopsy: needle design and clinical trials. *Radiology* 1986; **161**: 605–7.

3. Lufkin R, Teresi L, Hanafee W, New needle for MR-guided aspiration cytology of the head and neck. *AJR* 1987; **149**: 380–2.

4. Lufkin R, Jordan S, Lylyck P, Vinuela F, MR imaging with topographic EEG electrodes in place. *AJNR* 1988; **9**: 953–4.

5. Parker D, Smith P, Sheldon P et al, Temperature distribution measurements in two-dimensional NMR imaging. *Med Phys* 1983; **10**: 321–5.

6. Hall A, Prior M, Hand J et al, Observation by MR imaging of in vivo temperature changes induced by radiofrequency hyperthermia. *J Comput Assist Tomogr* 1990; **14**: 430–6.

7. Hall L, Talagala S, Mapping of pH and temperature distribution using chemical-shift-resolved tomography. *J Magn Reson* 1985; **65**: 501–5.

8. Dickinson R, Hall A, Hind A, Young I, Measurement of changes in tissue temperature using MR imaging. *J Comput Assist Tomogr* 1986; **10**: 468–72.

9. Ebner F, Temperature monitoring for tissue ablation by means of MRI. *Proc Interventional MRI Workshop, Marina Del Rey, CA, 1994*, 119.

10. LeBihan D, Delannoy J, Levin R, Temperature mapping with MR imaging of molecular diffusion: application to hyperthermia. *Radiology* 1989; **171**: 853–7.

11. Hindeman JC, *J Chem Phys* 1966; **44**: 4582.

12. Stollberger R, Thermal monitoring using the water proton chemical shift. *Proc Interventional MRI Workshop, Boston, 1994*, 12.

13. Goldhaber, D, Heat mapping with MRI. *Proc Interventional MRI Workshop, Marina Del Rey, CA, 1994*, 113–16.

14. Young I, Hand J, Oatridge A et al, Further observations on the measurement of tissue $T1$ to monitor temperature in vivo by MRi. *Magn Reson Med* 1994; **31**: 342–5.

15. Jolesz F, Bleier A, Jokab P et al, MR imaging of laser tissue interactions. *Radiology* 1988; **168**: 249–53.

16. Lewa C, Majewska Z, Temperature relationships of proton spin-lattice relaxation time $T1$ in biological tissues. *Bull Cancer (Paris)* 1980; **67**: 525–30.

17. van Vaals J, Brummer M, Dixon W et al, 'Keyhold' method for accelerating imaging of contrast agent uptake. *J Magn Reson Imaging* 1993; **3**: 671–5.

18. Lufkin R, Teresi L, Chiu L, Hanafee W, A technique for MR guided needle placement in the head and neck. *AJR* 1988; **151**: 193–6.

19. Lufkin R, Layfield L, Coaxial needle system for MR and CT guided aspiration cytology. *J Comput Assist Tomogr* 1989; **13**: 1105–7.

20. Lufkin RB, MR-guided needle biopsy with a high-field-strength MR system. *AJNR* 1991; **12**: 1268.

21. Duckwiler G, Lufkin R, Teresi L et al, Head and neck lesions: MR-guided aspiration biopsy. *Radiology* 1989; **170**: 519–22.

22. Duckwiler G, Lufkin R, Hanafee W, MR-directed needle biopsies. *Radiol Clin N Am* 1989; **27**: 255–63.

23. Wenokur R, Andrews J, Abemayor E et al, Magnetic resonance imaging-guided fine needle aspiration for the diagnosis of skull base lesions. *Skull Base Surgery* 1992; **2**: 167–70.

24. Trapp T, Lufkin R, Abemayor E et al, MR guided aspiration cytology of the head and neck. *Laryngoscope* 1989; **99**: 105–8.

25. Kondziolka D, Dempsey P, Lunsford L et al, A comparison between magnetic resonance imaging and computed tomography for stereotactic coordinate determination. *Neurosurgery* 1992; **30**: 402–7.

26. Schnall M, MR-guided breast biopsy. *Proc Interventional MRI Workshop, Boston, 1994*, 42.

27. Castro DJ, Lufkin RB, Saxton RE et al, Metastatic head and neck malignancy treated using MRI guided interstitial laser phototherapy: an initial case report. *Laryngoscope* 1992; **102**: 26–32.

28. Anzai Y, Lufkin RB, Saxton RE et al, Nd : YAG interstitial laser phototherapy guided by magnetic resonance imaging in an ex vivo model: dosimetry of laser–MR–tissue interaction. *Laryngoscope* 1991; **101**: 755–60.

29. Kahn T, Bettag M, Ulrich F et al, MRI-guided laser induced interstitial thermotherapy of cerebral neoplasms. *J Comput Assist Tomogr* 1994; **18**: 519–32.

30. Gewiese B, Beuthan J, Fobbe F et al, Magnetic resonance imaging-controlled laser-induced interstitial thermotherapy. *Invest Radiol* 1994; **29**: 345–51.

31. Anzai Y, Lufkin R, Castro D et al, MR imaging-guided interstitial Nd : YAG laser phototherapy: dosimetry study of acute tissue damage in an in vivo model. *J Magn Reson Imaging* 1991; **1**: 553–9.

32. Anzai Y, Lufkin RB, Hirschowitz S et al, MR imaging—histopathologic correlation of thermal injuries induced with interstitial Nd :

YAG laser irradiation in the chronic model. *J Magn Reson Imaging* 1992; **2**: 671–8.

33. Organ L, Electrophysiologic principles of radiofrequency lesion making. *Appl Neurophysiol* 1976; **39**: 69–76.

34. Sweet W, Mark V, Hamlin H, Radiofrequency lesions in the central nervous system of man and cat: including case reports of eight bulbar pain-tract interruptions. *J Neurosurgery* 1960; **17**: 213–25.

35. Tomlinson F, Jack C, Kelly P, Sequential magnetic resonance imaging following stereotactic radiofrequency ventralis lateralis thalamotomy. *J Neurosurgery* 1991; **74**: 579–84.

36. White J, Sweet W, Hackett T, Radiofrequency leukotomy for relief of pain, coagulation of medial frontal white fibers in stages by means of inlying electrodes. *Neurology* 1960; **2**: 317–30.

37. Anzai Y, Black K, DeSalles AA et al, Preliminary experience with MR-guided thermal ablation of brain tumors. *AJNR* **16**: 39–48.

38. Sinha S, Parker J, Anzai Y et al, MR compatible RF system: initial experience. *Proc 12th Ann Mtg Soc Magn Reson Med, New York, 1993.*

39. ter Haar G, Robertson D, Tissue destruction with focused ultrasound in vivo. *Eur Urol* 1993; **23**(supp 1): 8–11.

40. Warwick R, Pond J, Trackless lesions in nervous tissues produced by high intensity focused ultrasound. *J Anat* 1968; **102**: 387–405.

41. Madersbacher S, Kratzik C, Szabo N et al, Tissue ablation in benign prostatic hyperplasia with high-intensity ultrasound. *Eur Urol* 1993; **23**(supp 1): 39–43.

42. Gelet A, Chapelon J, Margonari J et al, Prostatic tissue destruction by high-intensity focused ultrasound: experimentation on canine prostate. *J Endourol* 1993; **7**: 249–53.

43. Yang R, Sanghvi NT, Rescorla FJ et al, Liver cancer ablation with extracorporeal high-intensity focused ultrasound. *Eur Urol* 1993; **23**(supp 1): 17–22.

44. Pomeroy O, Hynynen K, Singer S et al, MR guided treatment of breast fibroadenomas by high intensity focused ultrasound. *Proc Interventional MRI Workshop, Boston, 1994*, 62.

45. Sibille A, Prat F, Chapelon J et al, Characterization of extracorporeal ablation of normal

and tumor-bearing liver tissue by high intensity focused ultrasound. *Ultrasound Med Biol* 1993; **19**: 803–13.

46. Chen L, ter Haar G, Hill C et al, Effect of blood perfusion on the ablation of liver parenchyma with high-intensity focused ultrasound. *Phys Med Biol* 1993; **38**: 1661–73.

47. Hynynen K, Darkazanli A, Unger E, Schenck J, MRI-guided noninvasive ultrasound surgery. *Med Phys* 1993; **20**: 107–15.

48. Cline H, Hynynen K, Hardy C et al, MR temperature mapping of focused ultrasound surgery. *Magn Reson Med* 1994; **31**: 628–36.

49. Gilbert J, Rubinsky B, Roos M et al, MRI-monitored cryosurgery in the rabbit brain. *Magn Reson Imaging* 1993; **11**: 1155–64.

50. Onik G, Cobb C, Cohen J et al, US characteristics of frozen prostate. *Radiology* 1988; **168**: 629–31.

51. Onik G, Porterfield B, Rubinsky B, Cohen J, Percutaneous transperineal prostate cryosurgery using transrectal ultrasound guidance: animal model. *Urology* 1991; **37**: 277–81.

52. Onik G, Gilbert J, Hoddick W et al, Ultrasonic monitoring of hepatic cryosurgery: preliminary report on an animal model. *Cryobiology* 1984; **21**: 715 (abst).

53. Gilbert J, Onik G, Hoddick W, Rubinsky B, Real time ultrasonic monitoring of hepatic cryosurgery. *Cryobiology* 1985; **22**: 319–30.

54. Matsumoto R, Oshio K, Jolesz F, Monitoring of laser and freezing-induced ablation in the liver with T1-weighted MR imaging. *J Magn Reson Imaging* 1992; **2**: 555–62.

55. Gilbert J, Roos M, Wong S et al, NMR monitored cryosurgery in the rabbit brain. *Proc 11th Ann Mtg Soc Magn Reson Med, Berlin 1992*, 1010.

56. Rubinsky B, Gilbert J, Onik G et al, Monitoring cryosurgery in the brain and prostate with proton NMR. *Cryobiology* 1993; **30**: 191–9.

57. Rubinsky B, Shitzer A, Analysis of a Stefan-like problem in a biological tissue around a cryosurgical probe. *Trans ASME: J Heat Transfer* 1976; **98**: 514–19.

58. Bottomley P, Hardy C, Argersinger R, Allen-Moore G, A review of ¹H nuclear magnetic resonance relaxation in pathology: are T_1 and T_2 diagnostic? *Med Phys* 1987; **14**: 1–37.

59. Gage A, Current progress in cryosurgery. *Cryobiology* 1988; **25**: 483–6.

60. Rubinsky B, Onik G, Cryosurgery: advances in the application of low temperatures to medicine. *Int J Refrigeration* 1991; **14**: 1–10.

61. Unger E, Kartchner Z, Karmann S, Measurement of intratumoral ethanol concentrations with CT in patients undergoing percutaneous ethanol injection [abstract 78]. *Scientific Program 79th Scientific Assembly and Ann Mtg RSNA, Chicago, 1993*, 118.

62. Unger E, MR-guided alcohol ablation of the body. *Proc Interventional MRI Workshop Marina Del Rey, CA, 1994*, 150–9.

63. Sironi S, Livraghi T, DelMaschio A, Small hepatocellular carcinoma treated with percutaneous ethanol injection: MR imaging findings. *Radiology* 1991; **180**: 333–6.

64. Sironi S, Livraghi T, Angeli E et al, Small hepatocellular carcinoma: MR follow-up of treatment with percutaneous ethanol injection. *Radiology* 1993; **187**: 119–23.

65. Vogl T, Felix R, Head and neck tumors: MR guided laser-induced thermotherapy (ILTT). *Proc Interventional MRI Workshop Marina Del Rey, CA, 1994*, 145–7.

66. Yoshimi A, Lufkin R, Interventional MRI of the head and neck. *Proc Interventional MRI Workshop Marina Del Rey, CA, 1994*, 139–44.

67. Hall-Craggs MA, Paley WM, Mumtaz H, Bown S, Laser therapy of breast carcinomas: MR/histopathological correlation. *Proc Interventional MRI Workshop, Boston, 1994*, 61.

68. Pomeroy O, Hynynen K, Singer S, Frenna T, Hiramatsu H, Jolesz F, MRI guided treatment of breast fibroadenomas by high intensity focused ultrasound. *Proc Interventional MR Workshop, Boston, 1994*, 62.

69. Siebel R, Groenmeyer D, Interventional MR of the spine. *Proc Interventional MRI Workshop Marina Del Rey, CA, 1994*, 136–7.

15

Proton spectroscopy of the human brain

Martyn Paley

Introduction

Proton spectroscopy of the human brain has advanced rapidly over the past few years as reliable in vivo measurements have become feasible.[1–10] However, many reported studies have involved just a handful of patients and even fewer control subjects, and many confusing and conflicting results have appeared in the literature. It is only recently that large, well-controlled and in some cases coordinated multicenter trials have allowed the true potential of proton spectroscopy to be assessed. These suggest that proton spectroscopy has a vital role to play in the assessment of clinical trials, including monitoring of new therapies, but because of limited sensitivity it may have to play a less important part in the clinical management of individual patients without further technical progress. In addition, proton spectroscopy has proved to be more useful in 'diffuse' rather than 'focal' conditions of the brain because of limited spatial resolution.

This frustrating situation is largely because of the limited signal-to-noise ratio available using current MR technology. However, advances in acquisition techniques and radiofrequency coils have allowed voxel sizes as small as 1 ml to be regularly measured at locations throughout the brain. Although still a factor of a thousand worse than the highest-resolution MR imaging available, this represents an improvement of a factor between ten and one hundred times better compared with equivalent measurements using phosphorus spectroscopy. In addition, in many instances much of the information contained within a phosphorus spectrum may actually be inferred from the proton spectrum.

The challenge for magnetic resonance spectroscopists is to characterize the basic spectral patterns in control subjects and in disease states. This is complicated by the fact that a single acquired spectrum does not provide information on absolute concentration of a particular biochemical. Instead, it is necessary to make multiple measurements to take account of the basic magnetic relaxation processes (T_1 and T_2) as well as changes in concentration. This is obviously time-consuming in patients who may be ill or in pain and who may find it difficult to remain motionless for a period extending up to an hour or more. An alternative approach to absolute quantification that has been used extensively is to rely on the ratio of peaks in the spectrum corresponding to the different biochemical substances. This has the obvious disadvantage of missing overall changes in concentration of both chemicals, but can provide much useful information.

The approach taken in this chapter is firstly to provide a brief overview of observable biochemicals and acquisition methodologies, followed by a more detailed look at the findings from proton spectroscopy studies in HIV-infected and AIDS patients using data acquired at our own site. We have a cohort of HIV-infected individuals who volunteer to attend for regular MRI and MRS examinations as well as other clinical, neurological and neuropsychological tests.

A brief review of the major findings from other groups in other disease processes of the human brain is also included, although this is by no means exhaustive and reflects the situation as of late 1994. The reader is referred to other chapters for further details. Many of the latest contributions in proton spectroscopy are only in the form of conference abstracts to date, and so these have been referred to as necessary.

Observable biochemicals

Despite the problems mentioned above, considerable progress has been made in characterizing spectra in a diverse range of diseases and conditions. Observable biochemicals identified in spectra from the human brain using a standard 1.5 T MRI system are shown in Table 15.1 and some of the relevant molecular structures are shown in Fig. 15.1. This list is not exhaustive, and the number of compounds assigned will probably increase with improved understanding of the detailed biochemical processes involved.

N-Acetyl aspartate (NAA)

Perhaps the most important peak present in the proton spectrum is associated with N-acetyl aspartate (NAA), which has the interesting property of being located primarily within neurons.[10] This provides MR spectroscopy with a window into the status of the basic units that constitute the functional aspect of the human brain. NAA is a relatively small molecule, and it is the mobile CH_3 group that gives rise to the sharp single line located at 2.02 ppm.

A second peak is observed at 2.6 ppm that is typically 6–8 times weaker than the peak at 2.02 ppm. This peak is in fact a triplet, and undergoes complex modulation, depending on the exact echo time and localization sequence used for observation. Attempts have been made to assess the ratio of NAA to NAAG (N-acetyl aspartate glutarate),[11] which overlaps the NAA peak, by using the second NAA peak at 2.6 ppm. NAA is thought to have an in vivo concentration in white matter of 6–10 mmol/kg.

NAA persists in the brain for about 24 h postmortem in rat brain,[12] and increases in concentration in the brain with maturation.[13] Changes in the T_2 of NAA have been reported in disease states.[14]

Table 15.1 Major spectral peaks assigned in human brain proton spectra from white matter

Compound	Chemical shift (ppm)	Approximate concentration (mmol/kg wet weight)
N-Acetyl aspartate	2.02	7–10
N-Acetyl aspartate glutamate	2.05	2
Choline-containing compounds	3.22	1.5
Creatine-containing compounds	3.02	5–7
myo-Inositol	3.56	5–7
scyllo-Inositol	3.35	1
Glucose	3.55	1–3
Glutamate/glutamine	2–2.5, 3.4–3.7	6–10
Lipid	1.3	<0.5
Lactate	1.3	0.5
Alanine	1.48	<0.3

N-Acetyl aspartate glutamate (NAAG)

Up to 20% of the resonance close to 2.0 ppm is thought to be from N-acetyl aspartate glutamate, which is a dipeptide with an actual chemical shift of 2.045 ppm. It is thought to be present only in white matter at a concentration of about 2 mmol/kg, is not present in gray matter, and has a relatively uniform distribution.[15]

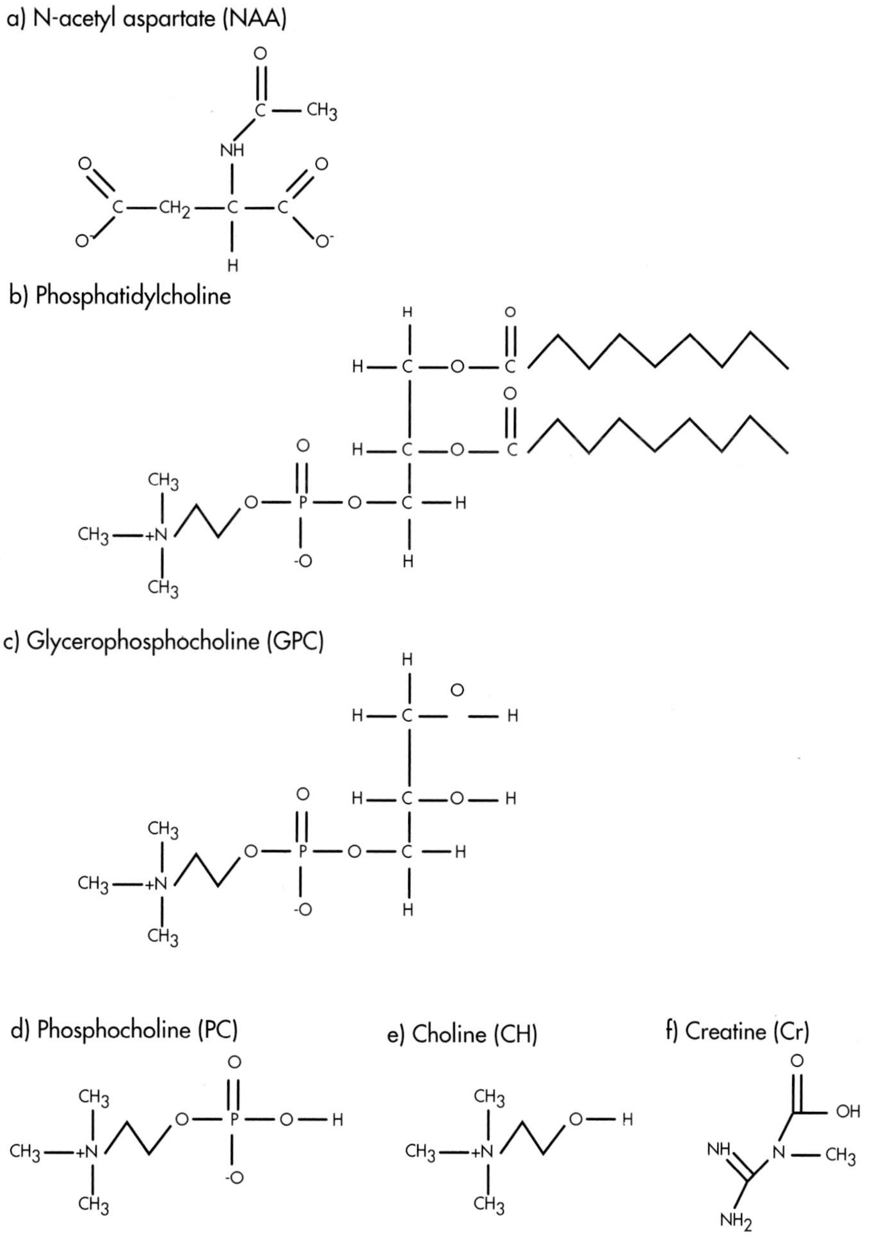

Figure 15.1

Schematic diagrams of important biomolecules for proton spectroscopy (a) N-acetyl aspartate (2.02 ppm). (b–e) some of the choline-containing compounds (3.22 ppm): (b) phosphatidylcholine; (c) glycerophosphocholine; (d) phosphocholine; (e) choline. (f) Creatine (3.02 ppm).

Choline-containing compounds

Choline-containing compounds visible in an in vivo MR spectrum include predominantly glycerophosphocholine (GPC) and glycerophosphoethanolamine (GPE), which form the phospholipid bilayer in cell membranes. Free choline, which is active metabolically, is present at much lower concentrations (micromolar), and so does not affect the MR spectrum directly. Thus the choline peak, which is a singlet resonance at 3.22 ppm, provides an indicator of cell density and may be able to provide information on cell swelling or the replacement of glial cells by astrocytes in reactive astrocytosis. Certainly the choline peak is often increased in tumors. Typical in vivo concentration of the choline compounds (making an assumption that nine protons contribute to the peak per molecule) is approximately 1.5 mmol/kg wet weight.[15]

Creatine-containing compounds

The creatine peak at 3.02 ppm consists of protons involved in the creatine kinase reaction, which is one of the basic metabolic processes within the human body. The proton spectrum observes the sum of protons on both sides of the reaction mechanism from phosphocreatine and creatine. Phosphorus spectroscopy looks at the phosphocreatine directly. The typical concentration of the creatine molecules in white matter has been estimated as 6 mmol/kg wet weight and slightly higher at 8 mmol/kg wet weight in gray matter.[15] The creatine peak has been proposed to be relatively constant in concentration with time owing to tight regulation of the creatine kinase reaction in normal function, but does have a regional variation.

myo-Inositol (MI)

myo-Inositol (MI) may only be observed at 3.6 ppm in short-echo-time (TE) spectra, since the peak is modulated by J-coupling, which severely attenuates the signal at later echo times. MI has been suggested to act as a cellular osmolyte that regulates transport across cell membranes.[15]

scyllo-Inositol

scyllo-Inositol has been identified as a singlet resonance at 3.35 ppm with a concentration of approximately 3 mmol/kg from six equivalent protons.[15]

Glucose

Glucose has a strongly coupled resonance with peaks appearing at 3.43 and 3.8 ppm due largely to tissue glucose at a concentration of approximately 1 mmol/kg wet weight. These resonances have been shown to correlate with glucose infusion studies in both rats[16] and humans.[17]

Glutamate (Gln)/glutamine (Glu)

Glutamate (Gln) is a storage form of glutamine (Glu), which is a basic neurotransmitter. Glutamate is found in relatively high concentration in human brain (6–10 mmol/kg wet weight). The Glx peak (Glu + Gln) located between 2.0 and 2.5 ppm in the short-TE spectrum has a very complicated modulation behavior. A recent report has suggested the novel expedient of using a low field strength to collapse some of the multiplet structure into a single much stronger peak.[18]

Lipid

Broad peaks at 0.9 ppm and 1.3 ppm are often identified in the proton spectrum from human brain, especially in and close to tumors. Initially it was thought that these peaks were the result of lipid contamination. However, careful work has shown that in fact they may often be identified with macromolecules resulting from breakdown of myelination in the white matter.[19]

Lactate

Lactate is not normally detected in spectra from the brains of adult volunteers using long- or short-TE spectra. Lactate is the result of anerobic glycolysis, and may often be identified in spectra from and close to lesions, but also in processes other than masses. The lactate peak is a doublet at 1.33 ppm, with a 135 ms modulation period corresponding to a J-splitting of approximately 7 Hz. In a $TE = 135$ ms spectrum the lactate is inverted, which makes it easy to identify. However, this is complicated by the fact that this peak overlaps the lipid peak described above. Techniques have been developed to selectively edit out the lactate from the lipid, but unfortunately most of these also reduce the signal-to-noise ratio substantially. However, the lactate peak has proved very useful, and provides access to some of the information normally only obtained from phosphorus spectroscopy. Lactate is present at a typical concentration of 1 mmol/kg in the normal adult.

Alanine

Alanine is not usually seen in normal in vivo human brain spectra, but gives a doublet at 1.48 ppm. It has been reported in vitro at concentrations of 0.3–0.9 mmol/kg wet weight.[15]

Spatial localization methods

Although acquisition methods and artifacts are described in detail elsewhere in this book, a quick review of commonly used gradient localization methods and their variants used for proton spectroscopy of the human brain will be discussed here, for completeness, with particular reference to some of their practical advantages and drawbacks.

Free induction decay: DRESS, SLIT-DRESS

Perhaps the simplest gradient localization scheme is DRESS,[20,21] which consists of a single plane-selective radiofrequency pulse followed by data acquisition. This technique may be used with a surface coil to provide a disk of material located deep within the brain without contamination from the overlapping lipids from the scalp. However, the localization is crude, and the method suffers from the fact that the peak of the echo that occurs at the center of the radiofrequency pulse cannot be sampled. This introduces a baseline roll artifact in the acquired spectra. The sequence may be run in slice-interleaved multislice mode (SLIT-DRESS!).

In order to suppress the much stronger water signal, it is necessary to precede this slice-selection procedure by a frequency-selective pulse. A long, low-amplitude Gaussian pulse may be used for this purpose (Fig. 15.2a).

Spin echo: PRESS, MESA

To avoid this sampling problem, the data collection can be improved by forming a spin echo using a 180° pulse following the initial 90° pulse. By arranging the slice-selection gradient to be perpendicular to the gradient applied during the 90° pulse, two dimensions of spatial localization are achieved. The signal in the echo comes from a column perpendicular to the two applied gradients. Now, since the T_2 decay times of many of the metabolites of interest in brain spectra are relatively long (>200 ms), it is possible to refocus the signal again using a second 180° pulse with a third gradient perpendicular to the previous two. The second echo is now formed from the small cubic region at the intersection of all three planes. This echo is then collected without any gradient pulses applied. In this way, complete voxel localization may be achieved. Water suppression may also be provided using a Gaussian pulse preceding the localization pulses. This is known as PRESS: point resolved selective spectroscopy[21] (Fig. 15.2b).

A variant on this technique, MESA[22] uses a binomial (1331) pulse to achieve water suppression and excitation of the relevant metabolites simultaneously. This is then followed by a train of three 180° pulses, each with a unique applied gradient direction. This ensures similar excitation profiles on all three axes and may be less sensitive to B_0 inhomogeneity, although it has the drawback of variable spectral response, making quantification difficult (Fig. 15.2c).

All spin echo localization schemes have the advantage of acquiring the full magnetization excited in the sample, although T_2 losses tend to be greater owing to the increased echo time needed to apply the 180° pulses and reform an echo for data collection. Typically, spin echo sequences are used with an echo time of 135 ms, at which time any lactate signal will be inverted making identification easier.

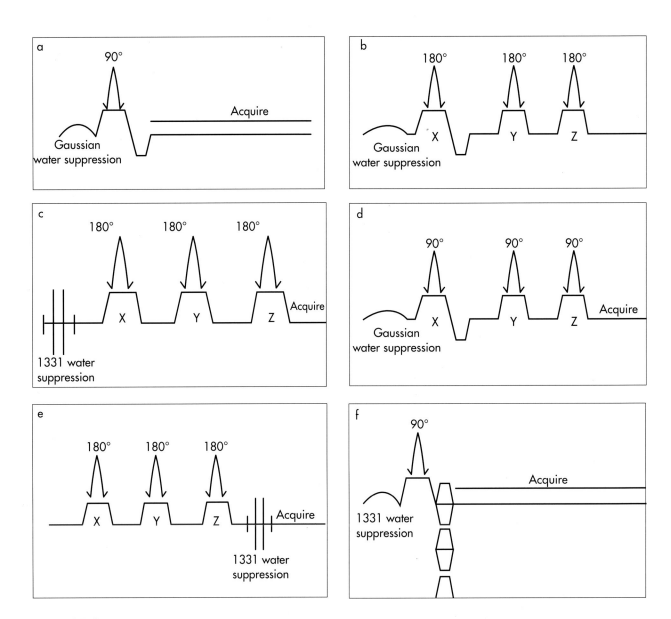

Figure 15.2

Sequence diagrams for several common spectroscopic
localization sequences: (a) DRESS; (b) PRESS;
(c) MESA; (d) STEAM; (e) ISIS; (f) 4DFT CSI.

Stimulated echo: STEAM

STEAM has been used to obtain shorter echo
times with good voxel definition.[23] STEAM uses
the property of a train of three identical radiofrequency pulses applied with three perpendicular
localization gradients within a time that is short
compared with T_2 to generate multiple signal
echoes. This has the disadvantage that the available signal is weaker, since it is split between
the multiple echoes formed. In fact, as much as
50% of the signal is lost in a stimulated echo

acquisition, which can be a serious difficulty for
observing weak metabolite species. However,
the advantage of being able to operate at shorter
echo times and detect metabolites that have
short T_2 or that have a highly modulated signal
at longer echo times may often outweigh this
disadvantage (Fig. 15.2d).

Another potential advantage of the sequence is
that the magnetization is stored in the longitudinal
direction (aligned with the magnet field) during
the period between the second and third pulses,
which means that T_2 losses do not occur. Instead,

the signals undergo T_1 changes with characteristically much longer T_1 times. The stimulated echo sequence may also be sensitive to diffusion and temperature effects—which can be either a problem or a solution, depending on the results desired! Interpretation of STEAM spectra must always take into account the complicated nature of the acquisition process.

ISIS

Another sequence used to achieve localization with very short echo times is ISIS.[24,25] ISIS uses combinations of three inversion pulses, which have the effect of restricting the signal to the desired voxel but leaving the signal in the Z direction and thus not suffering T_2 losses. A broadband binomial readout radiofrequency pulse with water-suppression capability can then read the signal from the region of interest (Fig. 15.2e).

ISIS requires a minimum of eight phase cycles to localize the signal, which makes shimming difficult (normally single-shot methods are preferred), and relies on accurate signal additions and subtractions, placing high demands on system stability and dynamic range. Other techniques have been proposed that leave the magnetization along the Z direction using many radiofrequency pulses,[25] which can localize within a single shot; however, these techniques are extremely difficult to calibrate and use in practice.

Despite these problems, ISIS does provide a way to access spectra at very short echo times, and thus has an important role to play.

Chemical shift imaging

All the localization schemes described so far only provide information from a single voxel located at the intersection of the three planes. Using phase-encoding strategies adopted from MR imaging, it is possible to encode information from multiple voxels simultaneously.[26] One, two or three dimensions of phase encoding may be applied. Data are transformed using up to a four-dimensional Fourier transform to extract chemical shift information from multiple positions. This is extremely efficient, providing many voxels in times usually only slightly longer than single-voxel techniques. The advantage is similar to that achieved with 3D techniques in MR imaging compared with 2D planar techniques. Each phase-encoding application acts as a signal average

(Fig. 15.2f). Another advantage of CSI is that the data may be retrospectively shifted to make the voxels align with tissues of interest, e.g. a lesion (this is a property of the Fourier transform, which allows data to be shifted using a phase change). A potential problem with CSI is the wraparound of high-intensity lipid signal from the scalp onto the data set. To prevent this, CSI is often combined with a voxel localization method such as PRESS or STEAM to restrict acquired signals to within the brain only.

In order for CSI to work effectively, extremely high field homogeneity must be maintained over the entire region from which data is being acquired. Usually this requirement is not met at the edges of the region, and so many spectra suffer from severe distortion, making quantification very difficult. Spatially dependent eddy currents also provide a technical obstacle to CSI, although this problem is less severe with newer-generation shielded gradients.

The vast quantity of data generated with CSI techniques make management, analysis and interpretation of CSI spectra a daunting challenge in the clinical setting. Before embarking on a CSI study, it is always worth considering whether the required information may be achieved more reliably using a pair of high-quality single voxels located in the appropriate regions. CSI, however, promises to be the localization technique of choice for the future when software and hardware advances allow the method to be applied rapidly and reproducibly.

Acquisition and analysis methodology

A typical proton spectroscopic experiment includes the following steps, each of which must be performed accurately if a spectrum with high resolution and high signal-to-noise ratio is to be successfully acquired. Many of the newer software packages automate most of these processes to simplify the procedure for the user. In fact, technologists and radiographers now routinely acquire in vivo spectra.

Voxel positioning

The first and most obvious task is to locate the spectroscopic voxel in the correct location within

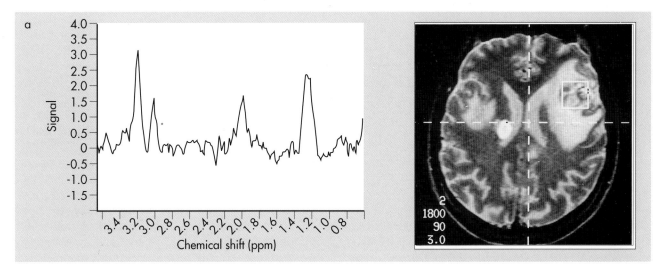

a

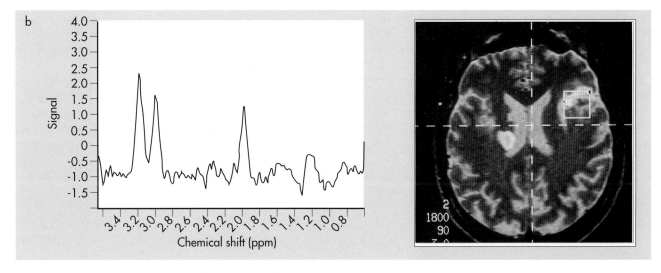

b

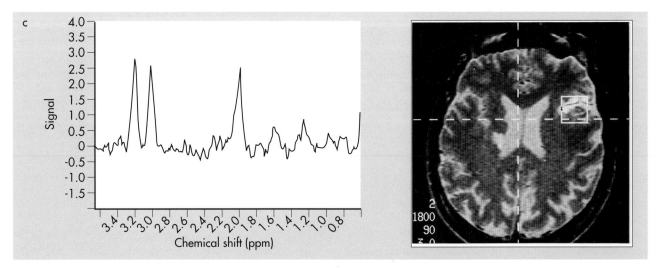

c

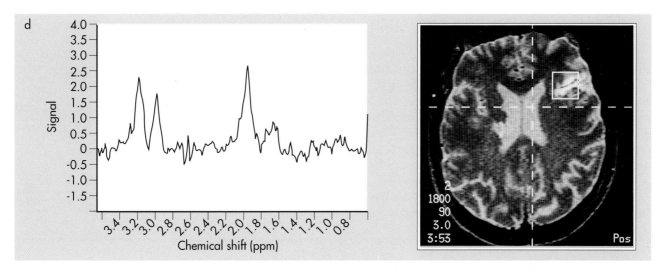

d

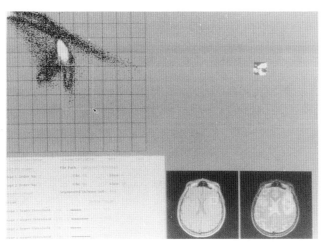

e

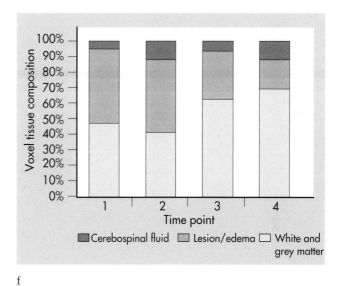

f

Figure 15.3

(a–d) Axial T_2-weighted MR images (TR/TE = 1800/90 ms) and proton spectra (TR/TE = 1600/135 ms) from an AIDS patient with a probable toxoplasmosis lesion 0, 29, 77 and 97 days after receiving anti-toxoplasmosis therapy. (e) Result of a scatter plot image segmentation procedure[45] from high-resolution 3 mm slice proton-density- and T_2-weighted images acquired through the voxel. (f) Relative calculated volumes of tissue contained within the voxel at the four different time points. It can be seen that the proportion of lesion reduces relative to normal tissue within the voxel over time. Contamination by CSF remains relatively constant at 3–5%. (From Paley et al.[27])

the brain. This may actually be quite difficult because of the large size of the voxel, which might include white matter, gray matter and cerebrospinal fluid (CSF) as well as lesion or abnormal tissue. It is obviously vital to obtain as 'pure' a voxel as possible. It is usually much easier to acquire good spectra if the voxel can be located to avoid contamination with lipid from the scalp or from pulsing CSF in the ventricles. Regions of the brain with large magnetic susceptibility variations, such as close to the sinuses, should also be avoided if possible.

A useful strategy that helps identify tissue included within a voxel is to acquire a set of high-resolution, thin-slice images through the region in which the voxel is to be placed. The position of the voxel is then displayed in each slice, and the images are sequentially reviewed until the best compromise position is found to maximize inclusion of the tissue of interest. Using image segmentation techniques, it is possible to quantify the composition of the spectroscopic voxel, which aids interpretation (Fig. 15.3).[27,28] This is particularly important in the case of lesions that may change composition with time or in response to treatment.

Shimming

Adjustment of the magnetic field homogeneity over the voxel is probably the most time-consuming aspect of an in vivo spectroscopy experiment, and usually represents the largest source of variation in the final result. Shimming is performed by repeatedly acquiring a signal from the voxel of interest, adjusting one of the field correction terms (typically X, Y, Z and Z_2 terms), and comparing the signal with the previous value until a maximum is achieved. The process is then iterated for each term until a final maximum value is obtained.

Water suppression

Most MR scanners have a limited range of amplitude over which they can successfully digitize the signal. In order to adjust the range for the weak metabolite signals, it is necessary to remove the much larger water signal, which dominates the in vivo spectrum. There are three main techniques used to suppress water.

Gaussian chemical shift selective pulses (CHESS pulses[29])

A narrowband pulse (usually around 50 Hz bandwidth) that only saturates the water pulse is applied prior to the localization sequence.

Binomial pulse sequences (e.g. 1331 pulse[30])

This sequence of radiofrequency pulses does not excite the abundant water peak, but only the metabolites of interest, again by having a specific spectral response function.

Use of inversion recovery and echo times[31]

The inversion time in a sequence with a preparatory inversion pulse may be adjusted so that the signal from brain water is minimized. This method is of limited applicability, since many of the metabolites of interest have T_1 times similar to those of the brain water. Use of long echo times (typically 405 ms) may also help to suppress water, since brain metabolites in general have longer T_2 times than water in the brain.

Radiofrequency calibration

Since the localization techniques described above typically use multiple radiofrequency pulses, it is critical that the amplitudes are carefully adjusted to minimize the production of artifactual signal during the data collection period. This is usually achieved by monitoring the signal as each pulse is varied in turn, and measuring the received signal. The signal strength is optimized by adjusting the amplitude of the pulses.

Averaging

In order to improve the signal-to-noise ratio from weak metabolites, it is usual to acquire multiple signals and average them together. This is based on the fact that the signal adds up directly, whereas the detected noise, being a random process, only adds up as the square root of the number of averages. Thus a 256-average spectrum has $\sqrt{256} = 16$ times better signal-to-noise ratio than a single signal acquisition.

Fourier transformation

In order to calculate the chemical shift data from the acquired time signal, it is necessary to perform a Fourier transformation. The time-dependent signal may be filtered to improve the signal-to-noise ratio by attenuating the noisier data acquired at later times relative to the peak signal prior to transformation. This method has the result of slightly degrading the resolution and thus producing a more blurred version of the spectrum. For chemical shift imaging, multiple Fourier transforms are required for each encoded spatial direction as well as the chemical shift direction.

Phasing

The data is actually detected as two components known as real and imaginary channels or in-phase and quadrature. Quadrature data is essentially two components of the signal shifted in phase by 90°, which provide information on whether the signal is above or below the resonance frequency. When the data has been transformed, it is usually at some arbitrary phase angle and so it is necessary to correct it to zero phase. This is achieved by multiplying each point in the spectrum by a simple mathematical factor derived from the sine and cosine of the phase angle. The spectrum is adjusted until the peaks appear as 'absorption mode' or real spectra. Although this is often seen as a qualitative step, it is possible to perform this using mathematical techniques that are not subjective.

Higher-order corrections are sometimes required to take account of frequency-dependent phase errors across the spectrum. In general, it is best to try and optimize the hardware and sequences so that these higher-order phase shifts are not introduced in the first place.

A useful way of phase-correcting errors introduced by eddy currents is to use the phase of a water spectrum acquired prior to the spectral acquisition. A similar phase multiplication technique is used. This method of course relies on the patient not moving between acquisition of the reference and the spectrum of interest.

Baseline correction

After phasing, it may be apparent that the spectrum is not sitting on a flat baseline, which makes quantification of spectral areas impossible.

This may be due to the effects of incomplete water suppression or to residual eddy current effects. A number of ways have been devised to reduce baseline artifacts. Many of these are semiqualitative, relying on the user to indicate estimates of where the baseline is situated (e.g. cubic spline fits). Other methods rely on low pass filter to produce a baseline correction from the data itself.

Curve fitting

Once the spectrum has been correctly phased it is possible to extract information of metabolite concentrations or peak ratios depending on the method used for acquisition. This may be achieved using simple numerical integration of the area under each spectral line. More sophisticated techniques use fitting of a model spectrum, usually consisting of Lorentzian or Gaussian lineshapes placed at the same frequency and with approximately the same amplitude and width as the spectral peaks. By adjusting these parameters and minimizing the least squares error between the model and the data, a best-fit spectrum is achieved (Fig. 15.4). Areas of the

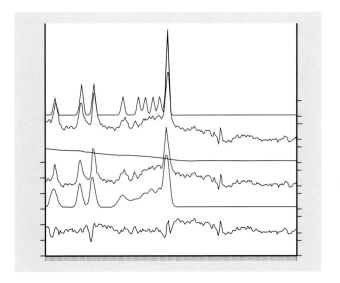

Figure 15.4

Curve fit of STEAM spectrum ($TR/TE/TM$ = 5000/20/30 ms) from an AIDS patient showing (top to bottom) the model spectrum, raw spectrum, low-pass-filtered baseline, baseline-corrected spectrum, fitted spectrum and the difference. (Reproduced, with permission, from Paley et al.[28])

peaks can then be calculated from the theoretically known area of the line. Of course, care must be taken to ensure that the theoretical model is a good representation of the data, otherwise the fit will be meaningless.

Relaxation time corrections

As mentioned in the introduction, proton spectroscopy is complicated by the fact that relaxation processes modify the spectral intensities, so that absolute concentration measurements cannot be made directly. Both changes in the number of molecules contributing to the signal and changes in relaxation times with disease complicate interpretation. This may be minimized by operating at a short echo time TE to minimize T_2 losses and at a long repeat time to minimize T_1 effects. However, spectra acquired on whole body systems are never completely free of relaxation time effects.

Attempts have been made to estimate the relaxation times in vivo to allow the interpretation of extended-TE spectra. However, these attempts are usually subject to large errors because of the extended time required to obtain multiple points on the relaxation curves. Also, it has to be realized that, as with MR imaging, the optimal 'contrast' between two metabolites in a clinical condition may not be found under fully relaxed conditions.

Absolute signal quantification

If fully relaxed short-TE spectra are acquired and an internal or external reference substance of known concentration is used then it is possible to estimate absolute concentrations of metabolites.

(See earlier chapter for more details of the problems involved.) Absolute measurements require careful control of all correction factors, and published results should be treated with due caution. Ratio data, although less informative, are probably more reliable at this stage of development, and should always be published and studied together with absolute measurements.

Measurements in control subjects

Without knowing the range of values to be expected in healthy control subjects and how these change with location in the brain and over time, it is meaningless to try and infer useful information about disease processes. Establishment of a control database is obviously of the highest importance for the advancement of human brain spectroscopy.

Spatial distribution

The spatial distribution of metabolites within the brain is of vital interest to clinicians who are trying to relate physical characteristics of the disease with behavioural, neurological and neuropsychological performance.[32] Table 15.2 gives results from voxels located in the parieto-occipital region from male control subjects measured at the Middlesex Hospital. These results tie in closely with those found in a recent multicenter trial.[33] Attempts have been made to characterize the spatial distribution of metabolites in the normal brain using CSI.[34] However, owing to the presence

Table 15.2 Typical values of metabolite ratios for control subjects using a spin echo localized sequence with $TR/TE = 1600/135$ ms

Middlesex site[33]		NA/Cr	NA/Cho	Cho/Cr
Parieto-occipital	$n = 49$ males	2.41 ± 0.37	2.45 ± 0.41	1.01 ± 0.23
Multicenter trial[45]				
Parieto-occipital	$n = 151$	2.16 ± 0.41	2.68 ± 0.56	0.81 ± 0.51
Basal ganglia	$n = 119$	1.87 ± 0.54	1.94 ± 0.63	0.95 ± 0.19

of some of the artifacts explained previously, these measurements are subject to large errors, especially in the periphery of the brain. The standard deviations of the multicenter trial results depended on how 'expert' the sites involved were at proton spectroscopy, illustrating the need for careful experimental technique. New automatic procedures may help reduce this 'expert' effect in future.[35] It has been shown by several groups that the NA/Cr ratio is markedly reduced in the cerebellum compared with the cortex.[36]

Age distribution

A number of published studies record how the NA/Cr ratio increases with maturation of an infant, reaches a plateau after a few years, typically at age 2, and perhaps shows a slight decline into old age.[13,37] NA/Cho ratio shows a similar behavior, whilst Cho/Cr remains relatively constant.

Sex distribution

Little work has yet been published looking at differences in metabolite ratios or concentrations between the sexes, although differences in brain weight and volume are well established. A multi-center trial recently found no significant difference between sexes for any metabolite ratios, but relatively high standard deviation due to intersite differences.[34]

Clinical applications

This section focuses on some of our results using proton spectroscopy in HIV infection/AIDS, and provides a brief summary of the work of other groups in further clinical applications of proton spectroscopy to the brain.

HIV/AIDS

In many ways, HIV infection and AIDS are ideal for study by proton spectroscopy. The patient group is well defined and relatively homogeneous in terms of age distribution and sex. In addition, many natural history studies have found patients to be cooperative and willing to return for repeat studies. The disease process occurs over an extended length of time (typically 10 years in asymptomatic mode), and so can be monitored throughout this period. Changes in the brain also tend to be of a diffuse nature, so that precise spatial analysis is not essential. Various markers of disease progression such as CD4 cell counts or β-microglobulin allow the prediction of disease progression when effects are likely to be observed, so that the frequency of monitoring can be increased appropriately.

Neurological disease is found in 30–40% of all AIDS patients, and this frequency is increasing as treatment for other complications such as *Pneumocystis carinii* pneumonia (PCP) have improved survival. The complication is that few, if any, neurological effects are observed during the latent period and most of the AIDS illnesses are contracted rapidly in the last 2–3 years following breakdown of the immune system.[38,39]

One of the aims of our investigation was to establish whether proton spectroscopy could be used as an early predictor for the onset of AIDS-related neurological disease, necessary for therapeutic and epidemiological purposes.

Preliminary reports[40,41] suggested that the NA/Cr ratio was reduced in neurologically impaired AIDS patients. In addition, direct neuronal counts following post-mortem examination of the brain indicated up to 35% loss in neuronal density in AIDS patients.[42,43] Our study attempted to investigate early-stage disease in a cohort consisting of an uninfected control group of low-risk and high-risk (of HIV infection) volunteers, asymptomatic HIV-infected volunteers, and immune-suppressed patients with AIDS-defining diagnoses.

Figure 15.5 shows typical $TR/TE = 1600/135$ ms spectra acquired from a 33-year-old male control subject and a 30-year-old male AIDS patient, showing characteristic changes with disease. The NA/Cr ratio is markedly reduced and the Cho/Cr ratio slightly increased in the AIDS patients.

Table 15.3 illustrates a summary of measurements for various patient groups. It can be seen that the most abnormal ratios are found for those patients with definite neurological signs, suggesting that proton spectroscopy may prove to be a sensitive marker of neurological status.[44–48]

MR spectroscopic abnormalities have also been identified with abnormal changes in signal from the white matter, with or without atrophy seen on MR imaging. These changes are referred to as HIV encephalopathy, and are thought to be a direct result of CNS infection by the human immunodeficiency virus itself. Changes in the spectra with gross atrophy of the brain that have been shown in late-stage disease[44] are not as highly correlated with spectral abnormalities as with HIVE.

Proton spectroscopy appears to offer good prospects in terms of monitoring the neuroprotective effects of drug therapies. Unfortunately, the drugs currently in use appear to have only short-term palliative effects.[49] A double-blinded study of

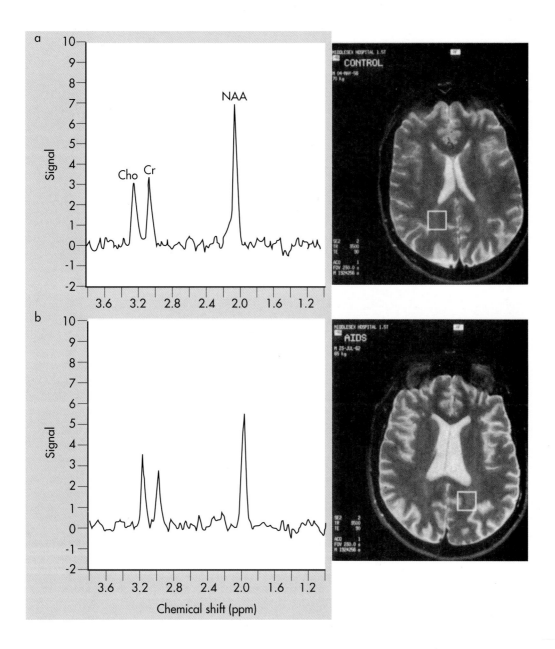

Figure 15.5

(a) Proton spectrum (*TR/TE* = 1600/135 ms, 256 acquisitions) and scout MR image (*TR/TE* = 3500/90 ms) showing the position of the volume of interest in a healthy 34-year-old man. The three main peaks are NAA, Cr/phosphocreatine (Cr) and total choline-containing compounds (Cho). (b) Proton spectrum and scout image (same parameters as (a)), obtained in a 30-year-old man with AIDS (CDC group IV). MR image shows cerebral atrophy and diffuse white matter changes of encephalopathy. There is a relative reduction of the NAA peak and a relative rise of the Cho peak when compared with the Cr peak. (Reproduced, with permission, from Chong et al.[45])

Table 15.3 Mean proton metabolite ratios compared with clinical, immunological and MRI classifications in HIV patients and normal controls

Group	n	NA/Cho	NA/Cr	Cho/Cr	NA/total
(a) Clinical classification of MRS results ($n = 92$)					
CDC II/III	22	2.21 ± 0.55	2.26 ± 0.23	1.08 ± 0.27	0.52 ± 0.04
CDC IV	70	1.94 ± 0.48	$*2.06 \pm 0.41$	1.10 ± 0.26	$*0.49 \pm 0.04$
(b) Immunological classification of MRS results ($n = 89$)					
CD4 > 200	18	2.39 ± 0.36	2.37 ± 0.28	1.01 ± 0.18	0.54 ± 0.02
CD4 < 200	71	$*1.89 \pm 0.47$	$*2.05 \pm 0.41$	1.13 ± 0.27	$*0.49 \pm 0.05$
(c) MRS in patients examined by a neurologist—focal lesions excluded ($n = 50$)					
No neuro signs	31	2.17 ± 0.44	2.25 ± 0.32	1.07 ± 0.23	0.52 ± 0.03
Neuro signs	19	$*1.67 \pm 0.40$	$*1.88 \pm 0.36$	1.19 ± 0.33	$*0.46 \pm 0.04$
Norm MRI – Neuro signs	19	2.29 ± 0.48	2.31 ± 0.26	1.05 ± 0.22	0.53 ± 0.03
Norm MRI + Neuro signs	6	1.90 ± 0.25	$*1.94 \pm 0.31$	1.04 ± 0.22	$*0.49 \pm 0.03$
Abn MRI – Neuro signs	12	1.98 ± 0.31	2.14 ± 0.39	1.01 ± 0.25	0.50 ± 0.03
Abn MRI + Neuro signs	13	$*1.56 \pm 0.42$	1.85 ± 0.39	1.25 ± 0.36	$*0.45 \pm 0.04$
(d) MRS results in patients with diffuse MRI abnormalities ($n = 70$)					
Normal MRI	36	2.25 ± 0.42	2.27 ± 0.33	1.03 ± 0.17	0.53 ± 0.04
Atrophy + WM change	15	$*1.61 \pm 0.37$	1.98 ± 0.28	$*1.27 \pm 0.29$	$*0.47 \pm 0.04$
Atrophy alone	14	1.98 ± 0.48	2.04 ± 0.49	1.07 ± 0.27	0.49 ± 0.05
WM change alone	5	1.73 ± 0.51	$*1.74 \pm 0.31$	1.07 ± 0.38	$*0.46 \pm 0.05$
(e) MRS results in the control group					
Control	23	2.54 ± 0.37	2.44 ± 0.38	0.98 ± 0.19	0.55 ± 0.03

$*p < 0.05$, corrected for multiple comparisons.

Zidovudine recently showed no significant change in metabolite ratios in early-stage disease between early and deferred use of the drug.[50]

It appears that the changes observed in HIV infection are not strictly alterations in neuronal density, since measurements indicate that in fact the T_2-relaxation time is increased in AIDS patients with abnormal MR imaging.[14]

Measurements in our cohort of HIV/AIDS patients suggest that the Cr resonance is stable over time on an absolute scale (ID Wilkinson, personal communication). Other groups have suggested from ^{31}P spectroscopy experiments that there is an overall loss in high-energy phosphates, including phosphocreatine, in AIDS.[51-53] These two observations appear to be contradictory unless there is a shift in equilibrium in the creatine kinase reaction

$$PCr^{2-} + Mg^{2+}.ADP^{3-} + H^+ \rightarrow Cr + Mg^{2+}.ATP^{4-}$$

Another important clinical problem in the management of AIDS patients is the timely diagnosis of toxoplasmosis (an inflammatory lesion) versus lymphoma (a tumor). Initial results seemed to indicate that, with short-TE spectra, toxoplasmosis gives rise to a large lipid peak and complete absence of other metabolites, whereas lymphoma typically yields a much increased Cho/Cr ratio. However, these results are not consistent, and atypical spectra are observed in many cases. A detailed analysis of the development of lesions over time might increase the ability to discriminate with proton spectroscopy, but this is usually impossible because of the necessity to provide the best treatment for each patient as soon as possible.

Other abnormalities observed in AIDS tend to be easier to discriminate with MR imaging. Progressive multifocal leukoencephalopathy (PML) has a characteristic spread through the white matter to the boundaries with the gray matter. Typical spectra often show lactate.[54]

Reports on small numbers of patients have indicated that the glutamate/glutamine and the myo-inositol regions may be early indicators in AIDS.[55,56] Our experience, again with relatively small numbers of patients, has not shown any statistically significant effects in this region or in the myo-inositol region, which has also been suggested as a marker for HIVE.[28]

In summary, proton spectroscopy has led to new insights into the development of neurological problems in AIDS, linking basic neuronal function with gross morphological and neurological status.[57] Monitoring of new neuroprotective agents will be an important task for future proton spectroscopy studies in AIDS, and preliminary data on reproducibility of spectroscopy in multicenter trials appears to hold promise in this respect.[58]

Multiple sclerosis (MS)

Unlike the diffuse processes often found in HIV infection, multiple sclerosis lesions are commonly focal, at least in the early phase of the disease. Lesions evolve and may disappear and/or reappear over a period of time. Thus tracking and monitoring individual lesions and establishing whether they are in the acute or chronic phase presents a major challenge to the clinical spectroscopist. In general, MS lesions are smaller than the localized spectroscopy voxel, resulting in considerable partial volume effects with normal brain tissue.

Despite these problems, many interesting studies have been published on multiple sclerosis. The general finding is a reduction in the NA/Cr ratio with increasing lesion age and an increase in lactate/Cr. Reversible changes in the NA/Cr ratio have been reported from acute MS lesions, which have been interpreted as illustrating that the neurons involved are not destroyed but are perhaps malfunctioning and that the spectral changes observed are changes in MR relaxation times rather than loss of cells.[59–61]

Peaks from lipids or protein macromolecules at 0.9 and 1.3 ppm have also been reported in short-*TE* spectra from MS lesions, which have been interpreted as reflecting myelin breakdown products.[13] This might provide further insight into the exact nature of the demyelination process when followed with time. One preliminary report has suggested the myo-inositol may be increased in multiple sclerosis lesions.[62]

Epilepsy

The major focus of proton spectroscopy has been in lateralization of the seizure focus in temporal lobe epilepsy.[63–67] Researchers have reported that the NA/Cr ratio is reduced in the damaged hippocampus. Combination of the spectroscopic data with quantitative T_2 imaging looks to be a promising method for presurgical planning.

As with MS, partial volume errors may cause considerable difficulty with acquisition and interpretation of spectra from epileptics. Additionally, the temporal lobe is difficult to shim, and thus well-resolved signals are hard to obtain. Motion of the patient, if fitting occurs during an examination, is an obvious problem. For this reason, a number of authors have used the ratio NA/(Cho + Cr), since it is not always possible to separate the choline and creatine resonances.

Parkinson's disease

Parkinson's disease is characterized by a progressive tremor and muscular problems that make controlled movement difficult or impossible. It is thought to be caused by degeneration of specific nerve cells with cell bodies located in the substantia nigra that lack dopamine (a transmitter of nerve impulses). Parkinson's disease has also been associated with increased iron in the basal ganglia, which would be expected to make shimming of proton spectra from this region difficult.

No significant reduction has been found in any of the metabolite ratios studied with the voxel sizes currently in use for voxels located within the corpus striatum. The NA/Cr ratio almost reached significant difference in a recent multicenter trial.[68] Future studies will concentrate on achieving sufficient sensitivity for more precise localization of small voxels within the substantia nigra.

Alzheimer's disease

Alzheimer's disease is the most common form of senile dementia; however, confirmation of the

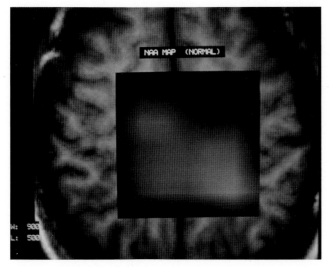

a

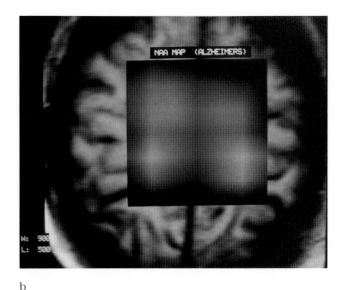

b

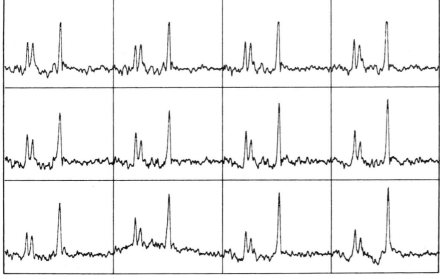

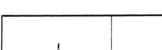

c

Figure 15.6

(a) Spectroscopic image formed from the NA resonance and overlaid on a transverse scout MR image for a control subject. The acquisition sequence was MESA-3D (TR/TE = 1500/270 ms, 8 × 8 matrix). The image has been interpolated to 64 × 64. (b) Raw data from central 3 × 4 voxels corresponding to (a). (c) Spectroscopic image of the NA resonance for an Alzheimer's patient. (Reproduced, with permission, from Paley et al.[72])

diagnosis is only possible at autopsy. A reliable method of diagnosing the disease during life would be very useful clinically. At post-mortem or with CT or MR imaging, cerebral atrophy is often observed, and so spectroscopic methods should take this complicating factor into account to avoid error. As with AIDS, the atrophic changes tend to be diffuse, although the frontal lobe is often implicated. Several theories implicate loss of metabolic choline in Alzheimer's disease, although this is typically at a much lower concentration than the choline compounds in membranes that dominate

the in vivo spectrum, and so is not observed directly.

A number of studies have shown a small but statistically significant reduction in the NA/Cr in the parietal lobe. CSI techniques have illustrated that changes in the frontal lobes appear to be the most severe.[69–72] Figures 15.6(a,b) illustrate maps of the N-acetyl resonance in a control subject and in a probable Alzheimer disease patient acquired using the MESA-3D sequence (TR/TE = 1500/270 ms, 8 × 8 matrix), showing relatively uniform distribution of NAA in both subjects. The fall-off at the edge of the

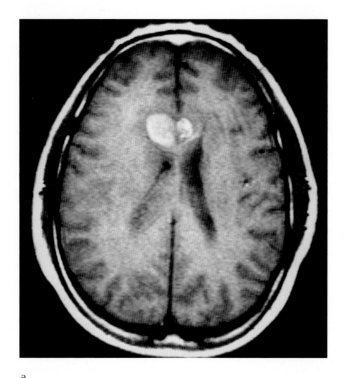

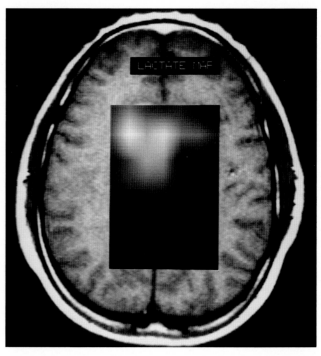

a   b

Figure 15.7

(a) T_1-weighted MR axial brain image ($TR/TE = 500/20$ ms) and (b) MESA-3D metabolite map ($TR/TE = 1500/270$ ms, 8×8 matrix) of lactate from a corresponding slice in the brain of a patient with a grade 2 astrocytoma. Good anatomical correlation of the lactate with the position of the astrocytoma is seen. (Reproduced, with permission, from Lampman et al.[22])

map is due to the shape of the localizing voxel applied concurrently with the phase-encoding localization scheme. Figure 15.6(c) illustrates the quality of the input data used to generate the map. The central 4×3 voxels are shown.

Primary and metastatic brain tumors

Improved diagnosis of tumor type, stage and response to various therapeutic regimens through characteristic spectral patterns has been a long sought after goal for proton spectroscopy of the brain. As with many other of the conditions described above, this has been frustrated by the heterogeneity exhibited by most lesions.[73–80] Typical spectral patterns include loss of NA (up to 100% relative to noise), increased Cho/Cr, and the appearance of lactate and/or lipid.

Figures 15.7(a,b) illustrate a T_1-weighted image ($TR/TE = 500/20$ ms) and MESA-3D metabolite map ($TR/TE = 1500/270$ ms, 8×8 matrix) of lactate from the brain of a patient with a grade 2 astrocytoma. Good anatomical correlation of the lactate with the position of the astrocytoma is seen.

Characteristic lipid peaks are also observed, often in the 'penumbra' of the lesion, perhaps reflecting peripheral breakdown of myelin. However, this is not always the case, and many lesions illustrate large lipid signals from their core region.

Hepatic encephalopathy

Reductions in myo-inositol and an increase in the Glx region have been found in spectra from the brains of patients with chronic hepatic encephalopathy.[81] myo-Inositol is an osmolyte found in the epithelial cells of the renal medulla and also in astrocytes.[82] Astrocytes are known to be the only cells capable of synthesizing glutamine. The changes observed in CHE have been interpreted as implying cell swelling.

Birth asphyxia

Birth asphyxia was one of the first clinical investigations carried out with in vivo ^{31}P spectroscopy.[83] The ratio of phosphocreatine to inorganic phosphate appears to correlate closely with outcome. Recent studies using proton spectroscopy have reported the appearance of lactate, which persists for many weeks after birth in asphyxiated infants. In addition, there is a reduction in the N-acetyl resonance relative to other metabolites, which presumably reflects neuronal loss or damage. Production of lactate is thought to result from anaerobic glycolysis, and the level of lactate does appear to correlate with outcome in preliminary studies.[84] If this observation is borne out then combined proton imaging and spectroscopy, with its increased sensitivity and ease of operation over ^{31}P spectroscopy, will provide a good method for monitoring children with birth asphyxia and predicting clinical outcome. Brain damage after near-drowning produces effects similar to birth asphyxia.

Stroke

Stroke patients may benefit from early diagnosis and intervention with neuroprotective agents. However, the practicality of putting stroke patients into a high-field MRI/S system within a few minutes or hours of the event provides a daunting but not insurmountable challenge.[85–89]

Proton spectral changes in stroke include an early drop in the N-acetyl resonance, which continues over the first one to two weeks. Also, lactate becomes elevated and may remain so for several weeks. It is not yet fully known if the drop in the NA resonance is partly due to changes in T_2 as well as neuronal loss. Some workers have reported seeing an increase in the NA signal after the patient has stabilized, suggesting that T_2 changes may be significant.

However, diffusion-weighted MR imaging also reflects changes rapidly after the stroke event, and, since it provides high spatial resolution, may turn out to be the most sensitive method for mapping damaged and 'viable' tissue.

SLE

Systemic lupus erythematosus (SLE) is a relatively common neuropsychiatric condition (1/2000 females in the USA) in which up to 75% of patients have nervous system involvement. It is a multisystem autoimmune disorder. Clinical findings include stroke, ischemic episodes, aseptic meningitis, movement disorders and various neuropathies. Patients are predominantly female (1 : 9, M : F), and often suffer from psychosis and affective disorders and have a high incidence of migrainous headaches. The pathogenesis of the condition is uncertain, and may result from vasculitis, thrombosis, auto-antibodies to neurons, and drugs used to treat the disease.

Using long-TE spectra (TR/TE = 1600/135 ms), the NA/(NA + Cho + Cr) ratio in parieto-occipital white matter in 42 patients has been shown to be significantly reduced compared with 14 female controls.[90] Using short-TE spectroscopy ($TR/TE/TM$ = 5000/10/30 ms) it appears that only voxels located in lesions with high signal on T_2-weighted MRI produced significantly reduced NA/Cr ratios from controls.[91]

Coronary artery bypass graft

Patients undergoing coronary artery bypass graft (CABG) surgery are often reported to have neurological deficit after surgery. This is thought to be due in part to the formation of micro-emboli during bypass, causing cerebral ischemia. A study of changes in the N-acetyl resonance may help shed light on whether this is due to neuronal loss or reversible damage. As with stroke, this is a difficult patient group to investigate immediately post-surgery, although some success has been achieved using MRI. A definitive study of proton spectroscopy in CABG has not yet been published, and the spectral characteristics are as yet unknown.

Future developments

In this section a number of suggestions will be made for system and technique developments that may improve the ease, reliability and sensitivity with which proton spectra are acquired in future.

One-touch spectroscopy protocols where the technologist simply chooses the appropriate timing, dimensions and position for the voxel(s) from the _appropriate locator images, and the system performs all other operations up to and including data analysis, will undoubtedly be possible. Such software is already available in preliminary forms from some of the major MRI/S manufacturers, but a number of outstanding problems such as automated baseline correction remain to be adequately addressed.

Automated shimming of multiple regions for multislice CSI experiments will require additional dynamic control of the shim hardware. Dedicated spectroscopy head coils have already been used, but the use of phased array and intracavity coils to improve signal-to-noise ratio remains in its infancy. Improved system stability (digital rf, rf feedback, reduced eddy currents and improved filtering) is an onward quest for the manufacturers.

Absolute quantification of metabolites will require detailed systematic analysis of the sources of error due to metabolite relaxation times, J-modulation effects, tissue compartmentation within a chosen voxel, rf coil sensitivity and motional artifacts, amongst others.

Mapping software that can rapidly produce metabolic images from CSI data will aid interpretation by nonspectroscopists, and, although these must be interpreted carefully, will undoubtedly be the way that spectroscopic data are presented in the future.

As mentioned in the introduction, an improved knowledge of concentrations and relaxation times in control and disease states will take many years to assemble. Multicenter trials using common protocols may help to improve this situation rapidly, and preliminary studies carried out so far are very encouraging in this respect.

Development of spectroscopic intracellular contrast agents and targeted labels have received little attention from the pharmaceutical manufacturers. It would seem to make sense in certain applications to shorten the T_1 relaxation times of the metabolites by known and equal amounts so that data could be acquired more quickly or averaged further within a given time. Cross-relaxation and dynamic polarization techniques may also provide a way forward in terms of absolute spectroscopic sensitivity.

current-generation hardware, it is a stable method technically as assessed from repeat measurements of volunteers, but large patient groups are usually required to show statistically significant changes (typically $n \geqslant 30$).

Long-echo-time spectra ($TE \geqslant 135$ ms) are useful for studies of background white matter, and are much easier to quantify than short-TE spectra, where overlapping peaks with increased linewidths and complex modulation patterns make interpretation much more difficult. However, short-TE spectra provide access to a number of biochemicals with short relaxation times, such as protein macromolecules, glutamate/glutamine, and myo- and scyllo-inositol, which provide a new window into the biochemistry of the brain.

The N-acetyl resonance as a marker that reflects neuronal viability will, it is hoped, prove to be a very useful tool in following the progress of patients on drug trials. This is particularly exciting for application to neurodegenerative diseases such as AIDS, where new combination therapies of antiretroviral drugs are just entering clinical trial.

The choline resonance provides a handle on rapid cell division/gliosis/astrocytosis, and the Cho/Cr ratio together with the lactate/Cr ratio looks promising for tumor grading if the partial volume problem can be successfully overcome through smaller voxels or image segmentation correction schemes.

Absolute concentration measurements are now being reported by a number of groups using either internal or external references. This appears to be a good step forward, but great care must be taken to avoid systematic errors and misinterpretation of changes between sites. It is probably wise at this time for authors of proton spectroscopy papers to present in addition sufficient data to enable all the standard metabolite ratios to be calculated.

In summary, proton spectroscopy is providing unique insights into in vivo biochemistry in a wide range of important clinical conditions. Much work remains to elucidate the subtleties and dynamics of spectral changes in normal and disease states, but it is clear that proton spectroscopy will develop into a very useful addition to the armoury of the practising neuroscientists of the 21st century.

Conclusions

Proton spectroscopy is now straightforward to apply in the clinical setting, and may easily be performed routinely by radiographers or technologists. With

Acknowledgements

I should like to acknowledge the help of my colleagues and former colleagues who helped in preparation of this chapter. These include Iain Wilkinson, W 'Kling' Chong, Roger Chinn, Margaret Hall-Craggs, Mike Harrison, the 'spectro-radiographers' at The Middlesex Hospital, UCLHT, London, England, and Dave Lampman, Jim Murdoch and Jim McNally at the Picker Clinical

Science Center, Cleveland, OH, USA. I should also like to acknowledge financial support from the Medical Research Council of Great Britain and to Siemens AG, Germany, in particular Rolf Sauter and his team, for their support of our proton spectroscopy research.

References

1. Gadian DG, *NMR and its application to living systems.* Clarendon Press, Oxford, 1982.

2. Behar KL, den Hollander JA, Stronski M et al, Detection of cerebral lactate by 1H NMR at relatively low field strengths (1.9 T). *Proc Natl Acad Sci USA* 1984; **81**: 2517.

3. Bottomley PA, Edelstein WA, Foster TH, Adams WA, In vivo solvent-suppressed localized hydrogen nuclear magnetic resonance spectroscopy: a window to metabolism? *Proc Natl Acad Sci USA* 1985; **82**: 2148–52.

4. Aue WP, Muller S, Cross TA, Seelig J, Volume selective excitation. A novel approach to topical NMR. *J Magn Reson* 1984; **56**: 350–4.

5. Prichard JW, Shulman RG, NMR spectroscopy of brain metabolism in vivo. *Annu Rev Neurosci.* 1986; **9**: 61–85.

6. Frahm J, Michaelis T, Merboldt KD et al, Improvements in localized proton NMR spectroscopy of human brain. Water suppression, short echo times and 1 ml resolution. *J Magn Reson* 1990; **90**: 464–73.

7. Bottomley PA, The trouble with spectroscopy papers. *Radiology* 1991; **181**: 344–50.

8. Cady EB, *Clinical magnetic resonance spectroscopy.* Plenum Press, New York, 1990.

9. Tofts PS, Wray E, A critical assessment of methods of measuring metabolite concentrations by NMR spectroscopy. *NMR Biomed* 1988; **1**: 1–10.

10. Birken DL, Oldendorf WH, N-acetyl-L-aspartic acid: a literature review of a compound prominent in 1H-NMR spectroscopic studies of brain. *Neurosci Biobehav Rev* 1989; **13**: 23–31.

11. Wilman AH, Allen PS, Observing NAA via both its N-acetyl and its aspartate group in in-vivo proton magnetic resonance spectroscopy. *Abstracts 2nd Ann Mtg Soc Magn Reson, San Francisco, 1994*, 1192.

12. Koller KJ, Zaczek R, Coyle JT, N-acetyl aspartate glutamate. Regional levels in rat brain and the effects of brain lesions as determined by a new HPLC method. *J Neurochem* 1984; **43**: 1136–42.

13. Toft PB, Christiansen P, Pryds O et al, T1, T2 and concentrations of brain metabolites in neonates and adolescents estimated with H-1 MR spectroscopy. *J Magn Reson Imaging* 1994; **4**: 1–5.

14. Wilkinson ID, Paley M, Chong WK et al, Proton spectroscopy in HIV infection: relaxation times of cerebral metabolites. *Magn Reson Imaging* 1994; **12**: 951–7.

15. Michaelis T, Merboldt KD, Bruhn H et al, Absolute concentrations of metabolites in the adult human brain in vivo: quantification of localized proton MR spectra. *Radiology* 1993; **187**: 219–27.

16. Gyngell ML, Michaelis T, Horstermann D et al, Cerebral glucose is detectable by localized proton NMR spectroscopy in normal rat brain in vivo. *Magn Reson Med* 1991; **19**: 489–95.

17. Gruetter R, Rothman DL, Novonty EJ et al, Detection and assignment of the glucose signal in 1H NMR difference spectra of the human brain. *Magn Reson Med* 1992; **27**: 183–8.

18. Prost RW, Li SJ, Erickson SE, Direct detection of glutamate/glutamine in-vivo. *Abstracts 2nd Ann Mtg Soc Magn Reson, San Francisco, 1994*, 307.

19. Davie CA, Hawkins CP, Barker GJ et al, Detection of myelin breakdown products by proton magnetic resonance spectroscopy (letter). *Lancet* 1993; **341**: 630–1.

20. Bottomley PA, Foster TB, Darrow RD, Depth resolved surface-coil spectroscopy (DRESS) for in vivo 1H, 31P and 13C NMR. *J Magn Reson* 1984; **59**: 338–42.

21. Bottomley PA, US Patent 4 480 228, 1984.

22. Lampman D, Murdoch JB, Paley M, In vivo proton metabolite maps using the MESA-3D technique. *Magn Reson Med* 1991; **18**: 169–80.

23. Frahm J, Merboldt KD, Hanicke W, *J Magn Reson* 1987; **72**: 502.

24. Ordidge RJ, Conelly A, Lohman JAB, Image-selected in vivo spectroscopy (ISIS). A new technique for spatially selective NMR spectroscopy. *J Magn Reson*, 1986; **66**: 283–94.

25. Luyten PR, den Hollander JA, ¹H MR spatially resolved spectroscopy of human tissues in situ. *Magn Reson Imaging* 1986; **4**: 237–9.

26. Brown TR, Kincaid BM, Ugurbil K, NMR chemical shift imaging in three dimensions. *Proc Natl Acad Sci USA* 1982; **79**: 3523–6.

27. Paley M, Wilkinson ID, Chong WK, Hall-Craggs MA, Image segmentation for correction of spectroscopic partial volume effects. *Abstracts 11th Ann Mtg Soc Magn Reson Med, Berlin, 1992*, 4318.

28. Paley M, Wilkinson ID, Chong WK et al, Short echo time proton spectroscopy in AIDS. *Abstracts 12th Ann Mtg Soc Magn Reson Med, New York, 1993*, 1561.

29. Haase A, Frahm J, Hanicke W, Matthaei D, CHESS. *Phys Med Biol* 1985; **30**: 341.

30. Hore PJ, Solvent suppression in Fourier transform nuclear magnetic resonance. *J Magn Reson* 1983; **55**: 283–300.

31. Bydder GM, Young IR, MR imaging: clinical use of the inversion recovery sequence. *J Comput Aided Tomogr* 1985; **9**: 659–75.

32. Hennig J, Pfister H, Ernst T, Absolute concentration of brain metabolites by localised in vivo proton spectroscopy. *Eurospin Q* 1991; **27**: 31–3.

33. Sauter R, Cerebral single volume proton spectroscopy on healthy volunteers. A multicenter pilot study, *Abstracts 12th Ann Mtg Soc Magn Reson Med, New York, 1993*, 1531.

34. Schneider M, Kolem H, Wicklow K et al, Evaluation of regional differences of the human brain in vivo by proton chemical shift imaging. *Abstracts 11th Ann Mtg Soc Magn Reson Med, Berlin, 1992*, 1926.

35. Webb PG, Napapon S, Kohler S et al, Automated single-voxel proton MRS: technical development and multisite verification. *Magn Reson Med* 1994; **31**: 365–73.

36. Frahm J, Bruhn HM, Gyngell ML et al, Localized proton NMR spectroscopy in different regions of the human brain in vivo. Relaxation times and concentrations of cerebral metabolites. *Magn Reson Med* 1989; **11**: 47–63.

37. Itoh S, Kimura H, Matsuda T et al, Evaluation of neuron population in human brain in normals aging using H1-MRS. *Abstracts 11th Ann Mtg Soc Magn Reson Med, Berlin, 1992*, 1927.

38. Harrison MJG, McAllister RH, Neurologic complications of HIV infection. In: *Kass handbook of infectious diseases* (ed JS Porterfield) 343–60. Chapman and Hall, 1991.

39. American Academy of Neurology AIDS task force, Nomenclature and research case definitions for neurologic manifestations of human immunodeficiency type 1 (HIV-1) infection. *Neurology* 1991; **4**: 778–85.

40. Menon DK, Baudouin CJ, Tomlinson D, Hoyle C, Proton MR spectroscopy and imaging of the brain in AIDS: evidence of neuronal loss in regions that appear normal with imaging. *J Comput Assist Tomogr* 1990; **14**: 882–5.

41. Menon DK, Ainsworth JG, Cox IJ et al, Proton MR spectroscopy of the brain in AIDS dementia complex. *J Comput Assist Tomogr* 1992; **16**: 538–42.

42. Everall IP, Luthbert PJ, Lantos PL, Neuronal loss in the frontal cortex in HIV infection. *Lancet* 1991; **337**: 1119–21.

43. Everall IP, Luthbert PJ, Lantos PL, Neuronal number and volume alterations in the neocortex of HIV infected individuals. *Abstracts 4th Int Conf. on the Neuroscience of HIV Infection: Basic and Clinical Frontiers, Amsterdam, 1992*, 71.

44. Chong WK, Paley M, Wilkinson ID et al, Cerebral ¹H-MRS in HIV infection and AIDS. *Abstracts 11th Ann Mtg Soc Magn Reson Med, Berlin, 1992*, 1942.

45. Chong WK, Sweeney BE, Wilkinson ID et al, Proton spectroscopy of the brain in HIV infection: correlation with clinical, immunologic and MR imaging findings. *Radiology* 1993; **188**: 119–24.

46. Chong WK, Paley M, Wilkinson ID et al, Localized cerebral proton magnetic resonance spectroscopy in HIV infection and AIDS. *AJNR* 1994; **15**: 21–5.

47. Meyerhoff DJ, MacKay S, Bachman L et al, Reduced neuronal marker (*N*-acetylaspartate) in HIV-infection. *Abstracts 11th Ann Mtg Soc Magn Reson Med, Berlin, 1992,* 1939.

48. Meyerhoff DJ, MacKay S, Bachman L et al, Reduced brain *N*-acetylaspartate suggests neuronal loss in cognitively impaired human immunodeficiency virus seropositive individuals: in vivo ¹H magnetic resonance spectroscopic imaging. *Neurology* 1993; **43:** 509–15.

49. Wilkinson ID, Hall-Craggs MA, Chong WK, Increase in NA/Cr metabolite ratio following anti-retroviral drug therapy in AIDS: a case study. *Abstracts 12th Ann Mtg Soc Magn Reson Med, New York, 1993,* 1561.

50. Hall-Craggs MA, Williams I, Wilkinson ID, Proton spectroscopy in a cross-section of HIV positive asymptomatic patients receiving immediate compared with deferred Zidovudine. *Abstracts 2nd Ann Mtg Soc Magn Reson, San Francisco, 1994,* 303.

51. Deicken RF, Hubesch B, Jensen PC et al, Alterations in brain phosphate metabolite concentrations in patients with human immunodeficiency virus infection. *Arch Neurol* 1991; **48:** 203–9.

52. Bottomley PA, Hardy CJ, Cousins JP et al, AIDS dementia complex: brain high energy phosphate metabolite deficits. *Radiology* 1990; **176:** 407–11.

53. Bottomley PA, Cousins JP, Pendrey DL et al, Alzheimer dementia: quantification of energy metabolism and mobile phosphoesters with ³¹P spectroscopy. *Radiology* 1992; **183:** 695–9.

54. Chinn RJS, Wilkinson ID, Hall-Craggs MA et al, Spectroscopic tissue diagnosis of CNS mass lesions in HIV infection. *Abstracts 2nd Ann Mtg Soc Magn Reson, San Francisco, 1994,* 133.

55. Jarvick JG, Lenkinski RE, Grossman RI et al, Proton MR spectroscopy in HIV-infected patients: characterization of abnormalities with imaging and clinical correlation. *Radiology* 1991; **181**(supp): 211 (abst 701).

56. Laubenberger J, Hennig J, Haussinger D et al, Proton spectroscopy of the brain in HIV-infected patients. *Abstracts 11th Ann Mtg Soc Magn Reson Med, Berlin, 1992,* 758.

57. Alonso J, Cozzone P, Paley M et al, Single volume proton MR spectroscopy on patients with AIDS: multicenter pilot study. *Abstracts 79th Ann Mtg RSNA, Chicago, 1993,* 985.

58. Paley M, Chong WK, Wilkinson ID et al, Cerebrospinal fluid–intracranial volume ratio measurements in patients with HIV infection: CLASS image analysis technique. *Radiology* 1994; **190:** 879–86.

59. Van Hecke P, Marchal G, Johannik K et al, Human brain proton localized NMR spectroscopy in multiple sclerosis. *Magn Reson Med* 1991; **18:** 199–206.

60. Arnold DL, Matthews PM, Francis G, Antel J, Proton MR spectroscopy in the evaluation of multiple sclerosis in humans in vivo: assessment of the load of the disease. *Abstracts 8th Ann Mtg Soc Magn Reson Med, Amsterdam, 1989,* 455.

61. De Stefano N, Francis G, Antel JP, Arnold D, Reversible decreases of *N*-acetylaspartate in the brain of patients with relapsing remitting multiple sclerosis. *Abstracts 12th Ann Mtg Soc Magn Reson Med, New York, 1993,* 280.

62. Zhu G, Allen PS, Koopmans R et al, A marked elevation of inositol in MS lesions. *Abstracts 2nd Ann Mtg Soc Magn Reson, San Francisco, 1994,* 1948.

63. Connelly A, Jackson GD, Duncan JS et al, The contribution of ¹H MRS to the presurgical assessment of temporal lobe pathology in patients with intractable epilepsy. *Abstracts 12th Ann Mtg Soc Magn Reson Med, New York, 1993,* 1463.

64. Matthews PM, Andermann F, Arnold D, A proton magnetic resonance spectroscopy study of focal epilepsy in humans. *Neurology* 1990; **40:** 958–9.

65. Layer G, Traber F, Muller LU et al, Spectroscopic imaging. A new MR technique in the diagnosis of epilepsy? *Radiology* 1993; **33:** 178–84.

66. Matthews PM, Andermann F, Arnold DL, A proton magnetic resonance study of focal epilepsy in humans. *Neurology* 1990; **40:** 985–9.

67. Jackson G, Achten R, Vainio P et al, Single volume proton MR spectroscopy in patients with intractable temporal lobe epilepsy: a multicenter pilot study. *Abstracts 12th Ann Mtg Soc Magn Reson Med, New York, 1993,* 1567.

68. Holshouser B, Komu M, Moller H et al, Single volume proton MR spectroscopy on patients with Parkinson's disease: a multicenter pilot

study. *Abstracts 12th Ann Mtg Soc Magn Reson Med, New York, 1993*, 235.

69. Klunk WE, Panchalingham K, Moossy J et al, *N*-acetyl-L-aspartate and other amino acid metabolites in Alzheimer's disease brain: a preliminary proton nuclear magnetic resonance study. *Neurology* 1992; **42:** 1578–85.

70. Kesslack JP, Drost DJ, Naruse D et al, Single volume proton MR spectroscopy in Alzheimer's disease patients: a multicenter pilot study. *Abstracts 12th Ann Mtg Soc Magn Reson Med, New York, 1993*, 235.

71. Moats RA, Ernst T, Shonk TK, Ross B, Abnormal cerebral metabolite concentrations in patients with probable Alzheimer disease. *Magn Reson Med* 1994; **32:** 110–15.

72. Paley M, Lampman D, Murdoch J et al, Spectroscopic imaging of Alzheimer disease: preliminary results. *Bull Clin Neurosci* 1990; **55:** 151–9.

73. Bruhn H, Frahm J, Gyngell ML et al, Noninvasive differentiation of tumours with use of localized H-1 MR spectroscopy in vivo: initial experience in patients with cerebral tumours. *Radiology* 1989; **172:** 541.

74. Luyten PR, Marcia AJH, Heindel W et al, Metabolic imaging of patients with intracranial tumours: H-1 spectroscopic imaging and PET. *Radiology* 1990; **176:** 797.

75. Alger JR, Frank JA, Bizzi A et al, Metabolism of human gliomas: assessment with H-1 MR spectroscopy and F-18 fluorodeoxyglucose PET. *Radiology* 1990; **177:** 633.

76. Segebarth CM, Baleriaux DF, Luyten PR, den Hollander JA, Detection of metabolic heterogeneity of human intracranial tumours in vivo by ¹H spectroscopic imaging. *Magn Reson Med* 1990; **13:** 62.

77. Arnold DL, Shoubridge EA, Villemeure JG, Feindel W, Proton and phosphorus magnetic resonance spectroscopy of human astrocytomas in vivo. Preliminary observations on tumor grading. *NMR Biomed* 1990; **3:** 184.

78. Demaerel P, Johannik K, Van Hecke P et al, Localized ¹H NMR spectroscopy in fifty cases of newly diagnosed intracranial tumours at 1.5 tesla. Preliminary experience at a clinical installation. *Acta Radiologica* 1991; **32:** 95.

79. Negendank W, Zimmerman R, Gotsis E et al, A cooperative group study of ¹H MRS of primary brain tumors. *Abstracts 12th Ann Mtg Soc Magn Reson Med, New York, 1993*, 1521.

80. Sijens P, Knopp M, Brunetti A et al, ¹H MRS in patients with metastatic brain tumours, a multicenter study. *Magn Reson Med* 1995; **33:** 818–26.

81. Kreis R, Ross BD, Farrow NA, Ackerman Z, Metabolic disorders of the brain in chronic hepatic encephalopathy detected with ¹H MR spectroscopy. *Radiology* 1992; **182:** 19–27.

82. Jungling FD, Huasinger D, Laubenberger J et al, ¹H MRS suggesting astrocyte swelling in chronic hepatic encephalopathy. *Proc 2nd Ann Meeting Soc Magn Reson, San Francisco, 1994*, 569.

83. Cady EB, Costello AMdeL, Dawson MJ et al, Non-invasive investigation of cerebral metabolism in newborn infants by phosphorus spectroscopy. *Lancet* 1983; **i:** 1059–62.

84. Peden CJ, Rutherford MA, Sargentoni J et al, Proton spectroscopy of the neonatal brain following hypoxic-ischaemic injury. *Dev Med Child Neurol* 1993; **35:** 502–10.

85. Berkelbach van der Sprenkel JW, Luyten PR, van Rijen PC et al, Cerebral lactate detected by regional proton magnetic resonance spectroscopy in a patient with cerebral infarction. *Stroke* 1988; **19:** 1556–60.

86. Graham GD, Blamire AM, Howseman AM et al, Proton magnetic resonance spectroscopy of cerebral lactate and other metabolites in stroke patients. *Stroke* 1992; **23:** 333.

87. Graham GD, Blamire AM, Rothman DL et al, Early temporal variations of cerebral metabolites in human stroke. A proton magnetic resonance study. *Stroke* 1993; **24:** 1891–6.

88. Duijn JH, Matson GB, Maudsley AA et al, Human brain infarction: proton MR spectroscopy. *Radiology* 1992; **183:** 711–18.

89. Petroff OA, Graham GD, Blamire AM et al, Spectroscopic imaging of stroke in humans: histopathology correlates of spectral changes. *Neurology* 1992; **42:** 1349–54.

90. Chinn RJS, Wilkinson ID, Paley M et al, Systemic lupus erythematosus: MR brain imaging, brain volumes and spectroscopy findings. *Proc Ann Sci Mtg RCR, Norwich, 1994*, 54

91. Davie CA, Barker GJ, McHugh NJ, Proton MRS of systemic lupus erythematosus involving the central nervous system. *Abstracts 12th Ann Mtg Soc Magn Reson Med, New York, 1993*, 1562.

16

Magnetoencephalography

Jeffrey David Lewine and William W. Orrison, Jr

Introduction

Magnetoencephalography (MEG) is a technique for the noninvasive characterization of brain electrophysiology.[1-5] Just as current flow within a wire produces a surrounding magnetic field, current flow within neurons produces a surrounding neuromagnetic field (Fig. 16.1). The magnetoencephalogram (also abbreviated to MEG) can be measured using special superconducting technologies. In some circumstances biophysical models can be used to infer the spatial location of neuronal populations that generate particular MEG signals of interest. Whereas MEG is not an advanced magnetic resonance (MR) technique per se, functional MEG information can provide a vital complement to structural and functional MR data in many clinical circumstances. MEG provides a millisecond-by-millisecond account of brain physiology, something unattainable by even the most rapid MR methods. When MEG and MR data are integrated to generate magnetic source localization images, clinicians are provided with an exquisitely detailed picture of the relationships between brain function, structure and pathology.

The very first biomagnetic studies utilized a two-million-turn induction coil to measure the magnetic field generated by the heart. These pioneering studies by Baule and McFee in 1963 demonstrated the potential for assessing electrophysiological activity in the body via completely noninvasive, noncontact methods.[6] Five years later, David Cohen, working in a specially designed magnetically shielded room, used special signal averaging techniques to make the first measurements of the brain's magnetic signature. These experiments clearly demonstrated a magnetic counterpart of the

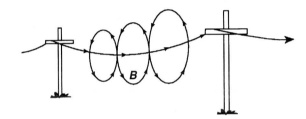

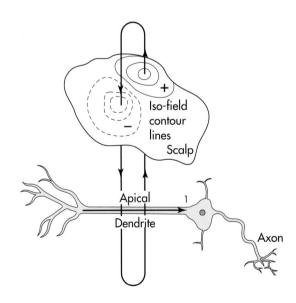

Figure 16.1

Currents in both wires and neurons produce surrounding magnetic fields **B**. Because of biophysical considerations, extracranial magnetic fields selectively reflect current flow in the apical dendrites of pyramidal cells oriented parallel to the skull surface. (Adapted from Lewine et al.[5])

well-characterized alpha rhythm of the electroencephalogram (EEG).[7]

Since these very first measurements of the magnetoencephalogram, biomagnetic investigations have focused primarily on basic research in sensory and cognitive neuroscience. Extensive reviews of these types of data are available elsewhere.[8,9] This chapter will focus on recent clinical advances made possible by the development of large array biomagnetometer systems capable of assessing large areas of the head simultaneously.

The development of the point-contact SQUID (superconducting quantum interference device) by James Zimmerman and his colleagues was a major advance in biomagnetic technology.[10,11] Operating at liquid helium temperatures of −269°C, the SQUID provides an unprecedented level of sensitivity to weak magnetic signals. Using SQUID technology in a shielded room, it is possible to record spontaneous brain rhythms without the need for signal averaging.[12] Signal averaging techniques may be used to process MEG signals obtained with superconducting technologies. Using this method, stimulus-evoked neuromagnetic signals can be extracted from the background noise.[13–15]

Early clinical research was hampered by the small size (1–7 channels) of the available sensor arrays. These had to be tediously repositioned repeatedly to provide adequate spatial sampling of neuromagnetic field patterns. The last five years have witnessed the development of 37-channel systems that have made clinical studies practical. New whole head systems developed in the last three years are beginning to find their way into the clinic.

MEG affords two major advantages over most other neuroimaging procedures, such as functional magnetic resonance imaging (fMRI), single photon emission computed tomography (SPECT) and positron emission tomography (PET). First, MEG provides a direct measure of brain electrophysiology, whereas fMRI, PET and SPECT measure changes in brain metabolism and hemodynamics that are secondary and tertiary to the neurophysiological changes of real interest. Since the exact nature of the coupling between brain electrophysiology, local metabolism and regional cerebral blood flow is only moderately understood, interpretation of these data is complicated. How this coupling varies from brain region to brain region is presently unclear, as is how it is affected by disease and pharmacological agents.[16] The second major advantage of MEG is its real-time resolution of brain activity. Information processing by the brain occurs on a scale of milliseconds. Regardless of how fast images can be taken with techniques such as PET and fMRI, the hemodynamic changes that are being measured take several seconds to develop.

Two imaging techniques have the ability to noninvasively assess brain electrophysiology with the requisite temporal resolution — MEG and EEG. The latter measures electrical potential differences established by extracellular currents between points of the skull surface. In many ways, MEG and EEG complement each other. Both methods provide direct, real-time measurements of brain electrophysiology; however, they have different spatial sensitivity profiles. Whereas MEG signals reflect current flow in the apical dendrites of pyramidal cells oriented tangentially to the skull surface, EEG reflects both tangential and radial activity. MEG signals pass through the tissues of the body without distortion. The differing electrical conductivity properties of the brain, cerebrospinal fluid, skull and scalp, however, result in significant distortion of the electrical potential pattern at the scalp surface (relative to that at the brain surface). As a consequence, without detailed knowledge of the exact shape and electrical properties of the skull and scalp, it is difficult to specify the locations of EEG sources with subcentimeter precision. Admittedly, electrical conductivity barriers cause some perturbation in the magnetic field pattern, but these effects are relatively small and inconsequential for most MEG applications.[17,18] Relatively simple source models can therefore be used to localize most MEG sources.

Basic principles of MEG

Any and all time-varying currents produce time-varying magnetic fields. The direction of the field is given by the 'right-hand rule'. When the thumb of the right hand points in the direction of current flow, the fingers curl in the direction of the magnetic field. Transmembrane, intracellular and extracellular currents of neurons all produce surrounding magnetic fields, but because the head resembles a spherical volume conductor, the extracranial magnetic field selectively reflects intracellular currents in neuronal elements oriented parallel to the skull surface.[19]

Postsynaptic currents contribute more than action currents, in part because postsynaptic currents are of longer duration (allowing for greater temporal overlap in signals generated by nearby cells). Also, the magnetic field generated by currents associated with the depolarizing lead

Table 16.1 Even the largest neuromagnetic signals — those associated with epileptic spikes — are more than one billion times smaller than the Earth's steady magnetic field. (Adapted from Lewine.[4])

Magnetic flux density (femtotesla)	Source
10^{11}	
10^{10}	Earth's magnetic field
10^{9}	
10^{8}	Urban noise
10^{7}	
10^{6}	Magnetized lung contaminants
10^{5}	Abdominal currents
10^{4}	Cardiogram, oculogram
10^{3}	Epileptic and spontaneous activity
10^{2}	Cortical evoked activity
10	SQUID noise
1	Brainstem evoked activity

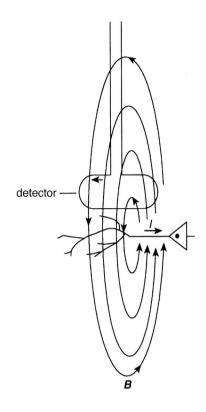

Figure 16.2

Neuromagnetic fields are measured using a detector made of niobium wire maintained in a superconducting state. Time-varying neuronal currents I give rise to a time-varying magnetic flux B that induces currents within the loops of the detection coil.

front of an action potential is mostly cancelled by the magnetic field of the currents associated with the repolarization tail of the action potential.

The magnetic field generated by a single neuron is almost negligible. Even when several thousand nearby cells are synchronously active, the summated extracranial magnetic field typically achieves a magnitude of only a few hundred femtotesla (1 fT = 10^{-15} T). This is over a billion times smaller than the Earth's magnetic field (Table 16.1). It is remarkable that devices with the requisite sensitivity are even available for routine clinical use.

When a time-varying magnetic field passes perpendicular to a loop of wire, it induces a current within the loop (Fig. 16.2). The induction coil is one of the key elements of the device used to measure neuromagnetic signals — the biomagnetometer. Because neuromagnetic fields are so weak, it is necessary to use coils made of superconducting materials. In most systems the coils are made of niobium wire, a substance that becomes superconducting at –258°C. In practice, the coil is kept in the superconducting state by immersing it in liquid helium contained within a cryogenically insulated vessel known as a dewar. When in a superconducting state, superconducting materials demonstrate essentially no resistance to the flow of electrical currents. This allows weak magnetic

fields to induce currents that are not quickly dissipated as heat by the resistance of the wire.

In clinical biomagnetometers the superconducting loop is inductively coupled to a superconducting quantum interference device (SQUID). The SQUID electronics produce a voltage output proportional to the current flowing in the detection circuit (Fig. 16.3). The SQUID is made of a ring of superconducting material interrupted by 'Josephson junctions'. A ring of superconducting wire interrupted by a large resistive segment behaves as though the entire ring is made of resistive material. If the ring is interrupted only by a microscopically thin section of resistive material (a Josephson junction), the entire ring still acts as a superconductor, provided that the amount of current in the ring is small. When the total current is below the critical current for the Josephson junction, electrons can 'tunnel' through the resistive segment without loss of energy. However, if the current level is above the

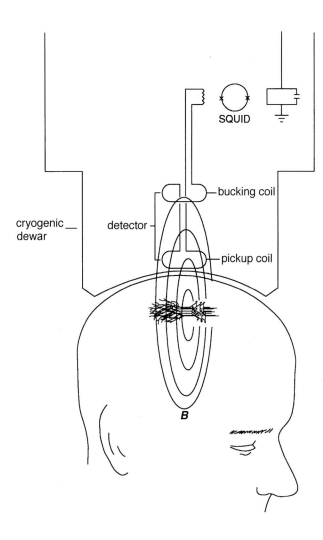

Figure 16.3

In clinical biomagnetometers, the detection circuit is inductively coupled to a SQUID. Neuronal currents give rise to a neuromagnetic field that induces currents in the detector. The magnetic field of these currents induces a current flow in the SQUID. The SQUID feedback electronics generate a voltage signal that is proportional to the original neuromagnetic flux. The superconducting devices are contained within a cryogenic dewar filled with liquid helium. (Adapted from Lewine et al.[65])

critical current, there is a significant voltage drop across the resistive segment.

These superconducting rings also act as induction coils, with changes in the magnetic field impinging on the ring causing a change in the magnitude of the current flowing in the ring. The detection circuit in biomagnetometers is inductively coupled to the SQUID, so that neuronally induced currents in the detection circuit generate magnetic fields that induce currents within the SQUID ring.

The electronics of the biomagnetometer are such that a small current is continually applied to the SQUID ring, with the feedback electronics acting to maintain the total current in the SQUID ring just below the critical current. When a magnetic field from current in the detection circuit induces an additional current within the SQUID ring, the total current exceeds the critical current and there is a significant voltage drop across the Josephson junction. The electronics measure this, and the feedback electronics readjust the applied current. The total current in the SQUID ring is again brought below the critical current. The magnitude of the required feedback current is continually monitored by the voltage it produces across a resistor in the feedback circuit. This serves as the output of the magnetometer system. In this fashion, the SQUID electronics transform a small, neuromagnetically induced current in the detection circuit into a large-amplitude voltage signal.

SQUID-coupled magnetometer systems are so sensitive to magnetic signals that they are easily overwhelmed by magnetic signals from noise sources, such as moving metallic objects or indoor electrical devices. It is therefore common practice to operate biomagnetometers in magnetically shielded rooms made of an alloy known as mu-metal. Mu-metal is used because of its high magnetic permeability (80 000 as compared with a permeability of 1 for air and other nonmetallic materials). An external magnetic field that impinges on the shielded room mostly flows through the high-permeability walls of the chamber rather than entering into the air-filled room. Typical rooms offer a shielding factor of less than 10 000, so the magnetic noise that manages to permeate the shielding remains orders of magnitude larger than the neuromagnetic signals of interest.

However, by modifying the configuration of the detection circuit, it is possible to isolate very small neuromagnetic signals. The magnetic field of an electric current decreases rapidly with increasing distance from the source (as a function of the square of the distance or higher, depending upon the exact current configuration). Near a magnetic source, the gradient of the magnetic field is steep (this gradient can be measured by two coils forming a 'gradiometer'). For example, the magnetic field at 7 cm is less than 10% of the field at 2 cm. Far from a source, the gradient of the magnetic field is shallow. The magnetic field at 1007 cm is more than 99% of that at 1002 cm. Hence, near the source, the output of the gradiometer is high (the two coils experience very different fields), but far from the source the output of the gradiometer is small, even if the overall field

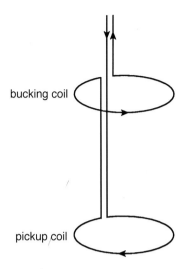

Figure 16.4

The detectors of most clinical biomagnetometers are configured as first-order axial gradiometers. The lower pick-up coil and upper bucking coil are wound in opposite directions. The device measures the first order d**B**/dx spatial gradient of the magnetic field rather than the absolute magnitude of the field.

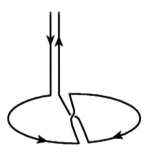

Figure 16.5

Some systems use planar gradiometers. For a planar gradiometer, the system output is maximal over the magnetic source.

strength at each coil is high. Consequently, the gradiometer is very sensitive to magnetic signals generated by neurons a few centimeters below the sensor, but insensitive to magnetic fields generated by hospital equipment several meters outside of the shielded room.

Biomagnetometer systems in general have their detectors configured as axial, first-order gradiometers (Fig. 16.4). These systems contain detectors

that consist of two coil loops, wound in opposite directions. The coils are connected in series, and sit one above the other, with a few centimeters separation. The current induced in the upper 'bucking' coil opposes that induced in the lower 'pickup' coil with the net current flow in the detection circuit reflecting the gradient (i.e. the first-order spatial derivative d*B*/dx) of the magnetic field. When the magnetic source is far away, the gradient at the coils is shallow, with the coils experiencing nearly identical magnetic fields. The induced currents in the pickup and bucking coils are hence nearly equivalent and mostly cancel each other, so that the overall output of the system is small, even if the absolute magnitude of the magnetic field is large. If the magnetic source is near the coils (within a few centimeters), the coils experience very different magnetic fields, and the output of the detection circuit is large, even if the absolute magnitude of the fields is small. By making the distance (baseline) between the pickup coil and the bucking coil about 5 cm, the output of the gradiometer is made to mostly reflect the magnetic field of nearby neuronal sources located below the detector.

Some systems utilize planar gradiometers, where the two coils are situated in the same plane (Fig. 16.5). The spatial sensitivity pattern of planar gradiometer configurations is narrower and shallower than that of axial gradiometers. Planar sensors detect fields from a more spatially restricted area, but because the baselines of planar gradiometers are generally short, they are less sensitive to deeper sources than standard axial configurations.

To date, the most extensive clinical experiments have been done using the 37-channel detector system of Biomagnetic Technologies Inc (BTi, Fig. 16.6), although other large array systems by BTi (Fig. 16.7), CTF Inc (Fig. 16.8) and Neuromag Ltd (Fig. 16.9) are obtaining increased clinical exposure.

The output of each sensor is a time-varying voltage waveform that reflects local changes in magnetic flux as a function of time. There are several neuromagnetic signals of interest, such as the various spontaneous brain rhythms described well in EEG (e.g. the alpha rhythm), which are also seen in MEG (Fig. 16.10). In many biomagnetic experiments, signal-averaging procedures are used to isolate time-locked information processing signals. For example, consider a typical experiment for localizing and mapping primary somatosensory cortex. Here an electrical stimulus is repeatedly applied to the median nerve while signals are recorded over the contralateral parietal lobe. Most

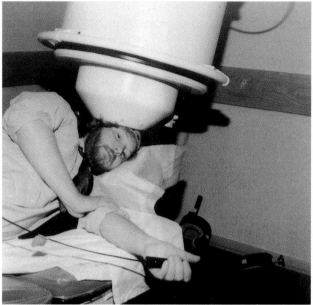

Figure 16.6

The BTi Magnes system contains 37 axial first-order gradiometers. It is easily positioned over brain regions of interest. (Picture courtesy of BTi, San Diego, CA.)

of the activity in each epoch is unrelated to processing the sensory stimulus, but a small portion of the signal does reflect activation of primary somatosensory cortex. The timing of this activation, relative to stimulus presentation, is constant from trial to trial, because of the fixed length of the neural conduction pathway from the hand to the brain. When data epochs spanning the stimulus event are averaged, the time-locked activity is extracted from the background noise (Fig. 16.11).

During an experiment, a 3D digitizer is used to define the exact spatial position of the detector coils within a head-centered coordinate frame. At each instant in time, it is therefore possible to define the spatial pattern of the magnetic field (Fig. 16.12). It is this spatial pattern that provides the critical information for localizing brain regions responsible for generation of the magnetic signals of interest.

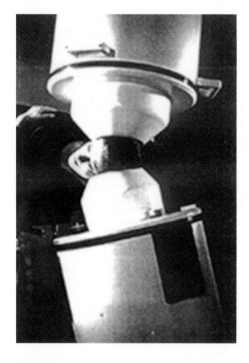

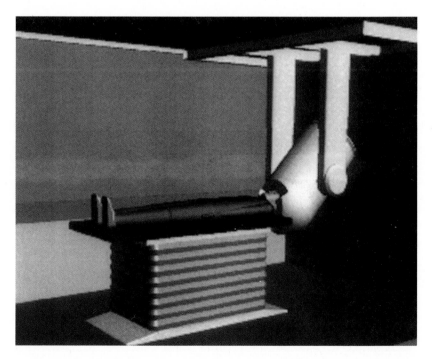

Figure 16.7

BTi has recently marketed a dual-probe system (left) that allows for simultaneous recordings over right and left hemispheres. The bottom, inverted dewar uses novel vacuum technology. This is leading to the development of a new whole head system, as conceptualized on the right. This new system will have 143 first-order axial gradiometers. Subjects will be able to sit upright or recline completely. (Pictures courtesy of BTi, San Diego, CA.)

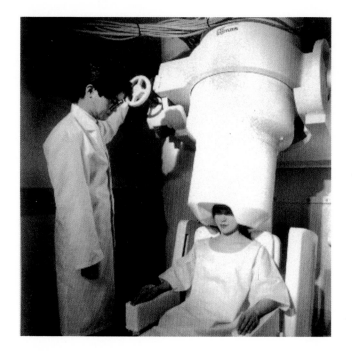

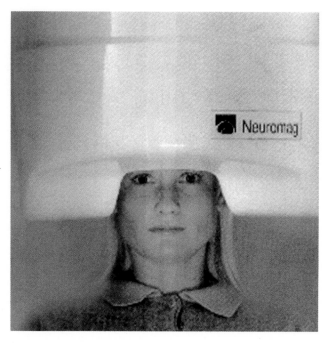

Figure 16.8

The CTF Inc whole head systems use first-order axial gradiometers. Systems are available with up to 140 detector channels. (Picture courtesy of CTF Inc, Vancouver, BC.)

Figure 16.9

The Neuromag Ltd whole head biomagnetometer contains 122 planar gradiometers.

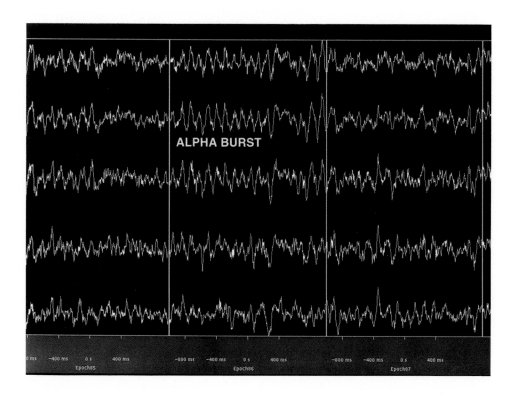

Figure 16.10

The output of each sensor channel is a time-varying voltage waveform that reflects temporal changes in the magnetic flux. Five channels from a BTi Magnes system are shown. The dewar was positioned over the occipital lobe, and a prominent magnetic 9 Hz alpha rhythm is seen, especially in the upper three channels in the first half of epoch 86.

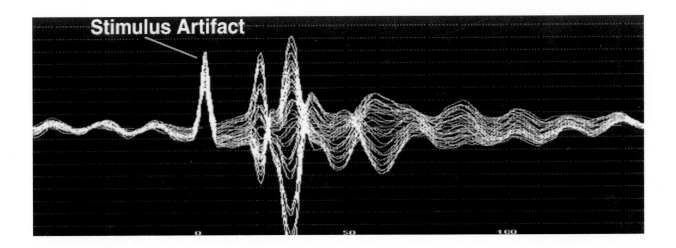

Figure 16.11

Signal averaging allows for the extraction of time-locked signal components. Data were collected with a 37-channel Magnes probe positioned over the right parietal lobe. Data epochs were collected in response to electrical stimulation of the left median nerve, and the epochs were signal-averaged. The resultant average evoked response is characterized by a quiet baseline, a large stimulus artifact (associated with the magnetic field of the stimulating current), and a series of neuromagnetic oscillations arising from the sensorimotor cortex. The waveforms from all 37 channels have been overlayed to emphasize that when some channels are detecting emerging flux (upward deflections) others are experiencing entering flux (downward deflections). (Adapted from Lewine et al.[5])

The magnetic field that any prespecified current produces at a particular sensor location can be exactly specified by a set of forward calculations using Maxwell's equations and the Biot–Savart law.[20] In contrast, the inverse problem of specifying the neuronal currents that generate a measured magnetic field pattern is ill-posed, because there are many intracranial configurations of current that all produce the same extracranial magnetic field pattern.[21] Only by making certain assumptions about the shape of the head and the nature of the underlying current configuration can the inverse problem be made mathematically tractable so that computer algorithms can be used to infer the location of the relevant neuronal activity.

The most common model used in the analysis of neuromagnetic signals is that of a dipole in a sphere. This model assumes (i) that the head can be modeled as a spherically symmetric volume conductor and (ii) that the recorded magnetic field can be modeled as though it were generated by a point-source, current dipole. The spherical assumption is not really essential, but it greatly simplifies the relevant calculations. Of course, the model provides only a first-order approximation of the geometry and electrical properties of real heads, but in most situations realistic deviations from sphericity cause only minimal errors in source modeling (except at anterior temporal regions where source location errors of more than 1 cm may be introduced by use of a spherical model).

The assumption that the magnetic field pattern of interest can be modelled as though it were produced by a current dipole is important to making the inverse strategy tractable. The current dipole is intended to provide a simplified biophysical representation of the actual currents that generate the recorded signal. Given this model, it is possible to employ computer algorithms to identify the location, orientation and strength of that dipole which best accounts (in a statistical sense) for the measured magnetic field pattern. These algorithms work as follows. First, a dipole is hypothesized to exist at a particular position, orientation and strength within the conductive volume. The Biot–Savart law is then used to forward-calculate the magnetic signal that this hypothetical dipole would generate at each of the detectors. At each detector, the difference between

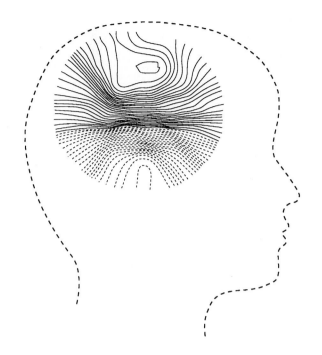

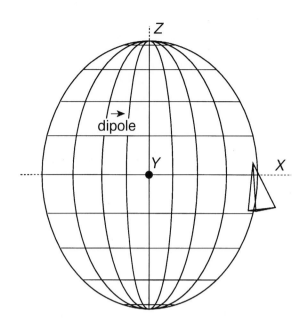

Figure 16.12

At each instant in time, the pattern of the neuromagnetic field can be described by an isofield contour map. The presented map corresponds to the peak of the 20 ms component of Fig. 16.11. Solid lines indicate emerging flux, dashed lines entering flux, in 10 fT steps. The data imply the existence of a dipole source located below the zero line (separating regions of entering and emerging flux).

Figure 16.13

Mathematical modeling of the magnetic field pattern allows for identification of the (X, Y, Z) spatial position, orientation and strength of the best-fitting current dipole. The head-centered coordinate frame is defined by three fiducials: the nasion (located at the bridge of the nose), and left and right pre-auricular points.

the forward calculated signal and the actually measured signal is determined. The value of this mismatch terms is then squared and summed across all of the detectors to generate an overall error term. A new dipole is then postulated at a different position, and its error term calculated. Using iterative minimization procedures, the computer algorithm continues to hypothesize dipoles until it determines the position, orientation and strength of that dipole that provides the smallest error term. The position, orientation and strength of this 'best-fitting' dipole are then taken as indicative of the position, orientation and strength of the relevant neuronal currents (Fig. 16.13).

In considering the validity of the dipole model, it is important not to confuse the model (a dipole) with that which is being modeled (a complex pattern of neuronal currents). The real key to the utility of the dipole model for source analysis is not the observation that the synaptic currents of individual neurons have a dipolar configuration; rather, it is the fact that dipolar components of the magnetic field decrease in magnitude less rapidly with distance than higher-order terms. Provided that the external neuromagnetic field mostly reflects activation of a single cortical region, and that the spatial extent of the active region is small compared with the distance to the detector coil, localization of the best-fitting dipole provides for excellent localization of the activated region. If multiple cortical regions simultaneously make significant contributions to the field pattern and a single dipole model is used erroneously, the dipole solution may fail to accurately characterize the neuronal activity.[22,23] Fortunately, in most of these

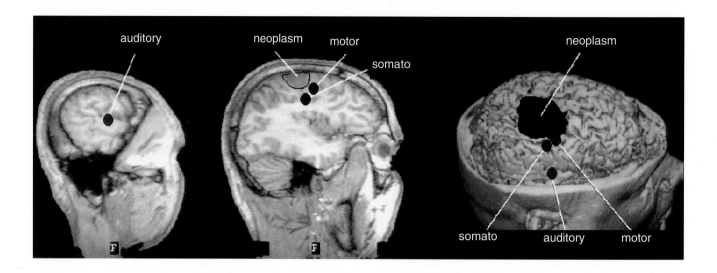

Figure 16.14

The fiducials used to define the MEG coordinate space can be easily identified on magnetic resonance (MR) images. This allows for generation of magnetic source localization images that plot MEG dipole locations on appropriate MR sections or three-dimensional reconstructions. These images show the spatial relationships between brain function, structure and pathology. This particular data set is from a patient with a parietal neoplasm. Dipole sources associated with activation of primary cortical regions are shown for auditory, somatosensory, and motor stimuli. (Adapted from Benzel et al.[33])

cases visual inspection of isofield contour maps, coupled with evaluation of the correlation between the dipole model and the field measurements, makes it possible to recognize when the dipole model is inappropriate. When needed, multiple dipole models can be applied, although these are mathematically more complex. A limitation of the dipole model is seen when neuromagnetic signals of interest are generated by activity of an extended cortical sheet, several square centimeters in area. Extended sheets often produce an apparently dipolar magnetic field pattern, and when a single-dipole model is used to describe this type of activity, the dipole may be erroneously localized deep in the white matter below the actual cortical site of activity. Nevertheless, these partly inaccurate localizations may still provide useful diagnostic information on the hemisphere and lobe of the critical activity.

Given the above complications, investigators must be knowledgeable in identification of those circumstances under which the dipole model is valid. Available empirical data indicate that the dipole model can be appropriately applied to neuromagnetic signals generated by the primary cortical regions involved in motor, somatosensory and auditory processing. The model is also valid for the characterization of some epileptic spikes, sharp waves and paroxysmal slow waves.

The head-centered MEG coordinate system in which dipole locations are specified is defined by left and right preauricular points and the nasion (located at the bridge of the nose). These fiducials are readily identified on magnetic resonance images. Using appropriate computer algorithms, it is possible to align MEG and MR coordinate frames so that MEG dipole sources can be plotted directly on the relevant anatomical images. The resulting magnetic source localization images thereby provide graphic details on the spatial relationships between brain structure, function and pathology (Fig. 16.14).

Clinical applications

As outlined below, magnetic source imaging (MSI) is particularly useful in:

(i)   the preoperative mapping of sensorimotor cortex in neurosurgical patients;
(ii) the characterization and localization of epileptiform activity; and
(iii) characterization of the abnormal spontaneous rhythms that are prominent in a wide range of neurological disorders.

Additional clinical applications are under development at clinical facilities throughout the world.

Preoperative mapping

Neurosurgical intervention in patients with neoplasms and vascular malformations is often complicated by the desire to effect complete removal of pathological regions without compromising nearby regions of healthy tissue critical for specific sensory, motor, or cognitive functions.[24,25] The sparing of sensorimotor cortex is particularly important because surgically induced hemiparesis markedly reduces the quality of postoperative life. Individual variability in brain morphology and physiology is such that MR anatomical guidelines for identification of sensorimotor cortex often fail, even in the evaluation of data from neurologically normal subjects.[26] In patients with space-occupying masses in frontal or parietal regions, the situation is even more difficult, and it is often impossible to use neuroanatomical imaging procedures (MR and CT) to identify the central sulcus (the divider between precentral motor and postcentral somatosensory cortices).

The traditional means for identifying sensorimotor cortex in neurosurgical patients is to record somatosensory evoked potentials directly from the cortical surface at the time of operation, or to electrically stimulate the brain during surgery (in order to localize motor regions).[27–30] There are several limitations to these invasive strategies. First, many patients with parietal or frontal lesions never actually get to surgery, because their lesions are incorrectly classified as inoperable on the basis of their spatial position alone. Intraoperative monitoring is not a risk-free procedure — it lengthens surgical time and increases the likelihood of infection. The quality of corticographic data is often dependent upon the location and extent of the craniotomy, and the data are not always easy to interpret, especially when the corticography grid partly overlies the lesion.[31] Finally, and most limiting, these intraoperative methods can only be applied after craniotomy and commitment to a

particular surgical approach. Clearly, detailed *preoperative* mapping of the spatial relationship between a lesion and the location of cortex responsible for specific brain functions would greatly assist in risk assessment, craniotomy site selection, and decisions regarding conservative versus aggressive approaches to the resection of the pathological tissue. As outlined below, MSI can easily accomplish this type of preoperative mapping in a reliable and efficient noninvasive manner.

The basic strategy in preoperative mapping examinations is to take advantage of signal averaging techniques. Stimuli designed to activate specific brain regions (e.g. tones for activation of auditory cortex and electrical pulses applied to the median nerve to activate somatosensory cortex) are presented a number of times, and data epochs spanning the stimulus event are signal-averaged to isolate time-locked brain responses.

Somatosensory cortex mapping by MEG is, in general, considered a relatively easy and straightforward procedure. Localization of the face area can be accomplished by tactile or vibratory stimulation of the lower lip or tongue. The hand area is localized by tactile, vibratory or electrical stimulation of the digits of the hand, or more commonly, by electrical stimulation of the median nerve. Electrical stimulation of the tibial nerve is typically used to localize the foot area of sensorimotor cortex.

In normals, dipole sources for the earliest components of somatosensory evoked responses consistently localize to the primary somatosensory cortex of the post-central gyrus (as identified by structural methods).[32] However, in patients with mass lesions in the region of the somatosensory cortex, the localizations may be removed from the anatomically anticipated locations (Fig. 16.15). For these patients, the availability of MEG somatosensory data can have a significant impact on surgical treatment.[33–36]

Direct MEG studies of motor function are more difficult to perform than somatosensory examinations, because they require that the patient be able to make smooth, well-controlled movements. Typically, the patient is asked to flex or extend one or more digits of the hand in a self-paced or visually cued fashion. Electromyography (EMG) can be used as a trigger for the MEG recordings, or the self-paced movement can trigger a photo-optic switch. The primary motor field is generally dipolar, and its source localizes to the anterior bank of the central sulcus. However, for some subjects, there is coincident activity in premotor and supplementary motor areas, which renders the

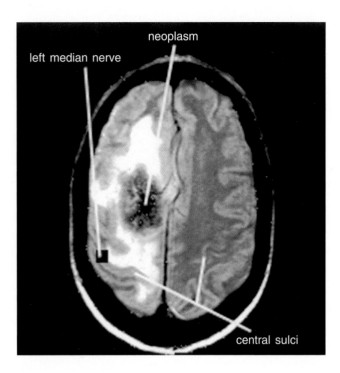

left median nerve

neoplasm

central sulci

Figure 16.15

Lesions can cause significant spatial displacement of
brain functional areas. In this case the right frontal
neoplasm and associated edema cause posterior
displacement of the central sulcus on the right, relative
to the left, as indicated by the posterior location of the
primary cortical response to stimulation of the left
median nerve.

dipole model inaccurate. In these cases, complex
spatio-temporal, multiple-dipole models are
needed to disentangle simultaneous activity in
multiple brain regions.[37]

Given the proximity of primary auditory cortex
to language areas, it can be useful to localize this
region in some neurosurgical patients. The presentation of a short-duration tone evokes a series of
neuromagnetic oscillations that correspond to P50,
N100 and P200 evoked potential components.
Dipole sources for the 100 ms component localize
to the auditory cortex of Heschel's gyrus and
demonstrate a tonotopic organization.[38]

Only a few presurgical studies of visual function
have been performed, since the magnetic field that
is evoked by transient visual stimuli is generally
too complex for standard dipole modeling.
However, using very small, short-duration stimuli

or small checkerboard patterns undergoing rapid
(>10 Hz) contrast reversals, it is sometimes possible
to isolate dipolar visual responses from the primary
visual cortex.[5]

Although the use of evoked-response methods to
evaluate cognitive functions (e.g. language, attention and memory) is being explored, these types of
examinations have yet to be sufficiently validated
to the point where they can be used in routine
clinical practice.

For motor, somatosensory and auditory processing, intraoperative monitoring has repeatedly
confirmed the millimeter accuracy of MSI inferences
on the location of the relevant primary cortical
areas.[33,35] It is noteworthy that the availability of
temporal information is often critical in these types
of examinations. For example, simple movement of
a finger generates activity in many brain regions,
including supplementary motor areas, premotor
areas, primary motor cortex and somatosensory
cortex. In cases where mass effects from lesions have
distorted the local neuroanatomy, the time sequence
of activation of brain areas provides the only clue as
to which region is the primary motor region.

In many cases MSI data have led surgeons to
alter their surgical approach to a lesion (in order
to better avoid eloquent cortex), and in many
instances, MSI has demonstrated that a lesion,
initially presumed to have been inoperable, could
be resected safely without induction of motor
deficits (Fig. 16.16). MSI functional mapping
experiments typically require less than 90 min,
including both the MEG and multislice volumetric
MR portions of the examination. In most instances,
magnetic source localization images can be made
available to surgeons within a few hours.

It is noteworthy that evoked response strategies
can be useful in the assessment of the abnormal
information processing that characterizes several
clinical conditions. In particular, analyses of
waveform component amplitudes and latencies
can be indicative of neurological dysfunction. For
example, in patients with multiple sclerosis (MS),
the pattern of activity evoked by electrical stimulation of the median nerve is found to be quite
abnormal (Fig. 16.17).[39]

Characterization of epileptiform transients

One of the oldest uses of MEG is in the study of
epileptic activity.[40–45] Epilepsy affects just under

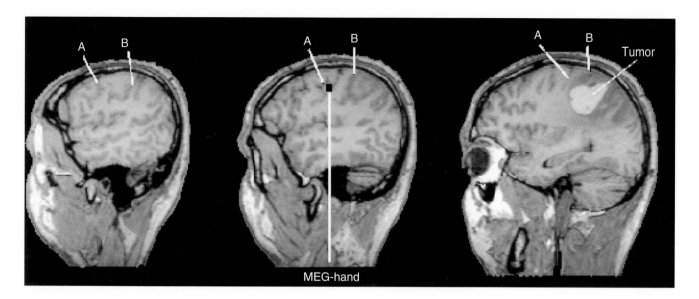

Figure 16.16

In several cases MEG data have altered surgical decisions. These data are from a 58-year-old male with a rapidly expanding astrocytoma. It is difficult from MR to discern if sulcus A or B is the central sulcus. When shown the full series of sagittal, axial and coronal MR images, each of six neuroradiologists concluded that sulcus B was most likely the central sulcus, with the tumor invading sensorimotor cortex. Three different neurosurgeons felt that this tumor could not be removed without causing severe hemiparalysis, and they each declined to perform a surgical intervention. Subsequent MEG examination involving stimulation of the right median nerve indicated the somatosensory hand representation to lie along sulcus A. That is, the MEG data indicated the central sulcus to be significantly anterior to the lesion. Surgery was performed, with intraoperative stimulation and recording procedures confirming the MEG inferences. The neoplasm was removed without inducing any motor deficits. (Adapted from Benzel et al.[33])

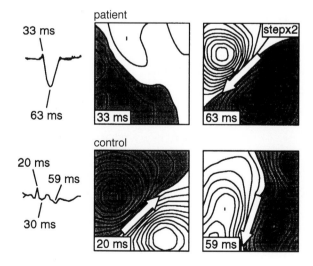

Figure 16.17

Somatosensory responses in patients with multiple sclerosis show different spatio-temporal properties than responses from neurologically normal control subjects. (Adapted from Karhu et al.[39])

1% of the general population, and for almost 20% of these patients, anticonvulsive medications are either contraindicated or ineffective. In these cases surgical treatment is often considered, but effective surgical intervention requires accurate knowledge of the location of the tissue responsible for seizure initiation. In some cases an obvious lesion may be present, but even when a lesion is identified, the site of an epileptic focus can be far removed (Fig. 16.18).[46]

Subdural grid and depth electrode monitoring is considered the 'gold standard' for localizing an epileptic focus prior to surgical resection, but the placement of the electrodes is a risky and expensive surgical procedure. Children generally do not tolerate invasive monitoring. Even for adult patients, there are only a few dozen medical centers with the expertise to perform these procedures. Hence,

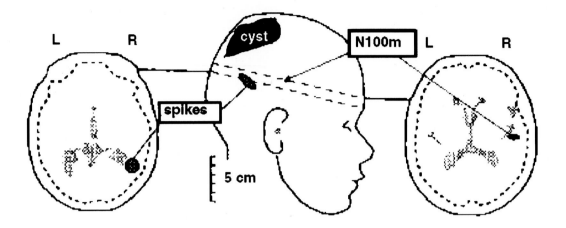

Figure 16.18

The cortical regions responsible for generation of epileptic spikes may be far removed from easily identified lesions of MR. In this case the seizure generation zone was found in posterior temporal cortex, several centimeters below a parietal cyst. The spike zone was also demonstrated to be posterior to primary auditory cortex, as identified by the source location of the N100m component of the auditory evoked response. At surgery, electrocorticography confirmed the location of the epileptic zone, and neuropathological examination of the tissue of the spike zone revealed abnormalities that were not apparent by MR imaging. (Adapted from Paetau et al.[46]).

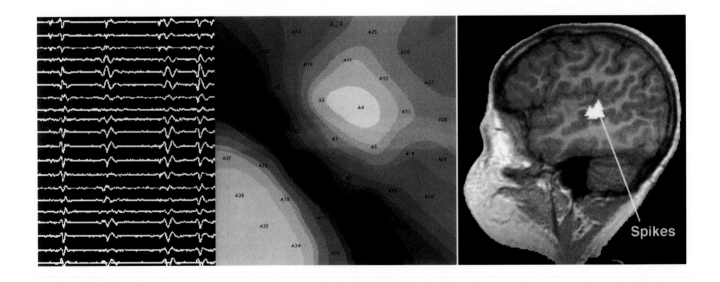

Figure 16.19

Many epileptic spikes (left panel) have simple dipolar magnetic field patterns (middle panel), with easily localizable sources (right panel). In other cases multiple dipole, spatio-temporal models may be required to localize the region of pathophysiology.

whereas some 350 000 Americans would probably benefit from surgical intervention, only 5000 epilepsy surgeries are performed in the USA each year, mostly because of the limited availability of the invasive localization procedures. Noninvasive procedures are therefore becoming increasingly important in the search for the epileptic focus.

The recent availability of large array biomagnetometers, combined with the development of MSI algorithms for aligning MEG and MR data, has brought MSI applications in epilepsy to the clinical forefront. MSI is particularly useful in the localization of generators of interictal spikes.[47–50] Although some spikes have complex magnetic field patterns not well characterized by single-dipole models, even these data can be analyzed by spatio-temporal dipole modeling algorithms now available for clinical use. These algorithms, in combination with the simpler single-dipole algorithms (which are appropriate for some spikes) can allow for sub-lobar localization of regions of epileptic pathophysiology (Fig. 16.19).

MEG evaluations currently focus primarily on interictal activity. The necessity for ictal electrophysiological observations by either MEG or EEG has not been resolved, but it appears that interictal MEG is at least as informative as other interictal techniques such as PET and conventional EEG. At some institutions, interictal MEG data are being used to guide the placement of depth probes. It remains to be seen if MEG can provide an adequate alternative to ictal depth electrode recordings. One promising area is in the distinction between mesial and lateral temporal lobe epilepsy. Patients with seizures originating in mesial/basal structures such as the hippocampus generally do quite well after resective surgery. In contrast, patients with lateral neocortical foci are only occasionally cured by partial temporal lobectomies. Recent work by Ebersole and colleagues indicates that MEG may allow easy separation of these patient populations.[51–53] Specifically, MEG dipole sources in patients later confirmed to have a mesial focus tend to be oriented in an anterior–posterior direction, whereas patients with neocortical foci tend to show dipole sources with a superior–inferior orientation.

MEG has shown particular promise in the evaluation of patients when it is difficult to determine if one of the two hemispheres is leading the other in spike formation.[54] An epileptic spike originating from one hemisphere will often generate a strong EEG signal over the other hemisphere. However, this is not typically the case for MEG. MEG data collected over the two hemispheres simultaneously can often demonstrate the temporal relationship between this bihemispheric epileptiform activity.

Characterization of abnormal spontaneous rhythms

The spontaneous MEG (and EEG) of normal individuals is usually dominated by signals in the 8–13 Hz alpha band. In cases where pathological conditions affect the brain, there is often an increase in the amount of slower brain activity in the delta (1–4 Hz) and theta (4–6 Hz) bands (Fig. 16.20). This slowing in the EEG is usually poorly localized, being present at many recording sites, though in some conditions the slowing can be quite focal. Interestingly, comparable slowing in the MEG is typically quite focal, and in some instances focal generators can be specified.[55–57]

Early efforts at the characterization of abnormal low-frequency magnetic activity (ALFMA) focused on ischemic disease (Fig. 16.21).[55–59] These types of investigations are now being expanded to include studies of epilepsy, trauma and psychiatric dysfunction.[57,59,60] In the typical study of ALFMA, a minimum of three minutes of continuous data are collected from multiple locations over the head, in order to provide for a whole head examination. The data are then filtered from 1 to 6 (or from 1 to 4) Hz to isolate low-frequency signals. Time points where the signal amplitude is unusually large (>200 fT) are identified and the magnetic field at these points is modeled by a single dipole. In most instances the dipole model for ALFMA is poor, so the source locations cannot be believed. Sometimes, however, the dipole model is quite good, with the correlation coefficient between the model and the actual field pattern being greater than 0.97. At these instances, the dipole model has some validity, although, even here, source localizations for ALFMA are probably accurate only to within a few centimeters (unlike source localizations for most stimulus-evoked signals, which are believed to be accurate to within a few millimeters). This is partly because averaging techniques are not used in these types of experiments, so the background noise level is high. An additional factor is that ALFMA often appears to reflect activity of an extended cortical region. In these cases the location of the dipole sources for the ALFMA are projected deep to the actual site of activation. This limitation of the analysis of ALFMA does not imply that the analysis is uninformative. Dipolar sources for 1–6 Hz activity are rarely found for normals (<10% of cases), but are common in many pathological conditions. When low-frequency activity is present in both MEG and EEG, the former provides better localization information than is typically available through routine EEG.

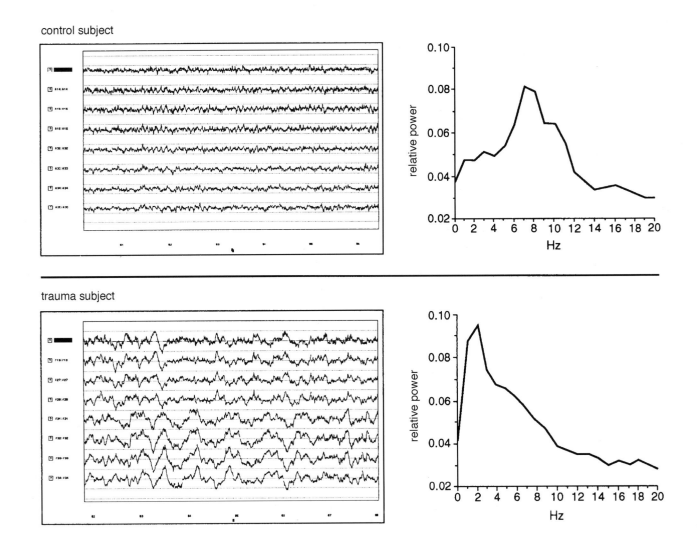

Figure 16.20

The spontaneous data records of normal control subjects are dominated by alpha activity in the 8–13 Hz band. Patients with brain dysfunction often demonstrate high-amplitude 'slow waves' with power spectra dominated by activity in the delta (1–4 Hz) or theta (4–6 Hz) band. The lower panel shows data from a patient with traumatic brain injury and a significant post-concussive syndrome. Prominent slow waves are seen, and the power spectra is dominated by 2–3 Hz delta activity. (Adapted from Lewine et al.[65])

ALFMA examinations may be beneficial in identifying those patients at risk for stroke, and can aid in the assessment of surviving brain tissue following a cerebrovascular accident (CVA). ALFMA can be identified and localized in about 40% of patients with a history of transient ischemic attacks, even after neurological deficits have cleared.[56–58,61] ALFMA is found in more than 80% of patients with cortical strokes, and the sources of this slow-wave activity localize selectively to the tissues along the margin of the lesion. This activity surrounding the infarcted tissue is believed to be indicative of the ischemic penumbra. The ability of the combined MEG and MR examinations to define both the region of encephalomalacia and the surrounding penumbra of ischemic tissue could assist in evaluating the potential for recovery and the planning of therapeutic intervention.[57,61]

Analyses of ALFMA can be important in the assessment of epileptic patients, especially because only 30% of these show interictal spiking,

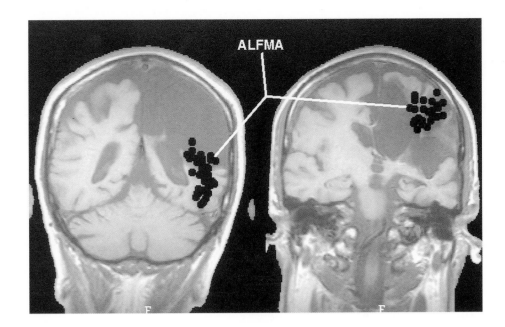

Figure 16.21

Abnormal low-frequency magnetic activity (ALFMA) is found in about 80% of patients with cortical infarcts. The sources of dipolar ALFMA (as indicated by the black circles) localize to the margins of the infarct in the ischemic penumbra.

whereas 80% show ALFMA.[57,62,63] In about 60% of these cases a single focus of ALFMA is identified. This is consistent with inferences from other noninvasive procedures (e.g. PET). In the remaining 40%, multiple regions of ALFMA are identified, with the most intense of these correlating with the suspected region of primary pathology (Fig. 16.22). In patients with both spiking and ALFMA the dipole sources co-localize, and in several surgical cases electrocorticography has confirmed the validity of slow-wave localizations and their relevance to epileptic pathology.[64]

Head trauma victims often suffer from a variety of post-traumatic syndromes characterized by neurological or psychological dysfunction. In cases of serious trauma radiological imaging (CT and MR) can reveal pathological conditions such as contusions or deep white matter injury, but in mild trauma traditional radiological examinations are often negative, even in patients with significant post-traumatic psychological changes. ALFMA is identified in about 60% of these cases of mild head trauma, whereas EEG and MR are typically abnormal in only about 30%. In cases of trauma from a focal impact with a blunt object, sources of ALFMA localize to sites coup or contra-coup to the

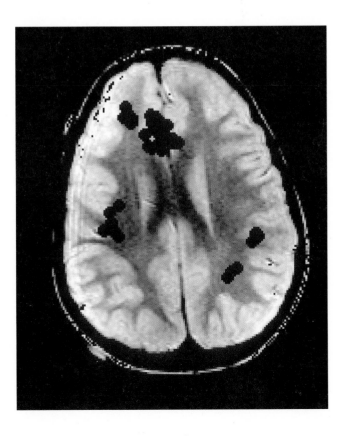

Figure 16.22

Epileptic patients occasionally show multiple foci of sources for ALFMA. In general, the most 'intense' source defines the location of primary pathology. These data, from a five-year-old girl with seizures, show ALFMA foci at right midline frontal, right temporal and left temporal-parietal locations. The right frontal activity shows the largest number of source localizations. Epileptic spikes were also recorded from this child, and all co-localized with the right frontal activity.

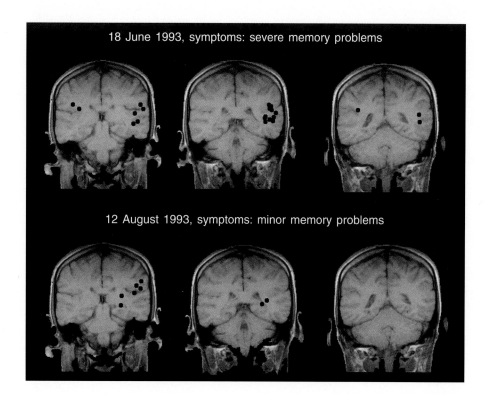

18 June 1993, symptoms: severe memory problems

12 August 1993, symptoms: minor memory problems

Figure 16.23

Source locations for ALFMA generally make clinical sense with respect to functional neuroanatomical considerations. For example, patients with temporal lobe ALFMA have memory problems, whereas those with bi-parietal ALFMA often show attentional problems. The data presented here are from a 17-year-old male who suffered head trauma in a bicycle accident. At the time of initial MEG examination (18 June 1993), the patient had severe memory problems. Extensive temporal lobe and insular ALFMA was found, especially on the left, which was the side of primary impact. Two months later, most, but not all, deficits had cleared. MEG revealed less ALFMA. (Adapted from Lewine et al.[65])

site of impact. There is a predictable neurofunctional relationship between the locations of sources for ALFMA and specific neuropsychological functions (Fig. 16.23). The persistence or alleviation of clinical symptoms correlates well with the persistence or alleviation of ALFMA.[65]

Examination of ALFMA may be useful in several other clinical conditions, including psychiatric dysfunctions, dementia, substance abuse and learning disabilities.[5] Whereas ALFMA examination is a sensitive index of pathophysiology, the presence of ALFMA is not specific for any particular clinical condition. This somewhat limits the utility of this type of examination, so efforts are underway to determine if characterization of slow-wave burst patterns, waveform morphology and/or source localization patterns can lead to more specific diagnostic tests.

Summary

Clinical applications for MEG continue to be explored at an ever-expanding number of sites throughout the world. Although large-array systems have been available for routine clinical use for less than five years, tremendous progress has been made in a variety of areas. Presurgical mapping and the evaluation of epileptic activity are probably going to remain the primary clinical applications of MEG in the immediate future, but new applications are developing rapidly.[66-69] The integration of MR and MEG data is now moving beyond the simple mapping of MEG data onto MR images to the point where neuroanatomical data are being used to specifically constrain inverse modeling procedures.[70] This should lead to more accurate and realistic characterization of the generators of neuromagnetic signals. The development of high-temperature SQUIDs and superconducting shielding is certain to play an important role in increasing the efficiency and efficacy of neuromagnetic procedures.

One particularly exciting new area for biomagnetic methods is in the assessment of fetal brain and cardiac activity. In some cases it is possible to show central nervous system mediation of cardiac activity, and in some cases fetal brain activity can be recorded directly. Overall, biomagnetic techniques may afford a unique opportunity to assess the developing nervous system and fetal well-being.[71,72]

In both the cognitive neuroscience research laboratory and the neuroradiology clinic, the ability of MEG to characterize brain activity in both time and space renders it one of the most useful brain imaging modalities.

References

1. Hari R, Ilmoniemi RJ, Cerebral magnetic fields. *CRC Crit Rev Biomed Eng* 1986; **14:** 93–126.

2. Williamson SJ, Kaufman L, Analysis of neuro-magnetic signals. In: *Handbook of electroencephalography and clinical neurophysiology.* Volume 1: *Methods and analysis of brain electrical signals* (eds AS Gevins, A Redmond) Elsevier, Amsterdam, 1987.

3. Hari R, The neuromagnetic method in the study of the human auditory cortex. In: *Auditory evoked magnetic fields and electric potentials* (eds F Grandori, M Hoke, GL Romani) Karger: Basel, 1990.

4. Lewine JD, Neuromagnetic techniques for the noninvasive analysis of brain function, In: *Noninvasive techniques in biology and medicine* (eds SE Freeman, E Fukushima, ER Greene) San Francisco Press, San Francisco, 1991.

5. Lewine JD, Orrison WW, Magnetoencephalography and magnetic source imaging. In: *Functional brain imaging* (eds WW Orrison, JD Lewine, JA Sanders, MF Hartshorne), Mosby Year Book, Inc., St. Louis, 1995.

6. Baule GM, McFee R, Detection of the magnetic field of the heart. *Am Heart J* 1963; **66:** 95–6.

7. Cohen D, Magnetoencephalography, evidence of magnetic fields produced by alpha rhythm currents. *Science* 1968; **161:** 784–6.

8. Sato S (ed), *Magnetoencephalography* (*Advances in Neurology*, Vol. 54). Raven Press, New York, 1990.

9. Hamalainen M, Hari R, Ilmoniemi RJ et al, Magnetoencephalography: theory, instrumentation, and applications to noninvasive studies of the working brain. *Rev Mod Phys* 1993; **65:** 413–98.

10. Zimmerman JE, Thiene P, Harding JT, Design and operation of stable rf-biased superconducting quantum interference devices and a note on the properties of perfectly clean metal contacts. *J Appl Phys* 1970; **41:** 1572–80.

11. Cohen D, Edelsack EA, Zimmerman JE, Magnetocardiograms taken inside a shielded room with a superconducting point-contact magnetometer. *Appl Phys Lett* 1970; **16:** 278–80.

12. Cohen D, Magnetoencephalography: detection of the brain's electrical activity with a superconducting magnetometer. *Science* 1972; **175:** 664–6.

13. Brenner D, Williamson SJ, Kaufman L, Visually evoked magnetic fields of the human brain. *Science* 1975; **190:** 480–2.

14. Brenner D, Lipton J, Kaufman L et al, Somatically evoked magnetic fields of the human brain. *Science* 1978; **199:** 81–3.

15. Teyler TJ, Cuffin BN, Cohen D, The visual evoked magnetoencephalogram. *Life Sci* 1975; **17:** 683–91.

16. Roland P, *Brain activation.* Wiley, New York, 1993.

17. Hämäläinen MS, Sarvas J, Feasibility of the homogeneous head model in the interpretation of magnetic fields. *Phys Med Biol* 1987; **32:** 91–7.

18. Meijs JWH, Bosch FGC, Peters MJ et al, On the magnetic field distribution generated by a dipolar current source situated in a realistically shaped compartment model of the head. *Electroenceph clin Neurophysiol* 1987; **66:** 286–98.

19. Okada Y, Neurogenesis of evoked magnetic fields, In *Biomagnetism, an interdisciplinary approach* (eds SJ Williamson, GL Romani, L Kaufman et al) Plenum Press, New York, 1983.

20. Cohen D, Hosaka HJ, Magnetic field produced by a current dipole. *J Electrocardiol* 1976; **9:** 409–17.

21. Sarvas J, Basic mathematical and electromagnetic concepts of the biomagnetism inverse problem. *Phys Med Biol* 1987; **32:** 11–22.

22. Okada Y, Discrimination of localized and distributed current dipole sources and localized single and multiple sources, In *Biomagnetism, applications and theory* (eds H Weinberg, G Stroink, T Katila) Pergamon Press, New York, 1985.

23. Supek S, Aine CJ, Simulation studies of multiple dipole neuromagnetic source localization: model-order and limits of resolution. *IEEE Trans Biomed Engng* 1993; **40:** 529–40.

24. Spencer DD, Spencer SS, Mattson RH et al, Access to the posterior medial temporal lobe structures in the surgical treatment of temporal lobe epilepsy. *Neurosurgery* 1984; **15:** 667–71.

25. Shapiro WR, Intracranial neoplasms, In: *The clinical neurosciences* (eds RN Rosenberg, RG Grossman) Churchill Livingstone, New York, 1983.

26. Sobel DF, Gallen CC, Schwartz BJ et al, Central sulcus localization in humans: comparison of MRI-anatomic and magnetoencephalographic functional methods. *AJNR* 1993; **14:** 915–25.

27. Morris HH, Lueders H, Hahn JF et al, Neurophysiological techniques as an aid to surgical treatment of primary brain tumors. *Ann Neurol* 1986; **19:** 559–67.

28. Penfield W, Boldrey E, Somatic motor and sensory representation in the cerebral cortex of man as studied by electrical stimulation. *Brain* 1937; **60:** 389–443.

29. Black PM, Ronner S, Cortical mapping for defining the limits of tumor resection. *Neurosurgery* 1986; **20:** 914–19.

30. Berger MS, Kincaid J, Ojemann GA et al, Brain mapping techniques to maximize resection safety and seizure control in children with brain tumors. *Neurosurgery* 1989; **25:** 786–92.

31. Sutherling WW, Crandall PH, Darcey TM et al, The magnetic and electric fields agree with intracranial localizations of somatosensory cortex. *Neurology* 1988; **38:** 1705–14.

32. Galen CC, Sobel DF, Lewine JD et al, Neuromagnetic mapping of brain function. *Radiology* 1993; **187:** 863–7.

33. Benzel EC, Lewine JD, Bucholz RD et al, Magnetic source imaging: a review of the Magnes system of Biomagnetic Technologies Incorporated. *Neurosurgery* 1993; **33:** 252–9.

34. Orrison WW, Lewine JD, Magnetic source imaging in neurosurgical practice. *Perspectives Neurol Surg* 1993; **4:** 141–8.

35. Galen CC, Sobel DF, Waltz T et al, Noninvasive pre-surgical neuromagnetic mapping of somatosensory cortex. *Neurosurgery* 1993; **33:** 260–8.

36. Lewine JD, Bucholz RD, Baldwin NG et al, Event-related magnetic fields and neurosurgical practice. In: *Biomagnetism: fundamental research and clinical applications* (eds C Baumgartner, L Deecke, G Stroik, SJ Williamson). Elsevier-IOS Press, Amsterdam, 1995, 120–4.

37. Weinberg H, Cheyne D, Crisp D, Electroencephalographic and magnetoencephalographic studies of motor function. In: *Magnetoencephalography* (*Advances in Neurology*, Vol 54) (ed S Sato) 193–206. Raven Press, New York, 1990.

38. Pantev C, Hoke M, Lehnertz K et al, Tonotopic organization of the human auditory cortex revealed by transient auditory evoked magnetic fields. *Electroenceph clin Neurophysiol,* 1988; **69:** 160–70.

39. Karhu J, Hari R, Makela J et al, Somatosensory evoked magnetic fields in multiple sclerosis. *Electroenceph clin Neurophysiol* 1992; **83:** 192–200.

40. Barth DS, Sutherling W, Engel J et al, Neuromagnetic localization of epileptiform spike activity in the human brain. *Science* 1982; **218:** 891–4.

41. Barth DS, Sutherling W, Engel J et al, Neuromagnetic evidence of spatially distributed sources underlying epileptiform spikes in the human brain. *Science* 1984; **223:** 293–6.

42. Rose DF, Smith PD, Sato S, Magnetoencephalography and epilepsy research. *Science* 1987; **238:** 329–35.

43. Sato S, Epilepsy research, NIH experience. In: *Magnetoencephalography* (*Advances in Neurology*, Vol 54) (ed S Sato) 223–30. Raven Press, New York, 1990.

44. Sutherling W, Barth DS, Magnetoencephalography in clinical epilepsy studies: the UCLA experience. In: *Magnetoencephalography* (*Advances in Neurology*, Vol 54) (ed S Sato) 231–46. Raven Press, New York, 1990.

45. Ricci GB, Italian contributions to magnetoencephalographic studies on the epilepsies. In: *Magnetoencephalography* (*Advances in Neurology*, Vol 54) (ed S Sato) 247–60. Raven Press, New York, 1990.

46. Paetau R, Kajola M, Karhu J et al, MEG localization of epileptic cortex — impact on surgical treatment. *Ann Neurol* 1992; **32:** 106–9.

47. Stefan H, Schnieider S, Abraham-Fuchs K et al, Magnetic source localization in focal epilepsy; multichannel magnetoencephalography correlated with magnetic resonance brain imaging. *Brain* 1990; **113:** 1347–59.

48. Stefan H, Schnieider S, Abraham-Fuchs K et al, The neocortico to mesio-basal limbic propagation of focal epileptic activity during the spike-wave complex, *Electroenceph clin Neurophys* 1991; **79:** 1–10.

49. Paetau R, Kajola M, Hari R, Magnetoencephalography in the study of epilepsy, *Neurophysiologie Clinique* 1990; **20:** 169–87.

50. Paetau R, Kajola M, Korkman M et al, Landau– Kleffner syndrome: epileptic activity in the auditory cortex, *NeuroReports* 1991; **2:** 201–4.

51. Ebersole JS, Squires K, Gamelin J et al, Simultaneous MEG and EEG provide complimentary dipole models of temporal lobe spikes. *Epilepsia* 1993; **34:** 531.

52. Ebersole JS, Squires K, Gamelin J et al, Dipole models of temporal lobe spikes from simultaneous MEG and EEG. *Abstracts, AEEGS, New Orleans, 1993.*

53. Ebersole JS, Squires K, Gamelin J et al, Dipole models of temporal lobe spikes from simultaneous MEG and EEG. *Abstracts, Biomag '93, Vienna, 1993,* 6–7.

54. Hari R, Ahonen A, Forss N et al, Parietal epileptic mirror focus detected with a whole-head neuromagnetometer. *NeuroReports* 1993; **5:** 45–8.

55. Vieth J, Magnetoencepalography in the study of stroke (cerebrovascular accident). In: *Magnetoencephalography* (*Advances in Neurology*, Vol 54) (ed S Sato) 261–9. Raven Press, New York, 1990.

56. Gallen CC, Schwartz BJ, Pantev C et al, Detection and localization of delta frequency activity in human stroke, In: *Biomagnetism: clinical applications* (eds M Hoke, SN Erne, YC Okada et al) Elsevier, Amsterdam, 1992.

57. Lewine JD, Orrison WW, Astur RS et al, Explorations of pathophysiological spontaneous activity by magnetic source imaging. In: *Biomagnetism: fundamental research and clinical applications* (eds C Baumgartner, L Deecke, G Stroik, SJ Williamson). Elsevier-IOS Press, Amsterdam, 1995, 55–9.

58. Vieth J, Kober H, Sack G et al, The efficacy of the discrete and the quantified continuous dipole density plot (DDP) in multichannel MEG. In: *Biomagnetism: clinical applications* (eds M Hoke, SN Erne, YC Okada et al) Elsevier, Amsterdam, 1992.

59. Vieth J, Grummich P, Kober H et al, Localization of slow and beta MEG waves associated with epileptogenic lesions. *Epilepsia* 1993; **34:** 532.

60. Reeve A, Knight J, Maclin E et al, Resting-state magnetoencephalography in schizophrenia. *Abstracts, International Congress for Schizophrenia Research, Colorado Springs, 1993.*

61. Reike K, Gallen CC, Sobel DF et al, Magnetic source imaging in cerebrovascular diseases. In: *Studies in biomagnetism: fundamental research and clinical applications* (eds C Baumgartner, L Deecke, G Stroink, SJ Williamson). Elsevier-IOS Press, Amsterdam, 1995.

62. Gallen CC, Iragi V, Tecoma E et al, Identification of epileptic regions via MEG focal slow wave localizations: comparison with EEG monitoring. *Abstracts, Biomag '93, Vienna, 1993,* 36–37.

63. Lewine JD, Orrison WW, Halliday A et al, MEG functional mapping in epilepsy surgery. In: *Neuroimaging in epilepsy: principles and practice* (eds GD Cascino, CR Jack) Butterworth–Heinemann, Boston, 1996. [In press].

64. Oommen KJ, Galen C, Hirschkoff E et al, Inter-ictal magnetic source imaging and ictal subdural strip EEG: a comparison in source localization. *Abstracts, AEEGS, New Orleans, 1993.*

65. Lewine JD, Sloan JH, Orrison WW et al, Neuromagnetic evaluation of brain dysfunction in post-concussive syndromes associated with mild head trauma. In: *Recovery after traumatic brain injury* (eds B Uzzell, H Stonnington, J Doronzo) Lawrence Erlbaum, New York, 1996. [In press].

66. Reite M: Magnetoencephalography in the study of mental illness. In: *Magnetoencephalography* (*Advances in Neurology*, Vol 54) (ed S Sato) 207–22. Raven Press, New York, 1990.

67. Hoke M, Feldman H, Pantev C et al, Objective evidence of tinnitus in auditory evoked magnetic fields. *Hearing Res* 1989; **37:** 281–6.

68. Lewine JD, Astur RS, Davis LE et al, Cortical organization in adulthood is modified by neonatal infarct: a case study. *Radiology* 1994; **190:** 93–6.

69. Armstrong RA, Janday B, Slaven A et al, The use of flash and pattern evoked fields in the diagnosis of Alzheimer's disease, In: *Advances in biomagnetism* (eds SJ Williamson, M Hoke, G Stoink et al) Plenum Press, New York, 1989.

70. George S, Lewis P, Ranken DM et al, Anatomical constraints for neuromagnetic source models. *Proc SPIE* 1991; **1443:** 37–51.

71. Blum T, Bauer R, Arabin B et al, Prenatally recorded auditory evoked neuromagnetic fields of the human fetus. In: *Evoked potentials III* (eds C Barber, T Blum) Butterworth, Boston, 1987.

72. Lewine JD, Orrison WW, Shaw P et al, Biomagnetic assessment of the integrity of the fetal central nervous system. *Abstracts, Soc. Neurosci.* 1994; **20:** 1695.

17

Future trends in imaging

Ian R Young

Introduction

It is fair to say that imaging, whether MR or any other type, is set for a period of extreme turbulence from which it will emerge successfully, though not without undergoing major changes. It is the purpose of this chapter to evaluate the future patterns not just of MRI but also of one or two modalities with the potential to have a significant impact on future clinical practice. There is no attempt, however, to evaluate the future roles of other currently established methodologies, except where direct comparisons are necessary.

One strategy in constructing a chapter of this kind is to analyze techniques on the basis of their physics and mechanisms; another is to define major areas of application, try to identify relevant techniques applicable to them, and then predict their place in the overall future scheme. This latter approach has been adopted here.

High-quality MR imaging represents the core of this book, and much of its value appears to have been fully established by now, with both its benefits and problems having been extensively studied. New imaging developments may influence existing ideas and protocols in MRI, but it is likely that these will become increasingly rare. There may well be a few more surprises in routine imaging such as the advent of FLAIR (fluid-attenuated inversion recovery),[1,2] which resulted in quite substantial improvements in lesion conspicuousity, but they will be few. Most innovations are likely to affect studies of body regions where MRI is currently not particularly effective, such as the abdomen and lungs, but, again, most of the principles needed to achieve better results in these areas have been identified, and it is now a matter of the development of known methods and improvement in their clinical implementation.

This chapter therefore concentrates on two major areas, and attempts to identify the ways in which they will develop, and the techniques available to assess their successful implementation. These two items are functional imaging and image guided therapy.

Functional imaging: an overview

While the name functional MRI (fMRI) has become very much associated with a particular form of experiment in which the brain's response to an external stimulus is studied, this is a very restrictive view of a diverse and expanding area.

Function is studied in MR through blood flow, behavior of contrast agent boluses, and by observation of physical properties such as tissue compliance, anisotropy (giving structural data), metabolic behavior (via spectroscopy) and information about interactions between free and bound protons obtained from magnetization transfer studies.

Function is also studied by many of the new techniques that may enter common practice, such as near infrared brain monitoring, magnetic source imaging (MSI) (or magnetoencephalography), applied potential tomography (APT) (also known as electric impedance tomography, EIT) and positron emission tomography (PET). There are other methods that may have some ability to detect useful functional changes in the future (such as microwave imaging), but their performance is so far from what might be useful that they are not further considered here.

The achievements and problems of MR are well documented elsewhere, so these will not be included in this section, even though they probably are as good as, if not better, indicators of function than most others yet available. However, many of the methods listed above detect functional changes through flow-related changes, and these will be reviewed briefly.

Function through metabolic changes

MR spectroscopy

In many ways, in vivo spectroscopy (MRS) has always seemed to be the answer to all tissue function questions. As a technique, it has provided more false dawns than any other, and yet research into its capabilities continues at much the same rate as it has for the past few years. It is reasonable to ask both whether there is genuine progress towards finding real clinical applications and why the technique has proven so intractable and difficult to implement.

Though it is easy to say that the data format is unfamiliar, and so radiologists will not accept it, this is facile. All clinicians are comfortable with graphical displays such as ECG data, and, if the justification were there, radiologists would find little difficulty in learning the different notation. MRS is, in principle, not significantly technically harder than MRI. The only significant extra step is a much greater need for care in shimming. (Water suppression — to be discussed in a moment — can be compared with operations like fat suppression or elimination in imaging, even if the ratio between what is to be discarded (at 60–80 M concentration) and what is sought (at mM concentrations) is much greater.)

The key issues affecting the success of MRS lie in the lack of sensitivity of the experiment (because there is so little of the metabolites present) and the difficulty of recognizing artifact (at least in part a problem derivative from the former one, since extensive averaging is invariably necessary in spatially localized spectroscopy). The former difficulty means that voxel sizes tend to be very large, so that it is much more by good luck than good judgment that the tissue content from which signals are being recorded is homogeneous. Partial volume problems are always significant, and can become very large. When chemical shift imaging (CSI) methods[3,4] are used, the need for all the spatial encoding to be done by pulsed phase encoding gradients only means that

spatial matrices are small, and there is substantial contamination of the apparent contents of one voxel by those of its neighbors. The method, too, is very vulnerable to motion artifacts,[5] as are some of the single voxel techniques (such as the ISIS[6] method quite commonly used for phosphorus studies). In proton spectroscopy failure to eliminate the very large water peak consistently and adequately is another source of contamination. Most methods of solvent suppression depend on field quality being very good (so that the water resonates at the same frequency from one place to another), since they are frequency-selective. Lipid signals, from peripheral fat and so on, are also a potential source of difficulties. While they may be localized in theory only to some defined voxels, motion artifacts of the same kind as those due to respiratory motion in the abdomen or pulsatility in blood affect the whole data array. The problem is that the artifacts can come from a signal ten thousand times as strong as that which is being sought, with the consequent certainty that they will predominate if allowed to be present.

Because of these factors, when CSI is in use, shimming has to be good over the whole volume to be imaged; it has to be good for single-volume acquisitions, but the necessary performance is not as demanding overall. The difficulty of shimming a small region, however, is that the signal available to work with is correspondingly smaller (even though practically all shimming, regardless of the final target of the experiment, is done using the water signal). Shimming, though increasingly aided by automation, requires skill and patience.

In some ways, therefore, it is almost surprising that spectroscopy produces useful results at all. Most of the early studies used phosphorus as the nucleus to be investigated,[7,8] and concentrated on muscle and hypoxia. First significant clinical claims were associated with infants suffering from birth asphyxia.[9] However, it seems likely that proton spectroscopy will emerge as being more useful.[10] Figures 17.1(a) and (b) illustrate data that

Figure 17.1

Spectra acquired from moderately (a) and substantially (b) brain-damaged neonates. The significant peak from an early diagnostic point of view seems to be the lactate one (Lac, arrowed). If this is elevated to three or more times the normal size during the first few (less than six) hours after birth, outcome is likely to be relatively unfavorable. With the potential development of drug therapies for the condition, such data could be vital in planning patient management. (Spectral acquisition parameters: 3D CSI; $TR = 1500$ ms, $TE = 130$ ms; $15 \times 15 \times 20$ mm^3 voxel size)

a

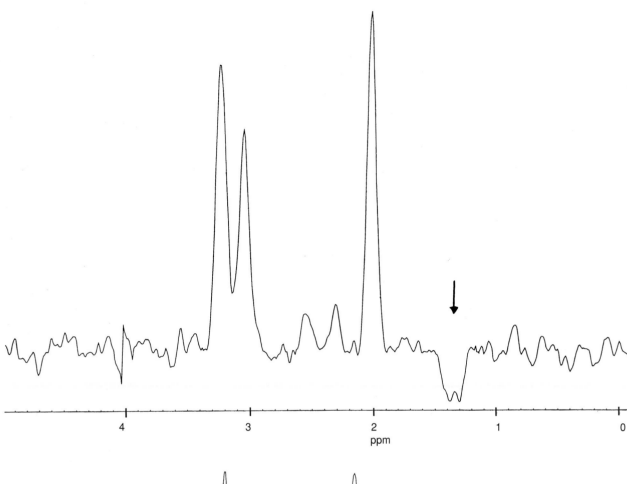

b

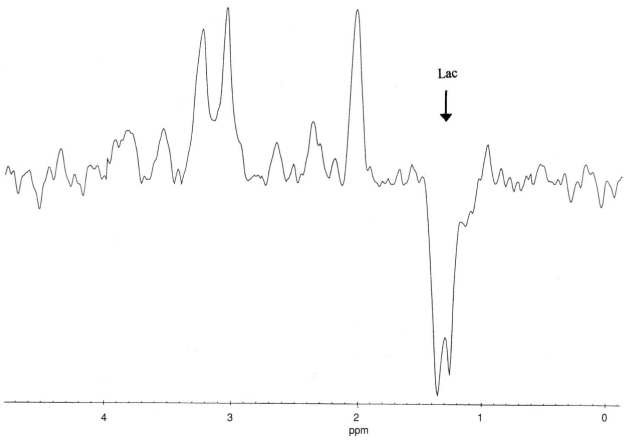

may well turn out to be clinically necessary in assessing patient management of neonates suffering from birth asphyxia where therapy is likely to have to be applied very soon after birth if it is to be successful.

Lactate production is certainly a very direct monitor of brain function, just as it is in muscle (seen directly by proton spectroscopy, or, through pH changes or the depletion of high-energy phosphates, rather less obviously by phosphorus spectroscopy). Other changes in the proton spectrum in disease are of less certain origin, though none the less potentially useful. There have been studies showing very early signs of the development of full blown AIDS in HIV-positive subjects,[11,12] and the very promising application of proton spectroscopy of the brain to monitor the progress and extent of patients suffering from liver encephalopathics.[13] This may well become the first application of spectroscopy to receive FDA approval.

Ultimately, carbon-13 spectroscopy may turn out to be as significant. While it has significant research utility in monitoring brain metabolism,[14] it may be that its use in observing lipid metabolism may be more immediately useful in providing information that could be of value to dieticians.[15]

The great advantage that spectroscopy possesses over other modalities that might compete with it (such as near-infrared – see below) is that it uses existing equipment. Any 1.5 T clinical imager is potentially capable of spectroscopy of any of the nuclei of interest. In the case of proton spectroscopy not even new rf coils and facilities are needed, though phosphorus and carbon spectrometers require new rf coils, and, desirably, a second rf channel to allow decoupling,[16] with the significant potential improvement both in signal-to-noise ratio and simplification of the spectra that this delivers.

Near-infrared studies of the brain

Possibly the nearest analog to MRS amongst the clutch of new modalities currently in the fairly early stages of their clinical application is in vivo near-infrared (near-IR) spectroscopy. In some ways it is a misnomer to describe it as 'new', since the original description of the method was published by Jöbsis in 1977.[17] The most apparent of its applications in regular clinical use is the pulse oximeter, which uses near-infrared light transmitted through a semitransparent part of the body like a finger tip or ear lobe. The metabolic components detected in

human studies are oxyhemoglobin, deoxyhemoglobin and cytochrome-aa3.

The technique depends on the differing absorption characteristics of the components at different light wavelengths. Thus if signals are detected at each of several spot wavelengths, a set of simple simultaneous equations can be solved to determine the relative concentrations of the components. Tissue is a very strongly scattering medium, so that the path of a beam of light through it is highly nondirectional. The distance the light traverses in passing from one point to another is very substantially larger than the geometrical distance between the two. Various techniques, using on the one hand the distortion of the shape of a very sharp laser pulse at the detector,[18] and on the other phase relationships between the incident and emergent light,[19] have been used to measure the effective light path. Typically, the actual mean optical path length is found to be four to six times the geometrical path length in tissue such as the brain[20] (distinctions between gray and white matter are impossible to make on the sort of distances studied).

Efforts are being made to image tissue (as in CT X-ray or MRI) using near-infrared. (Efforts have also been made at longer, microwave, wavelengths, though work on these seems to have sunk to a very low level at this time.[21]) The lack of any geometrically well-defined ray behavior, however, is making imaging an extremely difficult objective. Approaches are generally based on the idea that if a pulse of laser light with a very steap leading edge is projected into the tissue then those photons that emerge first must have taken the most direct available paths, and, as a result, their intensity relative to that of the incident beam must be some sort of indicator of the light absorption present in a reasonably well-defined path.[22] This detection process is very inefficient (in terms of energy input relative to useful energy output),[23] but some progress is being made. It seems unlikely that this approach can lead to images of comparable resolution and content to those of MRI within the foreseeable future.

Near-IR studies of the brain have been much the most productive in the neonate and very small infant. Here distances are short enough for transmitted light to reach a detector from an input source of acceptable power in spite of a typical absorption of near-IR radiation of an order of magnitude per centimeter.[24] As the brain develops, and the head grows and cortical bone hardens, the problems become greater. In principle, reflected light must be used, but the light observed is backscattered, which is disadvantageous for a start, since light is largely forward scattered in tissue. The source and detector optical systems are angled towards each other, and doubts have been expressed as to the degree of penetration of light through the skull into the brain parenchyma.[25]

Function through flow-related observations

Flow observation embraces a wide majority of techniques and experimental designs. These range from the direct observation of inflow and removal of tracers (in methods such as PET; using boluses of contrast agents such as Gd-DTPA in MRI studies) and more subtle studies involving the changes in blood oxygenation as well as motion that are at the basis of functional MRI.[26, 27]

More subtle observations of movement in the brain are the study of diffusion and its related phenomena, and of brain compliance, both by MRI. MRA, as already indicated, is not reviewed in this chapter.

Movement of tracers

Positron emission tomography (PET)

PET as a modern tomographic technique was first described in the mid-1970s,[28] so it is another modality that cannot be described as being 'new'. Its greatest strength is its enormous sensitivity, which means that it can be used to observe nanomolecular concentrations of metabolites in a manner unrivalled by other non-radioactive tracer modalities. It is thus capable of being used to study things like neurotransmitter behavior in the brain. Its disadvantage is that it uses radioactive nuclei as labels, many of which are of relatively short lifetimes. Complex and sophisticated 'hot' chemistry is frequently needed to label some of the more interesting and subtle probes of tissue behavior, and relatively few sites have developed the necessary resources to do this. PET is much more generally used, with much less exotic tracers, to monitor brain energetics, in much the same way as it had been hoped phosphorus MRS would do. Fluorine-18 is a relatively long-lived positron emitter, and this makes the logistics of obtaining and using it much easier.

Positrons emitted by the decay of radioactive nuclei travel some distance before they annihilate with electrons, with the emission of two 512 keV photons per annihilation, the coincidental detection of which in a ring of detectors determines both as coming from the same decay. The spatial resolution of PET is therefore restricted. The actual limit varies from nucleus to nucleus, but for oxygen-15, which is commonly used in the observation of brain function (as $H_2{}^{15}O$) it is of the order of 2 mm.[29] Modern PET scanners are now approaching quite close to the limit, and have increasing numbers of concentric rings of detectors to allow a rapidly improving close approximation of true volume imaging.

Much effort has been devoted to the use of PET as a means of observing the brain's response to external stimuli,[30,31] and many intriguing results have been reported, including some really quite complex patterns of response through multiple pathways. Unfortunately, achievable signal-to-noise ratio is not particularly high, and there is significant background from general blood flow, so that obtaining meaningful functional data from individual volunteers and patients has been difficult. Sophisticated statistical methods have been developed to allow data from populations to be treated together.[32] Inevitably, however, this has restricted the utility of the method in the study of individual patients, and clinical efficacy is some way from being demonstrated.

Functional MRI

Functional MRI (fMRI) has seemed to hold out the possibility that a number of the problems with PET can be overcome. For one, very important, thing, since it involves no radioactivity, there are no dose limitations, and frequent repeat examinations of individual subjects are possible.

While functional MRI is now being studied in a great many centers worldwide, there is still no very clear consensus as to the exact mechanisms that yield the effects which are observed. The BOLD (blood oxygen level dependent) contrast proposed by Ogawa et al[26] postulates that the signal differences seen are due to variations in the concentration of the paramagnetic blood component deoxyhemoglobin. In this model the metabolic increase in the cortex needed to sustain the electrical activity of the brain associated with the stimulus is supported by increased oxygen utilization, and an increase in the conversion of oxy- to deoxyhemoglobin. The system as a whole, however, responds to the demand by increased

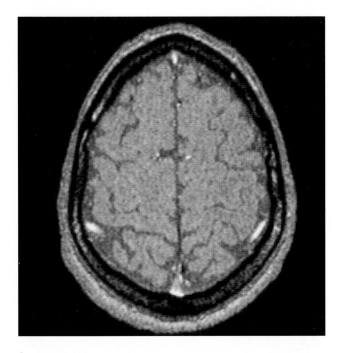

a

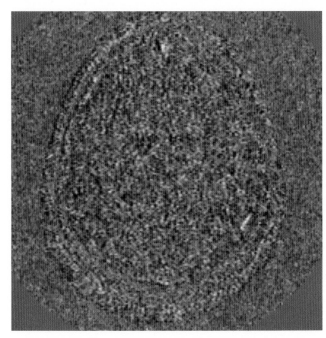

b

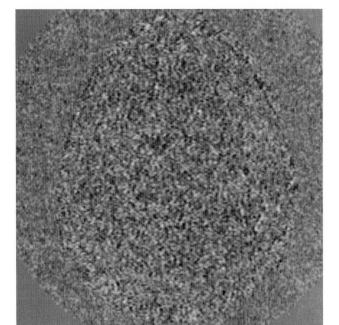

c

Figure 17.2

Images from an fMRI experiment. (a) Typical image, in this case acquired without stimulation, of the brain of a volunteer including the motor cortex, along the boundaries of which the cortex is expected to be involved on motor excitation. (GRE sequence; $TR =$ 50 ms; $TE =$ 20 ms (delayed); one image of a block of 192 with nominal slice thickness 1 mm, acquired at 1 T in a volunteer study). (b) Difference image, obtained by subtracting the image in (a) from the corresponding image in another volume acquisition acquired during motor activation by tapping fingers. (c) Difference image, after the two data sets had been filtered in all three dimensions (to correct for truncation effects) and co-registered as described by Woods et al.[42] The residual signal differences are now very small, and show little of the expected sensitization patterns seen in (b).

perfusion, supplying more blood than is necessary.[33] Thus the concentration of deoxyhemoglobin actually falls, rather than increasing, at first sight might be predicted. The consequence is an increase in the T_2^* of the blood, following, though modifying, the changes first reported by Thulborn et al[34] and an expectation of a greater signal in a delayed gradient recalled echo (GRE) image. This effect is predicted to be dependent on the square of B_0, and so is much enhanced at very high fields. Another effect, modelled by Callaghan[35] in his study of oil-bearing rock porosity, suggests that the effect of susceptibility changes in tubules outside them are directly dependent on field (assuming the correct relative orientation of tubule and field).

An alternative model (or, in some instances, complementary approach) attributes the enhanced signals that are seen to inflow effects, with blood that has experienced no previous excitation producing enhanced signals. Effects from, in particular, veins draining regions where there is excitation have also been suggested as sources of the enhanced signals that are observed.[36]

While there is a wide consensus as to the origin of changes seen in brain stimulation studies,[37-40] Hajnal et al[41] have expressed doubts as to what is happening. Figure 17.2 shows an example of the work that has led them to their conclusions. The first two images, (a) and (b), are typical of many fMRI studies. Figure 17.2(a) shows a typical baseline image (without stimulation) taken by a FLASH sequence with delayed GRE acquisition at 1.0 T. Figure 17.2(b) shows the residual signals when the unstimulated image in Fig. 17.2(a) is subtracted from the equivalent image when the subject was stimulated visually in both eyes with lights flashed with a frequency of about 8 Hz.

The pattern of stimulation is very familiar to those who have investigated the subject. If, however, the two sets of image data are filtered (using a sinc convolution) in all three directions to correct for the behavior of the point spread function in the band-limited data sets, and co-registered using the methods originally developed by Woods et al[42] for PET studies, before subtraction, the result is the very different one shown in Fig. 17.2(c). This shows only minor, and unconvincing, differences, not associated with the expected region where stimulation was expected.

Hajnal et al[41] point out that correlation of stimulation with image differences can be due to effects other than those that are sought. They cite small movements in response to stimulation as one potential example of this. The experimental difficulty is to distinguish desirable changes from others. The conventional approach that attempts to correlate response and stimulation is unable to resolve this, and recourse to statistical analysis (such as in statistical parametric imaging[32]) seems a useful alternative. Unfortunately this follows a pattern common to PET studies that ensures that diagnosis of individual patients is neglected as long as results from a population are meaningful.

PET has a huge advantage when compared with MR of sensitivity (typically operating with concentrations of metabolite four to six orders of magnitude less than those needed for whole body MR studies).[43] Even so, it is potentially vulnerable to the same sort of artifacts that can affect functional MRI.

Applied potential tomography (APT)

In applied potential tomography (APT) a belt carrying a number of electrodes (like ECG ones) is wrapped round the subject. Current is passed between a pair of electrodes, and voltages are measured at all the other electrodes. The choice of energized electrodes is then changed, and another set of data are acquired. The process is repeated until all diagonal pairs have been energized. In effect, this oversamples the data and resolution is limited. Currently, units have 16 electrodes (though ones with 64 electrodes are being built), with a theoretical planar resolution of 104 voxels. Voxel size is nonuniform across the plane, varying in size typically by a factor of 1.8 between regions near the electrodes (where they are smaller) and the center. The reconstruction is difficult, since it involves an inverse solution, in which a guess is made as to the distribution of conductivity and the signals expected at the electrodes are calculated. This results in a set of deviations relative to the observed values from which a better guess as to the conductivity distribution is made, and the process is repeated until further improvement is marginal. In practice, there is now a considerable volume of a priori knowledge of the likely result, and convergence can be accomplished very quickly. This technique is currently only capable of monitoring gross differences in tissue signals, and, even with the increase in the number of electrodes, it is unlikely that it will make a significant impact on clinical practice. Nevertheless, as illustrated in a recent book,[44] a determined minority will seek to find uses for the method.

Functional imaging by direct observation

There are only two techniques that look directly at the electrical signals that are the direct consequences of neuronal activation. These are electroencephalography (EEG) and magneto-encephalography (MEG) — which is also known as magnetic source imaging (MSI). The former will not be considered extensively here, since it is, arguably, less effective when used noninvasively. EEG detects surface potentials, and these are distorted by the presence of the skull. This is largely transparent to the low-frequency magnetic fields detected in MEG. However, only the component of the magnetic field normal to the skull (or other surface of the body) is detected, which means that the method is sensitive to currents parallel to the surface. In terms of the brain, this means that it is primarily activity in the sulci that is detected. (EEG tends to detect currents normal to the surface, and, in this sense, is complementary to MEG.) MEG is not a new technique, having been first described in the mid-1970s.[45] It uses superconducting quantum interference devices (SQUIDs) as detectors. These devices exploit the Josephson effect,[46] which is a phenomenon associated with a semiconducting junction in a superconducting loop. In effect, this forms a mechanism for quantizing magnetic flux, resulting in signals that can be detected.

Flux is coupled into the SQUIDs by detector coils, which are conventionally configured as gradiometers, designed to ignore flux from sources at a distance, while being sensitive to flux from sources close to. Various designs of gradiometer have been employed, and there has been some controversy as to the most effective design.[47] The basis of the discussion is whether it is preferable to have very considerable sensitivity for regions relatively close to the detectors, or to attempt to obtain better depth resolution.

SQUIDs are the most sensitive magnetic flux detectors known, with sensitivities (at unit signal–to–noise ratio) of greater than 10^{-10} of the Earth's magnetic field. As a result, MEG equipment is very vulnerable to ambient disturbances, and though, in principle, compensation systems can be designed that should eliminate the effects of distant disturbances completely, it is normal to install MEG equipment in very sophisticated screened and shielded rooms, with multiple layers of high-quality magnetically soft iron, and copper rf screens. The facilities needed tend to be at least as expensive as those associated with high-field MR systems.

The complexity of MEG systems has increased over the years, so that modern systems have over 100 detector channels. For brain studies, these are mounted in a helmet-shaped array at the foot of the cryostat. Currently systems use liquid helium, though high-temperature superconducting SQUIDs are improving steadily. The apparatus needed is becoming less cumbersome, but is still of substantial size.

The principal problem with MEG system implementation is reconstruction of the data. As with APT, the required process involves an inverse solution, which was shown many years ago to be nonunique.[48] The difficulty is that what is detected is the field produced by a small current dipole, and the field patterns produced by the many other dipoles in the same region as the putative dipole, which are of appropriate spatial arrangement and strengths, cannot be distinguished from it.

Reconstruction proceeds by assuming a signal source, then introducing others with appropriate locations and strengths until the observed field pattern is as well matched as possible. Currently sources cannot be too close to each other, and, currently too, no more than about six can be handled at the same time.[49] Clinical evaluation, and application of MEG techniques, is at a very early stage of development. Most of the interest has been concentrated on epilepsy,[50] but Orrison and his co-workers have been validating the performance of MEG with the help of neurosurgery,[51] using patients proceeding to subsequent operation.

Figure 17.3 illustrates typical results from a prototype 122–channel system (Neuromag, Helsinki). In the experiment the subject is stimulated through the right ear by a series of tones, spaced at about 1 s in time. Most of the notes are at 300 Hz, but there are also randomly introduced 600 Hz tones. It is expected that the left auditory centers will be stimulated by both tones, but there is a second center on the right-hand side that responds to a difference between consecutive tones. As Fig. 17.3(a) shows, there is a distinct difference in patterns between situations where the same tones follow each other and those where they differ.

Two things are apparent: the very high signal-to-noise ratio (though each data set was the average of 100 acquisitions) and the great temporal resolution. Each trace lasts for just 500 ms. Temporal resolution is one major potential advantage of the method, with time differences of around 1 ms being observable. Data can be reconstructed meaningfully with such a temporal resolution, and though the reconstruction process is difficult, modern computing power enables it to be completed within two to five minutes, even with 1 ms time increments.

Figure 17.3(b) shows the constant field contours reconstructed at the time of the peak signals from the array of SQUID detectors. Overlaid on these are arrows showing the direction of the current dipole calculated from the fields. The dipoles are located at the centers of the arrows — but their magnitude is representational only, and the arrows

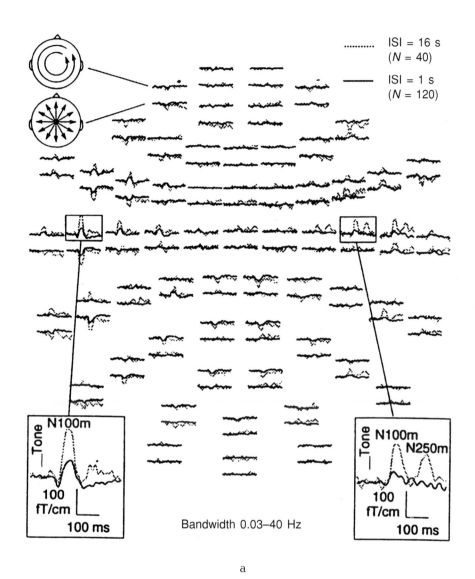

ISI = 16 s (N = 40)

ISI = 1 s (N = 120)

N100m

Tone

100 fT/cm

100 ms

N100m

N250m

Tone

100 fT/cm

100 ms

Bandwidth 0.03–40 Hz

a

Figure 17.3

Results of an MEG experiment. (a) Raw data derived from the SQUID detector array of a 122-channel Neuromag (Helsinki) system. There are two sets of data shown for each of the 122 channels for an experiment in which tones were fed to the right ear of a volunteer. One (heavier line) is the average of 100 'mismatch' events (where successive tone frequencies were different), and the lighter line is the average of 100 events where the tones were the same in successive activations. The appearance of additional signals on the right-hand side of the brain (as the SQUID signals are laid out to represent their locations relative to the brain) is apparent when the tones are mismatched. (b) The data are reconstructed, showing the contours of field intensity, and overlaid on a representation of the SQUID detector array shown located on the skull of the subject. The contours of field intensity are plotted at the peak of the signals in the case where successive tones are mismatched. Top, left and right hand views are shown. (Reprinted with permission from *Radiology* 1994; **192:** 307–17, Fig. 2.)

Left side   Top view   Right side

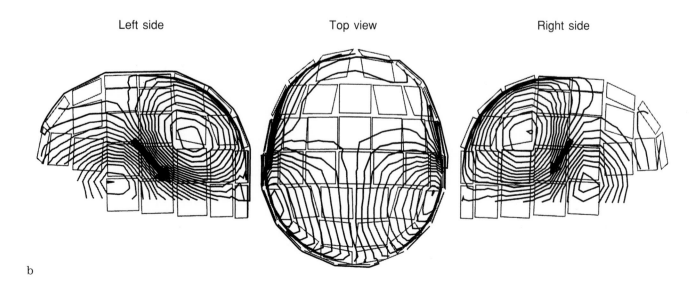

b

are no more than a statement that the responses of the particular volunteer are quite marked. MEG has yet to prove itself, and is certainly very expensive compared with EEG. However, it does observe function directly, and its performance is still improving. Hämäläinen et al[49] have published a major review, to which the reader may safely be referred for further information.

Image-guided therapy

The future of functional imaging is still open to debate — that of image guided therapy seems much more secure, even though its history is relatively short. The philosophy underlying the approach is surely unarguable — that observing the process of therapy is likely to result in better accuracy of location, more exact control of the extent of the applied treatment, and an earlier recognition of success or failure of the procedure.

There are, however, implications in the method that could profoundly affect radiological perceptions. The first of these concerns the magnets that are likely to be used. Intervention requires much greater access to patients than that needed for imaging only. This means that, if magnet cost is to be affordable, fields will be much lower than that usually considered desirable, particularly by neuroradiologists. Further, surgeons and other clinicians will have as much access to data as radiologists. Clearly, unless the latter move to expand their range of activities and interests, there is a danger of the speciality becoming marginalized. It cannot be assumed, with some complacency, that, though some areas of competency may be lost (by analogy with cardiology), there will be others that will remain unquestionably as parts of radiology. The predominant imaging methods of the future do not use X-rays, and neurosurgery and neurology are as open to the new methods as any other speciality.

Rationale for use of MR

Though MR has substantial apparent disadvantages as a vehicle for interventional work — it is expensive, while throughput is lower, and the bulk and shape of the magnet makes it hard to get near to the patient — it has some huge advantages that will justify the efforts that will be made to overcome the disadvantages. These are as follows:

(i)   It is perceived to have no safety problems, which means that procedures can be extended, and repeated, without concern, and that imaging can be as continuous as desired.

(ii)   It has a subtlety of soft tissue discrimination, which means that, though cortical bone is invisible, this is not the problem that it might at first sight seem. In any case, modern image processing means that a previously acquired set of X-ray data can be co-registered with the MR information.

(iii) It can be used to observe parameters such as metabolite concentrations, temperature and flow that are measures of the effectiveness of the therapy. Thus it has a potential range of applications that dwarf those of X–ray interventional procedures.

Equipment requirements

The dominant need in exploiting MR for interventional procedures is for the development of new magnets, though much other less substantial newly designed equipment will also be needed, largely to replace appliances containing ferromagnetic materials with units that are completely compatible with MR.

Initial steps in the development of new magnets include the complex double-doughnut arrangement developed by General Electric Company (Schenectady, NY),[52] which is cryogenic, operating without liquified gases at 0.5 T. This allows access to the patient from each side of the region of high-quality field. An alternate approach is the iron-yoked C-core design adopted by both Siemens (Erlangen, 'Magneton Open') and Picker Nordstar (Helsinki, 'Outlook'). Both of these are electromagnets operating at about 0.2 T. A third strategy uses permanent magnet machines, as developed by Toshiba America (operating at 0.064 T) and Hitachi (at 0.3 T). The latter two designs are iron cores as well, but the configuration used is essentially an H configuration (with iron on both sides of the region of good field), though the Toshiba magnet is implemented with four posts around the patient. The characteristic of all these systems is that the fields at which they operate are relatively low. However, ingenuity in the design of coils and sequences will mean that the loss in

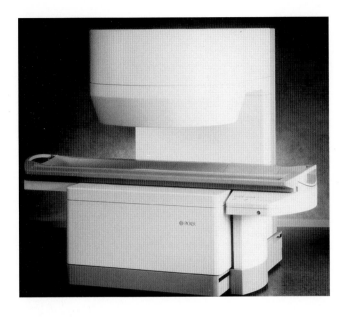

Figure 17.4

Photograph of a typical modern open magnet of the kind likely to be at the centre of the development of interventional MR procedures. (Courtesy of Picker Nordstar, Helsinki.)

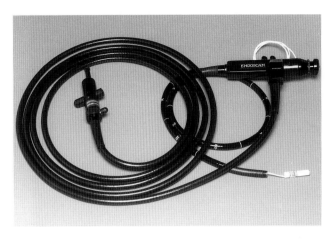

Figure 17.5

Photograph of a nonmagnetic endoscope (gastroscope), with a coil used with it also shown. The coil assembly (of the same diameter as the endoscope) is positioned ahead of the endoscope when inserted into the patient. The coil can also be pushed a distance rather ahead of the endoscopic nose, and the unit can then be operated normally, with both a visual channel and cleaning facilities. The normal pathway for a biopsy needle or other tool is used for the coil cable. The coil would need to be less than 3 mm in diameter to pass through the biopsy channel, which would mean that the field of view to which it is sensitive would be rather too small to be widely useful.

performance will be minimized. Cryogenic coils will be applied with increasing seriousness,[53,54] and 'keyhole' sequences[55] used to maximize image signal-to-noise ratio. Figure 17.4 shows a typical interventional magnet system (Picker Nordstar, 0.23 T magnet).

Other devices will need redevelopment for application in interventional MR. Displays, for example, will have to change from the traditional cathode-ray tube to liquid crystals or other forms unaffected by the fields, and will need, in turn, to be screened to prevent rf emissions contaminating the MR environment. All other tools and equipment to be used near the magnet, ranging from needles[56] to endoscopes,[57] will similarly need redesign to eliminate ferromagnetic materials and large areas of conducting material (which might affect machine rf fields). Figure 17.5 shows a nonmagnetic endoscope (which looks uncommonly like a conventional one) with an associated coil, which in this case is inserted just ahead of the endoscope itself, since it has to be large enough to give an adequate field of view.

Similarly, image handling will need to be much improved, with the need to integrate the outputs of multiple MR coil systems (e.g. array coils external to the body, and endo-rectal,[58] cervical,[59] endoscopic or other coils within it), with images from devices such as endoscopes, and previously recovered data from X-ray and other systems. Ultrasound data, particularly if focused ultrasound therapy is to be used, will also be available, together with output from surgical simulators.

Issues such as how to display data for clinicians will need resolution, including considerations such as the use of head-up displays of various kinds.

Therapy

Because of the sensitivity of MR to temperature changes, through T_1,[60,61] the diffusion coefficient,[62,63] and the chemical shift of the water line,[64,65] thermal therapies seem ideally suited to

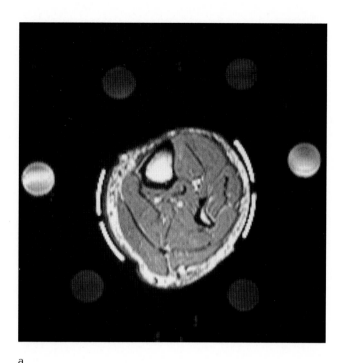

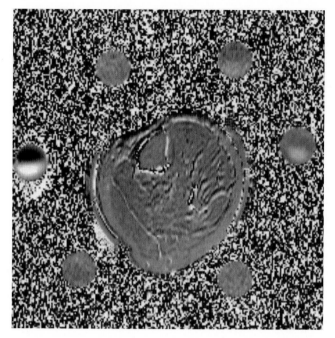

a   b

Figure 17.6

Temperature measurement in MRI. (a) Conventional magnitude image of the calf of a volunteer, which was cooled by water rigid pads (round skin). (b) Phase difference image, showing phase changes from an initial reference image, with one taken when the temperature in the region where signal differences are apparent was around 2.4°C different from that in the other image (as measured by implanted and superficial optical thermometer sensors (Luxtron)). The images were acquired at 1 T using a gradient recalled echo sequence with initial saturation of the slice, an effective TR = 225 ms and a TE = 60 ms.

monitoring by MR. Though accurate measurement of temperature is very difficult,[66] progress is being made, as illustrated by Fig. 17.6. The result shown here suggests a potential sensitivity of around 1°C at 1 T, though it is likely to rise as the field increases, since T_2 is effectively invariant over the range of fields used in imaging, and phase sensitivity is inversely proportional to field.

The therapies being most widely examined for use with MRI hyperthermia involve lasers[67,68] and focused ultrasound.[69] Other alternatives include rf hyperthermia,[70] cryosurgery[71] and chemical ablation.[72]

Other approaches include direct surgical intervention using an array of specially modified, though recognizably conventional, instruments,[73] and the monitoring of drug and other chemical therapies through MR.[74] Surgery may also be practised using frameless stereotaxic systems[75] in which an array of sensors (ultrasonic, infrared or radiofrequency methods are in use) are used to monitor tool movements, and the position of the patient's body is measured and referred to previously acquired three-dimensional image data sets. The motion of the patient is reflected in rotations and displacements of the images, and the location of the tools is superimposed on the images as well.

Simulation

One final important innovation involving images is that of simulation. In this, in rather the same way as with frameless stereotoxic methods, a surgeon is able to practise operations, ahead of the actual event, review past performances, and be trained on new procedures. Full simulation will take time to achieve, but it is reasonable to expect an ultimate sophistication approaching that of aircraft simulation.

Whether virtual reality (VR) will play a dominant role in image handling, manipulation and visualization is a matter of speculation. For this method, in which helmet-mounted displays are used to involve the wearer in what he/she is viewing apparently as though he/she was there, there are many putative uses, but, as yet, no serious real clinical applications.

pattern of practice of the speciality. Whether it will survive at all in its present form will be a measure of its flexibility and imagination in responding to the threats it faces.

Conclusions

At the time of writing, radiology is in a period of acute flux, with both cost pressures and technical innovations increasing threats to the existing

Acknowledgements

I acknowledge with gratitude the help of all my colleagues in the Robert Steiner MRI Unit at Hammersmith Hospital, and at Picker International. I also acknowledge gratefully the financial support of the Medical Research Council, which has made the work possible, and the help of the Helsinki University of Technology Low Temperature Group (MSI results and work), Professor BH Brown, University of Sheffield (APT data), and Professor DT Delpy, University College, London (near-infrared work).

References

1. Hajnal JV, Bryant DJ, Kasuboski L et al, Use of fluid attenuated IR (FLAIR) pulse sequences in MRI of the brain. *J Comput Assist Tomogr* 1992; **16:** 841–4.

2. Hajnal JV, De Coene B, Lewis PD et al, High signal regions in normal white matter shown by heavily $T2$-weighted IR sequences: a link between myelination, $T2$, susceptibility and diffusion effects? *J Comput Assist Tomogr* 1992; **16:** 506–13.

3. Brown TR, Kincaid BM, Ugurbil K, NMR chemical shift imaging in three dimensions. *Proc Natl Acad Sci USA* 1982; **79:** 3523.

4. Maudsley AA, Hilal SK, Parman WH, Simon HE, Spatially resolved high resolution spectroscopy by four dimensional NMR. *J Magn Reson* 1993; **51:** 147–52.

5. Young IR, Cox IJ, Coutts GA, Bydder GM, Some considerations concerning susceptibility, longitudinal relaxation time constants and motion artifacts in in vivo human spectroscopy. *NMR Biomed* 1989; **2:** 329–39.

6. Ordidge RJ, Connelly A, Lohman JAB, Image-selected in vivo spectroscopy (ISIS). A new technique for spatially selective NMR spectroscopy. *J Magn Reson* 1986; **66:** 283–94.

7. Radda GK, Bore PJ, Rajagopalan B, Clinical aspects of 31P spectroscopy. *Br Med Bull* 1984; **40:** 155–9.

8. Ross BD, Radda GK, Gadian DG et al, Examination of a suspected case of McCardle's syndrome by 31P nuclear magnetic resonance, *N England J Med* 1981; **304:** 1388.

9. Cady EB, Dawson JM, Hope PL et al, Non-invasive investigation of cerebral metabolism in newborn infants by phosphorus nuclear magnetic resonance spectroscopy. *Lancet* 1983; **i:** 1059–1062.

10. Cox IJ, Sargentoni J, Bryant DJ et al, 1H MRS and MRI of term infants with hypoxia-ischemic encephalopathy. *Proc 11th Ann Mtg Eur Soc Magn Reson Med Biol, Vienna, 1994,* 153.

11. Menon DK, Ainsworth JG, Cox IJ et al, Proton spectroscopy of the brain in AIDS dementia complex. *J Comput Assist Tomogr* 1992; **16:** 538–42.

12. Lenkinski RE, Jarvik JG, Leigh JS, Jr, Use of combined spectral parameters in the statistical analysis of MR spectroscopic studies of HIV infection. *Radiology* 1992; **185**: 299.

13. Kreis R, Ross BD, Farrow NA, Ackerman Z, Metabolic disorders of the brain in chronic hepatic encephalopathy detected with 1H MRS, *Radiology* 1992; **182**: 19–27.

14. Rothman DL, Novotny EJ, Shulman GI et al, *Proc Natl Acad Sci USA* 1992; **89**: 9603–6.

15. Moonen CT, Dimand RJ, Cox KL, The non invasive determination of linoleic acid content of human adipose tissue by natural abundance ^{13}C nuclear magnetic resonance, *Magn Reson Med* 1988; **6**: 140–57.

16. Luyten PR, Bruntink G, Sloff FM et al, Broad-band proton decoupling in human ^{31}P NMR spectroscopy. *NMR Biomed* 1989; **1**: 177–83.

17. Jöbsis FF, Noninvasive infrared monitoring of cerebral and myocardial oxygen sufficiency and circulatory parameters. *Science* 1977; **198**: 1264–7.

18. Delpy DT, Cope M, Van der Zee P et al, Estimation of optical pathlength through tissue from direct time of flight measurement. *Phys Med Biol* 1988; **33**: 1433–42.

19. Chance B, Harris M, Sorge J, Zhang MZ, A phase-modulation system for dual wavelength difference spectroscopy of hemoglobin deoxygenation in tissues. *Proc SPIE* 1992; **1204**: 481–91.

20. van der Zee P, Cope M, Arridge SR et al, Experimentally measured optical pathlengths for the adult head, calf and forearm and the head of the newborn infant as a function of inter optode spacing. *Adv Exp Med Biol* 1992; **316**: 143–53.

21. Young IR, A review of novel modalities having the potential for a future in radiology. *Radiology* 1994; **192**: 307–17.

22. Arridge SR, van der Zee P, Cope M, Delpy DT, New results for the development of infra red absorption imaging. *Proc. SPIE* 1990; **1245**: 91–103.

23. Cope M, Delpy DT, System for long-term measurement of cerebral blood and tissue oxygenation on newborn infants by near infra-red transillumination, *Med Biol Engng Comput* 1988; **26**: 289–94.

24. Delpy DT, Cope M, Van der Zee P, Arridge S, Wray S, Wyatt M. Estimation of optical path lengths through tissue from a direct time of flight measurement. *Phys Med Biol* 1988; **33**:1433–42.

25. Harris DNF, Cowan FM, Wertheim DA, NIRS in the temporal region — strong influence of the external carotid artery. *Adv Exp Med Biol* (in press).

26. Ogawa S, Lee T–M, Nayak AS, Glynn P, Oxygenation-sensitive contrast in magnetic resonance image of rodent brain at high magnetic fields. *Magn Reson Med* 1990; **14**: 68–78.

27. Kwong KK, Belliveau JW, Chesler DA et al, Dynamic magnetic resonance imaging of human brain activity during primary sensory stimulation. *Proc Natl Acad Sci USA* 1992; **89**: 5675–9.

28. Phelps ME, Hoffman EJ, Mullani NA, Ter-Pogossian MM, Application of annihilation coincidence detection to transaxial reconstruction tomography. *J Nucl Med* 1975; **16**: 210–24.

29. Phelps ME, Hoffman EJ, Song-Cheng Huang, Ter-Pogossian MM, Effect of positron range on spatial resolution. *J Nucl Med* 1975; **16**: 649–52.

30. Myers R, Spinks JJ, Lustra SR, Brooks DJ, Positron emission tomography. In: *Quantitative methods in neuroanatomy* (ed. MG Stewart) 117–61. Wiley, Chichester, 1992.

31. Playford ED, Jenkins IH, Passingham RE et al, Impaired mesial frontal and putamen activation in Parkinson's disease: a PET study, *Ann Neurol* 1992; **32**: 151–61.

32. Friston KJ, Frith CD, Liddle PF, Frackowiak RS, Comparing functional (PET) images: the assessment of significant change, *J Cereb Blood Flow Metab* 1991; **11**: 690–9.

33. Fox PT, Raichle ME, Focal physiological uncoupling of cerebral blood flow and oxidative metabolism during somatosensory stimulation in human subjects. *Proc Natl Acad Sci USA* 1986; **83**: 1140–4.

34. Thulborn KR, Waterton JC, Matthews PM, Radda GK, Oxygenating dependence of the transverse relaxation time of water protons in whole blood at high field. *Biochim Biophys Acta* 1982; **714**: 265.

35. Callaghan PT. Susceptibility-Limited Resolution in Nuclar Magnetic Resonance Microscopy. *J Magn Reson* 1990; **87**: 304–318.

36. Hopkins AL, Liai S, Haacke EM et al, High resolution 2D and 3D gradient field-echo functional imaging during finger motion demonstrates that the activation signal at 1.5 is not from cortical parenchyma. *Proc 10th Ann Mtg Eur Soc Magn Reson Med Biol, Rome, 1993*, 190.

37. Bandettini PA, Wong EC, Hinks RS et al, Time course EPI of human brain function during task activation. *Magn Reson Med* 1992; **25:** 390–7.

38. Kim S-G, Ashe J, Hendirch K et al, Functional magnetic resonance imaging of motor cortex: hemispheric asymmetry and handedness. *Science* 1993; **261:** 615–17.

39. Frahm J, Bruhn H, Merboldt K–D, Hanicke W, Dynamic MR imaging of human brain oxygenation during rest and photic stimulation. *J Magn Reson Imaging* 1992; **2:** 501–7.

40. Hennig J, Ernst Th, Speck O, Laubenberger J, Functional spectroscopy: a new tool for the observation of brain activation. *Proc 12th Ann Mtg Soc Magn Reson Med, New York, 1993*, 12.

41. Hajnal JV, Myers R, Oatridge A et al, Artifacts due to stimulus correlated motion in functional imaging of the brain. *Magn Reson Med* 1994; **31:** 283–91.

42. Woods RP, Cherry SR, Mazsiota JC, Rapid automated algorithm for aligning and reslicing PET images. *J Comput Assist Tomogr* 1992; **16:** 620–33.

43. Poke VW, Positron-emitting radioligands for studies in vivo — probes for human psychopharmacology. *J Psychopharmacol* 1993; **7:** 139–58.

44. Holder DS, *Clinical and physiological applications of electrical impedance tomography.* UCL Press, London, 1993.

45. Cohen D, Magnetoencephalography: detection of the brain's electrical activity with a superconducting magnetometer. *Science* 1972; **175:** 664–6.

46. Josephson BD, Possible new effects in superconductor tunnelling. *Phys Lett* 1962; **1:** 251–3.

47. Ahonen AI, Hämäläinen MS, Kajola MJ et al, A 122-channel magnetometer covering the whole head. *Proc Satellite Symp on Neuroscience and Technology, 14th Ann Conf. IEEE.*

Med Biol Soc, Lyon, 1992 (eds A Dittmer, JC Frosant) 16–20.

48. Helmholtz H von, UeberEinige Gesetze der Vertheilung Elektrischer Ströme in Körplichen Leitern, mit Anwerdung auf die Thierisch-Elektrischen Versuche. *Ann Phys Chem* 1853; **89:** 211–33, 353–77.

49. Hämäläinen M, Hari R, Ilmoniemi RJ et al, Magnetoencephalography — theory, instrumentation and applications to non-invasive studies of the working human brain. *Rev. Mod Phys* 1993; **65:** 413–97.

50. Sutherling WW, Crandall PH, Engel JJ et al, The magnetic field of complex partial siezures agrees with intracranial localization. *Ann Neurol* 1987; **21:** 548–58.

51. Orrison WW, Rose DF, Hart BL et al, Non-invasive pre-operative cortical localization by magnetic source imaging. *AJNR* 1992; **12:** 1124–8.

52. Roemer PB, Schenck JF, Jolesz FA et al, A system for MRI-guided interventional procedures. *Proc 2nd Mtg Soc Magn Reson, San Francisco, 1994*, 420.

53. Hall AS, Barnard B, McArthur P et al, Investigation of a whole-body receiver coil operating at liquid nitrogen temperatures. *Magn Reson Med* 1988; **7:** 230–6.

54. Hall AS, Alford McN, Button TW et al, Use of high temperature superconductor in a receiver coil for magnetic resonance imaging. *Magn Reson Med* 1991; **20:** 340–3.

55. Feinberg DA, Hoenninger JC, Crooks LE et al, Inner volume MR imaging: technical concepts and their application. *Radiology* 1985; **156:** 743–7

56. Lufkin R, Teresi L, Hanafee W, New needle for MR guided aspiration cytology of the head and neck. *AJR* 1987; **149:** 380–2.

57. Hall AS, Bryant DJ, Burl M, deSouza NM. Development of an MR compatible endoscope with an internal receiver coil for imaging the upper gastrointestinal tract. *Proc 2nd Mtg Soc Magn Reson, San Francisco, 1994*, 1581.

58. Martin JF, Hajek PC, Baker LL et al, *Radiology* 1986; **161:** 318.

59. Baudouin CJ, Soutter WP, Gilderdale DJ, Coutts GA. Magnetic resonance imaging of the uterine cervix using an intra–vaginal coil. *Magn Reson Med* 1992; **24:** 196–203.

60. Parker DL, Smith V, Sheldon P et al, Temperature distribution measurements in two-dimensional NMR imaging. *Med Phys* 1983; **10:** 321–5.

61. Dickinson RJ, Hall AS, Hind AJ, Young IR, Measurement of changes in tissue temperature using magnetic resonance imaging, *J Comput Assist Tomogr* 1986; **10:** 468–72.

62. Le Bihan D, Delannoy J, Levin RL, Temperature mapping with MR imaging of molecular diffusion: application to hyperthermia. *Radiology* 1989; **171:** 853–7.

63. Morvan D, Leroy-Willig A, Malgouyres A et al, Simultaneous temperature and regional blood volume measurement in human muscle using an MRI fast diffusion technique. *Magn Reson Med* 1993; **29:** 371–7.

64. Hindman JC. Proton resonance shift of water in the gas and liquid states. *J Chem Phys* 1966; **44:** 4582–92.

65. Ishihara Y, Calderon A, Watanabe H et al, A precise and fast temperature mapping method using water proton chemical shift. *Proc 11th Ann Mtg Soc Magn Reson Med, Berlin, 1992,* 4804.

66. Young IR, Hand JW, Oatridge A, Prior MV, Modelling and observation of temperature changes in vivo using MRI. *Magn Reson Med* 1994; **32:** 358–69.

67. Castro DJ, Lufkin RB, Saxton RE et al, First human case treated by MRI guided laser therapy. *Laryngoscope* 1992; **102:** 26–32.

68. deSouza NM, Puni R, Coutta GA et al, Use of magnetic resonance imaging for the intra-operative monitoring of laser treatment of benign prostatic hypertrophy. *Proc 2nd Mtg Soc Magn Reson, San Francisco, 1994,* 1585.

69. Cline HE, Hynynen K, Watkins RD et al, A clinical MR guided focused ultrasound surgery system. *Proc 2nd Mtg Soc Magn Reson, San Francisco, 1994,* 425.

70. Hall AS, Prior MV, Hand JW et al, Observation by MR imaging of in vivo temperature changes induced by radio frequency hyperthermia. *J Comput Assist Tomogr* 1990; **14:** 430–6.

71. Gilbert JC, MR Guided cryo ablation. In: *Syllabus of a Workshop on Interventional MRI, Los Angeles, 13/14 August 1994, organized by UCLA School of Medicine,* 20–31.

72. Gröenmeyer D, Seibel R, MR endoscopy for interventional microinvasive therapy. In: *Syllabus of a Workshop on Interventional MRI, Los Angeles, 13/14 August 1994, organized by UCLA School of Medicine,* 32–34.

73. Gröenmeyer D, Seibel R, MR appearance of ethanol ablation. In: *Syllabus of a Workshop on Interventional MRI, Los Angeles, 13/14 August 1994, organized by UCLA School of Medicine,* 81–82.

74. Wolf W, Presant CA, Albright MJ et al, F-19 MR spectroscopy of 5-FU as a method for non-invasive monitoring of drug targeting and delivery. *Radiology* 1987; **169:** 84.

75. Barnett GH, Korimos DW, Steiner CP, Weisenberger J. Intraoperative localization using an armless, frameless sterotactic wand. *J Neurosurgery* 1993; **78:** 510–14.

Index